A SHORT COURSE IN
MEDICAL
TERMINOLOGY

Senior Acquisitions Editor: Jonathan D. Joyce
Product Development Editor: John Larkin
Production Project Manager: David Saltzberg
Senior Marketing Manager: Leah Thomson
Design Coordinator: Holly McLaughlin
Compositor: Absolute Service, Inc.
Printer: RR Donnelley & Sons

Printed in China

Library of Congress Cataloging-in-Publication Data

Collins, C. Edward., author.
  A short course in medical terminology / C. Edward Collins. — Third edition.
     p. ; cm.
  Includes bibliographical references and index.
  ISBN 978-1-4511-7606-3 (alk. paper)
  I. Title.
  [DNLM: 1. Terminology as Topic—Problems and Exercises. W 15]
  R123
  610.1'4—dc23
               2013029203

To purchase additional copies of this book, call our customer service department at **(800) 638-3030** or fax orders to **(301) 824-7390**. International customers should call **(301) 714-2324**.

Visit Lippincott Williams & Wilkins on the Internet: http://www.LWW.com. Lippincott Williams & Wilkins customer service representatives are available from 8:30 am to 6:00 pm, EST.

4 5 6 7 8 9 10

RRS1603

C. EDWARD COLLINS

Text and Academic Authors Association,
St. Petersburg, Florida

A SHORT COURSE IN
MEDICAL
TERMINOLOGY

THIRD EDITION

 Wolters Kluwer | Lippincott Williams & Wilkins
Health

Philadelphia · Baltimore · New York · London
Buenos Aires · Hong Kong · Sydney · Tokyo

This book is dedicated to
Lisa Babcock, **NP**, *and*
Sheila Thompson, **RN**,
two remarkable health care professionals,
each of whom exemplifies all that is good
in the health care professions.

———

C. EDWARD COLLINS

New to This Edition

This new edition builds on the foundation established in the first and second editions. The reader will find the writing style of this edition easy to follow, given that the main focus of the text is restricted to medical terminology and its purposes. New exercises, along with more questions to existing exercises, have been added. These exercises will continue to appeal to the varying learning styles and preferences of students.

In consideration of the importance of those classical word origins that make up most medical terms, this edition includes an exercise early in each chapter to reinforce student acquisition of these term elements. A small amount of extra attention paid to them will pay rich dividends later on. Each chapter also contains an added but very brief "quick check" feature about halfway through as a kind of "speed bump" to help students know whether they might be rushing through the text too quickly and, perhaps, need to pause and review before continuing.

Approach and Content Organization

As mentioned, learning to use different combinations of word elements to form new terms yields rich rewards. Therefore, the text is divided into two parts: Part One, Introduction to Medical Terminology, reveals the foundation of medical terms and thereby provides a way to remember their meanings. Part Two, Body Systems, offers an overview of each system and introduces terms that identify the structure and function of that system along with terms naming system disorders and treatments.

- Part One, Introduction to Medical Terminology, consists of Chapters 1 and 2, which identify not only the kinds of word elements that form medical terms but also how these elements reveal their meanings.
- Part Two, Body Systems, begins with Chapter 3, which introduces the human body and briefly discusses terms related to the body's organization—from cells to organs—as well as the terms needed to locate specific points in the body. All the chapters of this third edition incorporate appropriate exercises within the text to immediately reinforce important information. Chapters 3 through 15 are structured in the following way:
  - *Learning Objectives*
  - *Introduction*
  - *Word Elements*
  - *Structure and Function*
  - *Disorders and Treatments*
  - *Abbreviations*
  - *Study Table*
  - *Additional Exercises*
  - *Chapter Quiz*

Other Resources

Online ancillary materials complement the text and, like the textbook proper, appeal to various student learning styles.

Student Resources:
- Question Bank, with a variety of exercise types to reinforce chapter material
- Educational Games, such as crossword puzzles, hangman, and word-building challenges
- Audio Glossary

- Flash Cards, including Flash Card Generator
- Chapter Quizzes
- Final Exam

Instructor Resources:

- PowerPoint slides and Lesson Plans include useful information to facilitate presentation of material by instructors.
- Test Generator, with more than 500 questions to test students' knowledge of terms, their meanings, and abbreviations
- Handouts include additional puzzles and games for additional student practice.

Author's Preface

To the Instructor

As requested by reviewers, the approach in this third edition differs somewhat from that of the second edition, the main difference being a greater emphasis on term elements. As noted in the preface of the first edition, there are two ways to approach the study of medical terminology: one way relies heavily on the subjects of anatomy, physiology, and diagnostics. However, most physicians will tell you that 7 or more years of intensive university study afforded them little more than a cursory understanding of those subjects and the medical terms associated with them.

The second way of approaching medical terminology is the direct way: learning medical terms *as terms*, with only minimal reference to the concepts that underpin related technical subjects. This approach follows from a realistic vision of a medical vocabulary's purpose, which is real-world communication with colleagues and patients.

Another change will be evident in the case study exercises, which have been redesigned to highlight the role medical terminology plays in communication. Both of these changes relate to a general affective behavior paraphrased directly from Benjamin Bloom's famous taxonomy of educational objectives:

> **INTERNALIZING VALUES:** The graduate leaves with a value system that is pervasive, consistent, predictable, and most importantly, characteristic of an attitude of service to patients.

The first 21 words are Bloom's; the final four are mine. When health care in the United States is compared to that in other countries, it usually comes out on top. However, although health care may be more problematic elsewhere, it is not perfect here either. The Institute of Medicine, the *Journal of the American Medical Association*, *The New England Journal of Medicine*, *The New York Times*, *USA Today*, and the *Washington Post* have all recently reported that health care errors are a major cause of injury and death in the United States. This problem must certainly exist in part because negative behaviors were missed or ignored during the training of medical professionals at every level.

In summary, health care workers make mistakes for a number of reasons, the following two being most prominent among them: first, as students, they were "welcomed into the club" instead of being taught about the centrality of the patient; second, their training didn't prepare them to carry out communication tasks, which is, in most cases, fully half of the job.

Although the focus of this edition has changed, the general layout remains nearly the same as that of the second edition. That is to say, each body chapter introduces Word Elements, terms relating to body parts and functions, and terms naming disorders and treatments. The pharmacology heading in each chapter has been eliminated in favor of an appendix containing a table of commonly prescribed drugs, a highly valued feature of the first edition.

To the Student

Learning medical terms is easy for those who approach the subject from a proper viewpoint. What does that mean? First of all, it means that medical terms do not make up a separate language. Medical terms are simply words that can be added to one's vocabulary, nothing more and nothing less. Also, as with all other words, medical words are meant to convey information.

As one entering a medical profession, you will be communicating with other medical professionals and with patients. Therefore, your job will include choosing words and sentence structures that convey accurate information and reflect a professional attitude. That is to say, both your communication skill and your attitude toward patients will affect everyone with whom you come in contact. Learning medical terminology is easy, as you are about to discover. Learning to use it wisely requires a little more work, and another purpose of this textbook is to put you on track for acquiring that skill, too.

Given these goals, this book will not talk down to you. As health care workers, you will need technical skills. However, those skills constitute only a framework for performing physical tasks. Your verbal, social, and personal skills, on the other hand, combine with your technical knowledge to make you a health care professional. To attain that level, you should begin the practice of looking up unfamiliar English words. You should also reflect on new words until they truly become yours. A knowledge of medical terms is important, but that knowledge, like technical skill, is only a beginning. Confidence follows from fully developed verbal skill, which helps you project a mien that signals maturity and ensures success as a professional.

C. Edward Collins
Text and Academic Authors Association
St. Petersburg, Florida

User's Guide

A Short Course in Medical Terminology, Third Edition, was developed to provide an easy, efficient, and effective way to learn medical terminology. This User's Guide introduces the features of the book that help the learning experience.

A **logical organization** guides students through the basics of medical terminology, word elements, and word analysis.

Part One, Introduction to Medical Terminology, introduces the basics of word building and sets the foundation for learning terms.

PART ONE
Introduction to Medical Terminology

1 Analyzing Medical Terms

LEARNING OBJECTIVES
Upon completion of this chapter, you should be able to:
- Recognize each of the four elements of medical terms: roots, suffixes, prefixes, and "combining forms."
- Divide medical terms into word elements.
- Explain what the phrase combining form means.
- Recognize the importance of proper spelling, pronunciation, and use of medical terms.
- Define the commonly used roots, suffixes, and prefixes introduced in this chapter.
- Discuss the purpose of medical terminology.

INTRODUCTION

The quickest way to learn medical terms is to relax and enjoy the experience. Most medical terms consist of word fragments—we'll call them elements—from Latin and Greek. The good news is that there are only 300 or so elements making up thousands of medical terms. For that reason, learning what medical terms mean is learning what the elements mean and noting how they fit together to form terms.

Attacking the subject head-on and cramming is another way to learn medical terminology, of course, but that consumes more energy and a lot more time. In fact, approached the right way, medical terminology may be the easiest subject in your program. Learning it takes a bit of thought and an open mind, but it need not involve sweating or ripping out your hair in frustration.

In this chapter, you will also learn an important truth, which is that communication skill is needed to use medical language effectively. For example, you will learn that medical terms are words rather than symbols, and you will come to understand why words have a power that symbols lack. You will also be able to discuss the concept of "language sense," ways of acquiring it, and the specific advantages it gives to health care workers.

This chapter then introduces you to some of the elements that form medical terms. When you have finished the chapter, you will be able to distinguish between three kinds of elements: **roots**, **suffixes**, and **prefixes**. You also will have learned a few medical terms and have built a foundation for learning many more.

1

PART TWO
Body Systems

...Body's Organization

...BJECTIVES
...ion of this chapter, you should be able to:
...levels of body organization.
...anatomical position and cite the directional terms used in relation to the body.
...lanes of the body.
...ody cavities.
...visions of the abdomen and back.
...fine, and pronounce the new terms introduced in this chapter.

...dy construction will help you retain the medical terms you are learning by ...of where things are. It is also useful to know the distinction between the ...*logy*. Anatomy comes to us from the Greek word *anatome*, which means ...ve recognized the element -tome, which indicates that anatomy has some- ...Physiology, on the other hand, is one of the many "ology" words; in this ...ow the body's parts work together. In short, anatomy reveals the "what it is" and physiology the "how it works."

The "what it is" begins with chemicals that act together to form cells. The cells process the food we eat and the air we breathe. Cells also reproduce themselves, each cell according to the DNA code it contains.

WORD ELEMENTS OFTEN USED IN TERMS RELATED TO BODY ORGANIZATION

Table 3-1 lists many of the elements making up terms related to the body as a whole. Not surprisingly, many of them have to do with what constitutes a major category or where things are located.

LEVELS OF ORGANIZATION

The body has four levels of organization: cells, tissues, organs, and systems; each level is defined subsequently under its own heading (Fig. 3-1).

31

Part Two, Body Systems, offers an overview of each system and introduces terms that identify the structure and function of that system along with terms that name system disorders and their treatments.

LEARNING OBJECTIVES

Upon completion of this chapter, you should be able to:

- Recognize each of the four elements of medical terms: roots, suffixes, prefixes, and "combining forms."
- Divide medical terms into word elements.
- Explain what the phrase combining form means.
- Recognize the importance of proper spelling, pronunciation, and use of medical terms.
- Define the commonly used roots, suffixes, and prefixes introduced in this chapter.
- Discuss the purpose of medical terminology.

Each body system chapter opens with a statement of **learning objectives**.

An introduction and a tabular presentation of **word elements** specific to each body system are presented next.

TABLE 5-1	WORD ELEMENTS COMMON WITHIN SKELETAL SYSTEM TERMS	
Element	**Type**	**Meaning**
-algia	suffix	pain
amphi-	prefix	both sides
ankyl/o	root	stiff, fused, closed
arthr/o	root	joint
brachi/o	root	arm
calcane/o	root	calcaneus, heel bone
carp/o	root	wrist
cervic/o	root	neck

Word Elements Exercise FILL IN THE BLANKS

Study Table 5-1 before attempting to complete this exercise. When you are confident that you know the meanings of each of the elements introduced in the table, fill in the blanks.

ELEMENT	MEANING
1. lord/o	_____
2. zygo-	_____
3. carp/o	_____
4. ped/o	_____
5. os/te/o	_____

Word Element Exercises offer students an opportunity to quickly review the elements before moving on to new material.

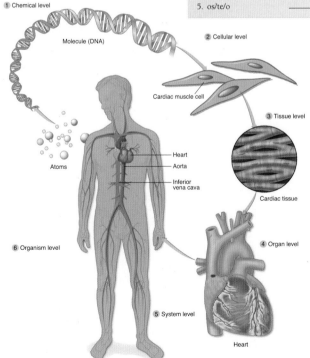

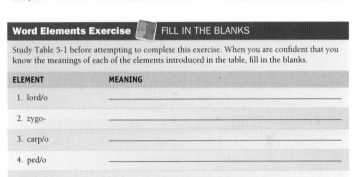

Full-color illustrations are included as needed to help visual learners.

Quick Check: Structure of the Skin, Hair, and Nails

Fill in the suffixes, and write the resulting word in the TERM column. The word that appears in boldface type in the MEANING column is a clue.

PREFIX	ROOT	SUFFIX	TERM	MEANING
sub-	cutane/o	_____	_____	**adjective** meaning "below the skin"
no prefix	melano	_____	_____	a pigment-producing cell
no prefix	seb/o	_____	_____	**adjective** referring to sebum, which may be described as an **oil or fat**

Quick Checks Exercises help reinforce the students knowledge of term elements before studying disorders and treatments of the body systems.

Sidebar information appears throughout to highlight interesting facts about medical terms and words in general.

Why can't we use the words floating, false, and true instead of fluctuantes, spuriae, and verae when talking about ribs? We can, and we do. However, the medical phrase for floating ribs is **costae fluctuantes**. Rib pairs 8, 9, and 10, together with the "floating ribs" 11 and 12, are sometimes collectively called **costae spuriae**, which means (false ribs). The first seven pairs of ribs are called **costae verae** (true ribs). If you know the English words fluctuate, spurious, and verify, you can associate them with these terms as a help in remembering them. If you are unfamiliar with those English words, look them up in a good dictionary and make them part of your general vocabulary.

Abbreviation Table 🔊 THE SKELETAL SYSTEM	
ABBREVIATION	**MEANING**
ACL	anterior cruciate ligament
C (C1, C2, etc.)	cervical
CT	computed tomography
CTS	carpal tunnel syndrome
Fx	fracture
L (L1, L2, etc.)	lumbar
LE	lower extremity
RA	rheumatoid arthritis
ROM	range of motion
S	sacral
T	thoracic
THR	total hip replacement
TKA	total knee arthroplasty
TKR	total knee replacement
Tx	traction

All body system chapters include an **Abbreviations Table**, which lists common abbreviations and their meanings.

Study Table — COMMON SUFFIXES

SUFFIX	MEANING	EXAMPLES
-ac, -al, -an, -aneous, -ar, -ary, -eal, -eous, -iac, -iatric, -ic, -ical, -oid, -otic, -ous, -tic, -ular	converts a root or a noun term to an adjective	geriatric, orthopedic, ocular, dental, cutaneous, cyanotic, atrial, cardiac, ureteral
-cele	protrusion, hernia	rectocele
-centesis	surgical puncture	thoracentesis
-cyte	cell	leukocyte
-desis	surgical binding	arthrodesis
-dynia, -algia	pain	arthrodynia
-ectasis, -ectasia	expansion or dilation	angiectasis
-ectomy	surgical removal	appendectomy
-edema	excessive fluid in intracellular tissues	angioedema
-emesis	vomiting	hematemesis
-emia	blood	uremia
-genic	origin, producing	osteogenic
-gram	written or pictorial record	electrocardiogram
-graph	device for graphic or pictorial recording	electrocardiograph
-graphy	act of graphic or pictorial recording	electrocardiography
-ian, -iatrist, -ist, -logist, -logy, -ics, -iatry, -iatrics	specialty of, study of, practice of	geriatrist, pediatrician, gynecology
-iasis	a suffix used to convert a verb to a noun indicating a condition	cholelithiasis
-ism	a condition of; a process; or a state of	dwarfism, gigantism
-itis	inflammation	appendicitis
-lith	stone, calculus, calcification	pneumolith
-lysis	disintegration	hemolysis
-malacia	softening	osteomalacia
-megaly	enlargement	gastromegaly
-meter	device for measuring	audiometer
-metry	act of measuring	audiometry
-oid	resembling or like	android
-oma	tumor	gastroma
-opsy	visual examination	biopsy
-osis	abnormal condition	osteoporosis, arthrosis
-pathy	disease	cardiopathy

All body system chapters include a **Study Table** summarizing terms for reinforcement of the material in an easy-to-reference format.

Chapter Exercises appear within the text as appropriate to maximize learning, with additional ones near the end of each body system chapter. Exercises include matching, crossword puzzles, word building, fill in the blank, spelling, true/false, case studies, and figure labeling.

EXERCISES

EXERCISE 1-1   DEFINING TERMS

Combine the suffix -logy with the proper root to indicate the following medical specialties:

1. Specialty dealing with heart disease _____

2. Specialty that deals with the problems of aging and diseases in the elderly _____

3. Specialty dealing with blood diseases _____

4. Specialty dealing with skin ailments _____

5. Specialty dealing with nervous system disorders _____

6. Specialty dealing with mental disorders _____

EXERCISE 1-2   ANALYZING TERMS

Analyze the following terms by putting the roots and suffixes in the appropriate columns. Then write a definition for each term.

	ROOT	SUFFIX	WORD TYPE AND DEFINITION
1. neuropathy	_____	_____	_____
2. psychology	_____	_____	_____
3. pathogenic	_____	_____	_____
4. neuralgia	_____	_____	_____
5. systemic	_____	_____	_____
6. psychiatrist	_____	_____	_____
7. pediatrician	_____	_____	_____
8. iatrogenic	_____	_____	_____
9. cardialgia	_____	_____	_____
10. neuritis	_____	_____	_____

◄ CHAPTER 1 QUIZ

Complete the following sentences with the appropriate terms or definitions

1. The prefix *peri-* denotes _____.

2. The suffix *-logy* means _____.

3. The word root derm/o refers to _____.

4. The medical term *osteoarthritis* contains two _____ and one _____.

5. The suffix *-logy* is derived from the Greek word _____, which means _____.

6. Tendonitis refers to the _____ of a _____.

7. A prenatal exam is one that occurs _____ birth of a child.

8. _____ is indicated by the suffixes -algia and _____.

9. Inflammation is indicated by the suffix _____.

10. The study of mental and emotional disorders is called _____.

A **Chapter Quiz** concludes each chapter to test comprehension of the material. Answers to the chapter quizzes are provided in Appendix A.

Reviewers

The author and publisher would like to thank the following individuals who helped to review this textbook:

Vicki Aube, AAS, CST
Surgical Technology Instructor
Tennessee Technology of Applied Technology
Knoxville, Tennessee

Pamela Caesar, AAS, BSc
Allied Health Assistant Professor
Prince George's Community College
Largo, Maryland

Cynthia Carr, MS, OTR/L
Occupational Therapy Associate Professor
Governors State University
University Park, Illinois

Joyce Davis, PhD
Exercise Science Professor
Elon University
Elon, North Carolina

Marianne Demsky, MPH
Lead Medical Terminology Instructor
John Hopkins Hospital
Baltimore, Maryland

Mary Fabick, MSN, MEd
Nursing Associate Professor
Milligan College
Milligan College, Tennessee

Michelle Farnworth, BA
Medical Administration Instructor
American Career Institute/American
    International College
Framingham, Massachusetts

Craig Harradine, DC
Nursing Instructor
Apollo College
Boise, Idaho

Lu Herbeck, BS
Health Sciences Faculty
Minnesota School of Business & Globe College
Richfield, Minnesota

Nancy Hislop, BS
Medical Assisting Instructor
Globe Education Network
Woodbury, Minnesota

Krista Hoekstra, MA, BS, RN
Director of Nursing and Health Sciences
Pine Technical College
Pine City, Minnesota

Joanne Holly, RN, MS, CMA (AAMA)
Allied Health Program Director
Midstate College
Peoria, Illinois

Carol Iaconelli, MS
Assistant Director of Nursing, Instructor, and
    Nurse Practitioner
Cumberland County College
Vineland, New Jersey

Patti Kalvelage, MOT
Senior Lecturer
Department of Occupational Therapy
Governors State University
University Park, Illinois

Louise Lee, MPAS
Assistant Professor
Physician Assistant Studies
Massachusetts College of Pharmacy and
    Health Sciences
Boston, Massachusetts

Donna Long, MSM, RT(R)(M)(QM)
Radiology Program Director
Ball State University/Clarian Health
Indianapolis, Indiana

Catharine Muskus, MS
Clinical Assistant Professor
University of Vermont
Burlington, Vermont

Sandra Olanitori, MS
Nursing and Allied Health Advisor/Faculty
Norfolk State University
Norfolk, Virginia

Dr. Bernard Pegis, MD
Family Practice Physician
Front Royal, Virginia

Debra Poelhuis, MS
Radiography Program Director
Montgomery County Community College
Pottstown, Pennsylvania

Roberta Pohlman, PhD
Biological Science Associate Professor
Wright State University
Dayton, Ohio

Jennifer Potter, BA, AA
Medical Assisting Practicum Coordinator
Cumberland County College
Vineland, New Jersey

Constance Sanderson, MA
Medical Office Specialist
Des Moines Area Community College
Ankeny, Iowa

Rebecca Schultz, PhD
Associate Professor of Exercise Science
University of Sioux Falls
Sioux Falls, South Dakota

Lisa Smith, AAS
Medical Coordinator
Minnesota School of Business
Waite Park, Minnesota

Susan Gurzynski-Wells, MS
Health Services National Education Manager
TechSkills, LLC
Irving, Texas

Margaret Yoder, AS, BSN, MHA
Nurse Education Associate Professor and
  Program Coordinator
Quinsigamond Community College
Worcester, Massachusetts

Michelle Yuhasz
Allied Health and Nursing Instructor
Lorain County Community College
Elyria, Ohio

Acknowledgments

With sincere gratitude, I wish to acknowledge all the hard work done by the members of the editorial staff of Wolters Kluwer: *viz*, David Troy and Jonathan Joyce for providing expert advice and direction, John Larkin for managing the program, and Teresa Exley for overseeing the production process. In addition, Mary Larsen, who worked on the second edition's ancillaries, revised them for this third edition, very ably handling that massive job.

Special thanks go, also, to Dr. Sean D. Collins of Thomas Aquinas College, Santa Paula, California, for his careful scrutiny of the manuscript. As a Great Books scholar, Dr. Collins was able to shed light on many interesting points related not only to those words from the classical languages that are the foundation of medical term elements but also to the historical impact language itself has had in the development of all the sciences, including medicine.

Table of Contents

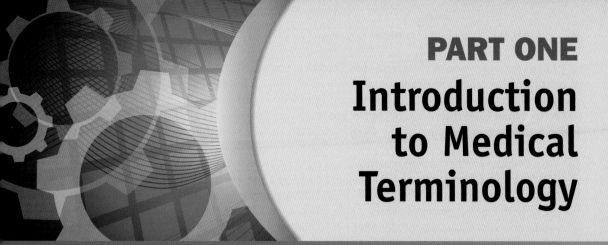

PART ONE
Introduction to Medical Terminology

1   *Analyzing Medical Terms*

LEARNING OBJECTIVES

Upon completion of this chapter, you should be able to:

- Recognize each of the four elements of medical terms: roots, suffixes, prefixes, and "combining forms."
- Divide medical terms into word elements.
- Explain what the phrase combining form means.
- Recognize the importance of proper spelling, pronunciation, and use of medical terms.
- Define the commonly used roots, suffixes, and prefixes introduced in this chapter.
- Discuss the purpose of medical terminology.

INTRODUCTION

The quickest way to learn medical terms is to relax and enjoy the experience. Most medical terms consist of word fragments—we'll call them elements—from Latin and Greek. The good news is that there are only 300 or so elements making up thousands of medical terms. For that reason, learning what medical terms mean is learning what the elements mean and noting how they fit together to form terms.

Attacking the subject head-on and cramming is another way to learn medical terminology, of course, but that consumes more energy and a lot more time. In fact, approached the right way, medical terminology may be the easiest subject in your program. Learning it takes a bit of thought and an open mind, but it need not involve sweating or ripping out your hair in frustration.

In this chapter, you will also learn an important truth, which is that communication skill is needed to use medical language effectively. For example, you will learn that medical terms are words rather than symbols, and you will come to understand why words have a power that symbols lack. You will also be able to discuss the concept of "language sense," ways of acquiring it, and the specific advantages it gives to health care workers.

This chapter then introduces you to some of the elements that form medical terms. When you have finished the chapter, you will be able to distinguish between three kinds of elements: **roots**, **suffixes**, and **prefixes**. You also will have learned a few medical terms and have built a foundation for learning many more.

Let us examine some medical term characteristics. First of all, they are words, not symbols, such as metric units or other quantifiable representations of reality. It follows that they are part of each language in which they occur and are not, as some people believe, part of a foreign language. Most of them are derived from Latin and Greek, of course, but so also are 75% of *all* English words. The plain truth is that accurate communication in any specialty field depends on something called language sense.

Aren't words, whether spoken or written, simply arbitrary symbols for things and actions? No, the idea that a word is a symbol for a sound made by a speaker is based on the observation that choosing a name for something is often arbitrary. However, a further observation, noted by more thoughtful persons, reveals that words take on a life of their own and that, therefore, words and symbols are essentially different. If further illumination of this truth is needed, one might consider what happens when someone steals someone else's identity or shouts "Fire!" in a crowded theater.

LANGUAGE SENSE

Language sense is knowing what words mean and forecasting the effects their combinations will produce. Semanticists and other linguists are fond of reminding us that "the word is not the thing." That obvious truth has been widely misinterpreted to mean that a word naming a thing, quality, or action is unimportant. The truth of the matter is that although the word naming a thing is not the thing named, it has real connections to whatever it names and, much more importantly, *the word is itself a thing*. In fact, words are not mere things; they are among the most important things in the world.

What are words? While it is true that words are not the things they name, a much more important truth is that words *themselves* are things. Indeed, they are the things that paint mental pictures, create abstract thought patterns, support intellectual inquiry, and promote both physical and emotional responses, which, when taken together, reflect the very essence of human existence.

A character in the 18th-century play *The Rivals*, by Richard Sheridan, illustrates perfectly what language sense is not. In one of her lines, the character named Mrs. Malaprop uses the word "allegories" when what she has in mind is "alligators." Not knowing the difference between an allegory and an alligator exemplifies a complete lack of language sense, of course, but the fuzzy thinking of Mrs. Malaprop is far more common than one might imagine. Are such errors prominent in the health care field? Indeed they are. As stated in an article by Barbara Starfield,[1] in the *Journal of the American Medical Association*, Volume 284, No. 4, errors by health care workers are the third leading cause of death in the United States.

Is malaprop really a word? The word malaprop (sometimes also "malapropism") is a real English word, named for a character in the Sheridan play noted in the text. It refers to an error that comes about when we fail to pay full attention to the words we use. Comedian Norm Crosby used many malaprops in his routine, in which he made such statements as, "All I wanted was a little love and affliction . . . " (love and affection). It's easy to pick out malaprops when they are intentionally humorous, but the confusion this kind of error can cause is not funny, especially in instances in which a life may be endangered.

---

[1]Barbara Starfield, MD, MPH. Honors and awards: the David Luckman Memorial Award from the State University of New York Downstate Medical Center in 1958; the HHS Secretary's Special Recognition Award in 1991; the Distinguished Investigator Award from the Association for Health Services Research; the American Public Health Association's Martha May Eliot Award in 1995; the Morehouse School of Medicine Excellence in Primary Care Award in 2002; and the AAFP's John G. Walsh Award for Lifetime Contributions to Family Medicine in 2005.

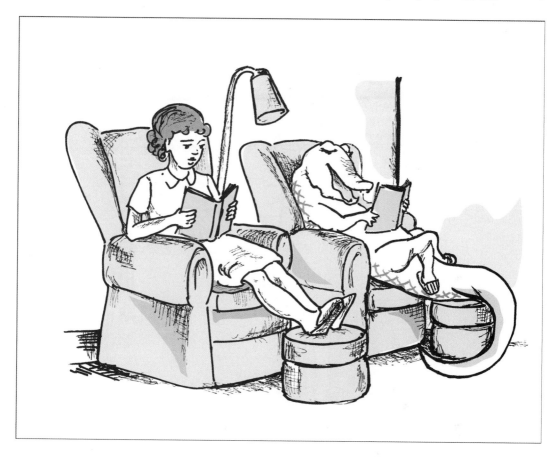

Language sense, then, is learning to attend to words and language structures in a serious way. It involves learning to listen; to understand meanings; and to know how, when, and when not to use certain words and structures.

One of several advantages in studying medical terminology from a language perspective, rather than as a subpart of a technical course, is that learners come to see an important truth: Medical terms are not mere references to cold, hard realities; they have the power not only to describe the health, failure thereof, or restoration thereto of real people, they also influence outcomes in direct proportion to the accuracy of their use and conveyance.

ACQUIRING LANGUAGE SENSE

What does language sense have to do with learning medical terms? First, words have parts, and examining those parts forces the learner to see and hear words in a new way (i.e., to become conscious of words as words). Second, the ability to use words well involves learning the phonetic and grammatical codes that make complex communication possible.

Language deconstructionism, prevalent in schools at every level and particularly in the education departments of many colleges, holds that only spoken language is pure and that written language is distorted by traditional ways of thinking. The irony is, of course, that deconstructionists expound these ideas in books, making them a lot like the man who goes to a bar every night to get drunk and preach the evils of drink to the other patrons. Unlike bar patrons, most of whom would be smart enough to ignore a pedantic drunk, patrons of deconstructionism have to be shown that the existence of books exalting the deconstruction of language is contradictory.

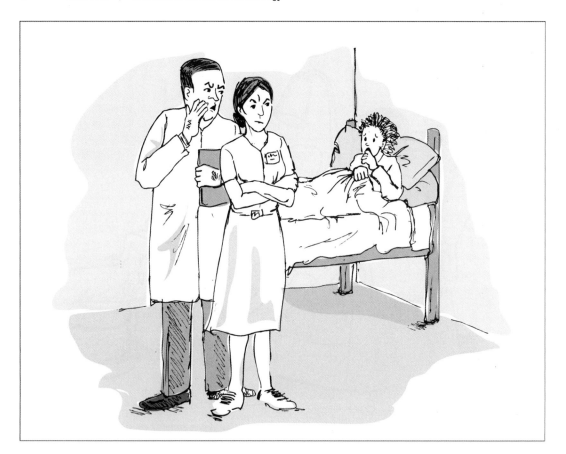

"Without education we are in horrible and deadly danger of taking educated people seriously."
—*Gilbert Keith Chesterton*

So, what does any of the foregoing have to do with medical terminology? Medical terminology is one's first exposure to clinical culture. The notion that one learns a special vocabulary to become a "member of a club" reflects deconstructionist views that, depending on the particular deconstructionist you encounter, may include the following:

- Communication with nonmembers is, at best, a necessary evil.
- Slang and other shortcuts are okay.
- Outsiders are obstacles to be ignored or overpowered unless your purpose is to impress them with your expertise.

Such attitudes work against professionalism and give insult to the vast majority of health care workers, whose first priority is helping sick people get well.

THE PARTS OF MEDICAL TERMS

Nearly every medical term contains one or more **roots**. It may also contain one or more **suffixes** and one or more **prefixes**. That is to say, a single medical term may consist of one part or several, but every part of a term behaves in one of three ways: root, suffix, or prefix. The good—and maybe surprising—news is that these three elements also make up all other English words. The even better news is that as an English speaker, you already know a lot of these elements, especially prefixes and suffixes.

Let's change the order of listing the word parts slightly and arrange them with prefixes coming first, roots second, and suffixes last, as they appear in that order in a word that contains all three. That is to say, a prefix (if one is present) appears at the beginning of the term, and a root (again, if a prefix occurs) is next and in the middle (if a suffix appears). Suffixes (when they appear) are always the endings of words.

Some words contain all three (e.g., anticlerical). The prefix is **anti-** (against), the root is **cleric** (clergyman), and the suffix **-al** makes the word an adjective. This word is thus an adjective meaning "against the clergy."

EXAMPLE: His <u>anticlerical</u> attitude colors everything he says.

Some words contain only one part (e.g., cleric [a root]). The word cleric is a noun that refers to a member of the clergy.

EXAMPLE: Mr. Witherspoon is a <u>cleric</u> who knows a great deal about antiquity.

Other words contain other combinations (e.g., anticlericalism [the prefix **anti-** again; **cleric**, a root; and two suffixes: **-al**, an adjective suffix coupled with **-ism**, a suffix that turns the word back into a noun]). Anticlericalism refers to the belief that any political influence of the clergy ought to be curtailed or abolished altogether.

EXAMPLE: <u>Anticlericalism</u> reached dramatic proportions in Spain during that nation's civil war in the 1930s.

Here is a medical term that has two roots: psychopath (**psycho** and **path**). *Psychopath* is a medical term that has become a common English word. It refers to a person who has a severe psychological disorder. One might contend that path is a suffix because in the term psychopath, it comes last. If we consider that the element *path* comes to us from the English word **pathos**, which means sorrow, suffering, or tragedy, then maybe we ought to identify it as a root. However, as it comes at the end of some terms, is it not also a suffix? The best answer to that question is, "Who cares?" You may call it a root or a suffix, and it doesn't really matter as long as you know what it means and where it goes in a particular term. The bottom line is that prefix, root, and suffix identification is a convenient way to look at and decipher terms; and most of the time, assigning the labels of prefix, root, and suffix to a word's parts leads to an acceptable definition. If the elements vary a little now and then, don't despair; the universe will go on.

ANALYZING TERMS

Learning to pick out prefixes, roots, and suffixes, as is done for you in Table 1-1, will permit you to define many, or even most, medical terms. Before going any further, we must deal with what has been traditionally referred to as a fourth word element: the **combining form**. Many, perhaps most, medical terminology instructors treat medical terms as having a fourth word element called the "combining form." However, the awkwardness of the phrase combining form (form of what?) sometimes confuses students. A combining form is simply a root that includes one or more vowels tacked onto the end of it to make a root–suffix combination pronounceable, as in the word *psychology*. The main root is psych (mind), and the suffix is -logy (study of). But psychlogy doesn't flow as well as psychology, and we insert the "o" to create a more English-sounding word.

So, as the example shows, the combining form concept is all about vowels, consonants, and pronunciation. A problem thus arises. That problem is that we remember a word (or a word part, for that matter) in two ways: by recalling the sound it makes when we hear it spoken and by the sound a visual combination of its letters makes when we see it written.

When I asked a colleague at a conference how she pronounced the root **iatr**, which means physician, she said, "eye-a-tro." Another conferee volunteered, "eye-at-ur," and a French friend of mine insists on, "eye-att-re" with a clipped final vowel sound, as in *Louvre*. Read the following to see an example of the problems of treating roots as though their spellings are given from the gods.

TABLE 1-1	ANALYSIS OF EXAMPLE WORDS			
Term	**Prefix**	**Root(s)**	**Suffix(es)**	**Term Meaning**
cardialgia		cardi (heart)	-algia (pain)	pain in the heart; also, heartburn (a digestive disorder)
cardiology		cardio (heart)	-logy (study of)	study of the heart and its disorders
carditis		card (heart)	-itis (inflammation)	inflammation of the heart
diagnosis	dia- (across; through)	gnosis (Greek word meaning "knowledge")		discovery of the cause of signs and symptoms
iatrogenic disease		iatro (physician); gen (origin, cause)	-ic (adjective suffix)	disease caused by health care (whether an individual worker, particular institution, or the system as a whole)
psychopath		psycho (mind); path (disease)		person with a (serious) mental disease

My morning star colored by the gelatin effect of the hazed hue precipitator, known to many as Pophx and to others as Mdth. But to most as Ropltz. This was an unspeakable truth.[2]

The lesson here is that calling a root something other than a root (e.g., a combining form after you have added a vowel to it) robs everyone of the most important way we remember roots, and that is by the sounds they make when we say them out loud.

In other words, every so-called combining form is also a bona fide root in itself. So, where does that leave the fourth word element, the combining form? If you and/or your instructor are accustomed to it and if it has become a part of your understanding of medical term construction, by all means use it. If you see it as an obstacle to learning medical terms, then forget about it. This book will, in deference to those who regard the concept of the combining form helpful, introduce roots with their potential combining vowels added with forward slant bars separating them from the rest of the root:

EXAMPLE: card/i/o

By the way, it would make equal sense to introduce them as follows:

EXAMPLE: card; cardi; cardio (All three are, phonetically speaking, roots.)

You can learn a great deal from Table 1-1. To begin with, the terms **cardialgia**, **cardiology**, and **carditis** not only show the three forms of the root for heart (**card**, **cardi**, and **cardio**) but also introduce you to three important suffixes: -**algia**, -**logy**, and -**itis**.
- -algia = pain
- -logy = study of
- -itis = inflammation

These three suffixes occur in many medical terms. For example, when you learn a new root, such as **neur/o**, which means nerve, you will know the meanings of **neuralgia**, **neurology**, and **neuritis**:
- neuralgia   pain in a nerve
- neurology   the study of the nervous system; also the specialty dealing with diagnosis and treatment of nervous system disorders
- neuritis   inflammation of a nerve

Discerning readers may have noted that the suffix -logy is in the same category as the suffix -path. Although they both may be regarded as suffixes, we might also note that -logy is a root that comes to us from the Greek word *logos*, meaning "word"—not as in "a" word so much as in "the" word, that is, an explanation of things. That final meaning is why we define it as "study of" in Table 1-1. You may also recognize this root in common English words such as logic, logical, logician, etc.

---

[2]This nonsensical bit of "wisdom" comes from a parody of Kahlil Gibran's *The Prophet*. It appears in a book called *The Profit* by Kehlog Albran, a very funny and brilliantly conceived little volume by Martin A. Cohen and Sheldon Shacket, published by Price/Stern/Sloan, Los Angeles, 1973.

Heraclitus, a philosopher who lived in the sixth century BC, used the Greek word *logos* in a special way. He used it to mean "the word," not *a* word but *the* word. That is, he used it to refer to that which underlies and explains all of reality. Following from Heraclitus' usage, *logos* also came to mean rationality, which is why logic is the English word that refers to the rules and practices governing rational thought.

In summary, you now know the first part of the definition of every term ending with any of the three suffixes introduced in the table: for -algia, the definition will begin with "pain in . . . " It is important to note here that a second suffix, "-dynia," also denotes pain. These two suffixes are sometimes interchangeable and sometimes not. Eventually, you will become familiar with instances in which one or the other is appropriate or at least most common. For -logy, the definition will usually begin with "study of . . . " For -itis, the definition will begin with "inflammation of . . . "

The term **diagnosis** introduces the prefix **dia-**, which means through, across, or between. You may have noticed that dia- appears in words you already know and use frequently, such as diameter, a straight line running *through* the center point of a circle; diagonal, a straight line running between opposite corners of a rectangle; and dialogue, people speaking words to each other across a space.

The word dialogue provides an example of how words change meaning when speakers or writers misunderstand their origins. This word has also come to refer to a conversation between two people because someone mistakenly interpreted the prefix to be di, meaning two, and other writers and speakers followed suit.

The medical term **diagnosis** refers to the determination of the presence of a disease or other disorder *through* consideration of signs, symptoms, and medical test results. That definition might seem to stretch the point of the word "through" until you learn that *gnosis* is the Greek word for knowledge: in other words, diagnosis is a procedure leading to a judgment through knowledge. The verb **diagnose** represents a departure in one respect from the etymology of the term diagnosis. As with all back-formed verbs, clarity is easily lost. In this case, fuzziness comes about because the noun "knowledge" names that which we know, whereas declaring (a verb) that we know it is something else entirely.

Iatr/o is a root that means physician, and **gen/o** (from a Greek word *gennao*, that simply meant the production of something) refers to origin or cause. The addition of **-ic** to gen yields **genic**, an adjective suffix meaning "originating from" or "caused by." Thus, an iatrogenic disorder is, literally speaking, "a disorder caused by a physician." In general use, the term *iatrogenic* refers to a disorder, disease, or ailment caused by any medical treatment or practitioner.

Another form of the root iatr/o is **iatr**, which may be coupled with other roots and several suffixes: **y**, **ic**, **ics**, **ist**, and **ician**. Here are examples of words formed from iatr, y, ic, ist, and ician:

psychiatry	psych + iatr + y	specialty dealing with disorders of the mind (in this case the y **does not** act as an adjective suffix)
psychiatric	psych + iatr + ic	adjective form of psychiatry
psychiatrist	psych + iatr + ist	specialist in psychiatry
geriatrics	ger + iatr + ics	specialty in disorders of the elderly
pediatrician	ped +iatr +ician	specialist in children's disorders

The root psycho comes from the Greek word *psyche*, which means soul or mind. The suffixes, **-ist** and **-ician** mean practitioner, and the suffixes **-y** and **-ics** mean practice. The final two items in the list introduce two new roots: **ger/o** and **ped/o**, the meanings of which you may deduce from the meanings of the terms **geriatrics** and **pediatrician**. The root ger/o (also sometimes **ger/onto**) comes from the Greek word *geron*, which means old man. The root **ped/o** is probably derived from the Greek word *pais*, which means child.

See Tables 1-2, 1-3, and 1-4, which list a sampling of roots, suffixes, and prefixes. There are many other word elements, and you will learn about them in subsequent chapters. Those listed in the tables will enable you to get started by building and defining terms.

TABLE 1-2   LIST OF SOME COMMON WORD ROOTS TO BEGIN BUILDING TERMS

arthr/o	joint
card/i/o	heart
derm/o/ato	skin
gen/o	origin, cause, formation
ger/o/onto	old age
hem/a/ato	blood
iatr/o	physician
muscul/o	muscle
natal	birth; born
neur/o	nerve
os/teo	bone
path/o	disease
ped/ia	child
phren/o	diaphragm, mind, or seat of passions
psych/o	mind
skelet/o	skeleton
tend/o, ten/o	tendon

TABLE 1-3   LIST OF SUFFIXES TO BEGIN BUILDING TERMS

-al	adjective suffix
-algia	pain
-dynia	pain
-gen, -genesis[a]	origin, cause, formation
-ic	adjective suffix denoting of
-itis	inflammation
-logy	study of
-pathy	disease
-scope	viewing, an instrument used for viewing

[a]The roots *gen, genic, path, pathy, logy,* and several others you will encounter later are common endings of many medical terms and have long been identified as suffixes. You should feel free to think of them as suffixes since that will help you understand terms in which they are the final syllable.

TABLE 1-4   LIST OF PREFIXES TO BEGIN BUILDING TERMS

epi-	upon, following, or subsequent to
micro-	small
peri-	around
pre-	before
post-	after

EXERCISES

EXERCISE 1-1 DEFINING TERMS

Combine the suffix -logy with the proper root to indicate the following medical specialties:

1. Specialty dealing with heart disease _____

2. Specialty that deals with the problems of aging and diseases in the elderly _____

3. Specialty dealing with blood diseases _____

4. Specialty dealing with skin ailments _____

5. Specialty dealing with nervous system disorders _____

6. Specialty dealing with mental disorders _____

EXERCISE 1-2 ANALYZING TERMS

Analyze the following terms by putting the roots and suffixes in the appropriate columns. Then write a definition for each term.

	ROOT	SUFFIX	WORD TYPE AND DEFINITION
1. neuropathy	_____	_____	_____
2. psychology	_____	_____	_____
3. pathogenic	_____	_____	_____
4 neuralgia	_____	_____	_____
5. systemic	_____	_____	_____
6. psychiatrist	_____	_____	_____
7. pediatrician	_____	_____	_____
8. iatrogenic	_____	_____	_____
9. cardialgia	_____	_____	_____
10. neuritis	_____	_____	_____

◀ **CHAPTER 1 QUIZ**

Complete the following sentences with the appropriate terms or definitions

1. The prefix *peri-* denotes _____.

2. The suffix *-logy* means _____.

3. The word root derm/o refers to _____.

4. The medical term *osteoarthritis* contains two _____ and one _____.

5. The suffix *-logy* is derived from the Greek word _____, which means _____.

6. Tendonitis refers to the _____ of a _____.

7. A prenatal exam is one that occurs _____ birth of a child.

8. _____ is indicated by the suffixes -algia and _____.

9. Inflammation is indicated by the suffix _____.

10. The study of mental and emotional disorders is called _____.

2 | *Common Suffixes and Prefixes*

LEARNING OBJECTIVES

Upon completion of this chapter, you should be able to:

- Recognize suffixes.
- Recognize prefixes.
- Define all of the suffixes and prefixes presented in this chapter.
- Analyze and define new terms introduced in this chapter.
- Pronounce, write, and spell each term introduced in this chapter.

INTRODUCTION

Chapter 1 presented the four word elements used in medical terminology: roots, suffixes, prefixes, and "combining forms." This chapter focuses on suffixes and prefixes.

As noted in Chapter 1, a suffix is the element that comes at the end of a word. The word suffix comes from the Latin word *suffixum*, which may be translated as "to attach under or to the end of." Although the suffix is located last in a medical term, it often comes first in its definition. For example, appendicitis means "inflammation (*-itis*) of the appendix." Therefore, the suffix, in this case -itis, provides us with the first word of the defining phrase. The term *gastrectomy* is another example. It is defined as "removal of the stomach." The definition begins with the meaning of the suffix, -ectomy, which means "removal of."

Chapter 1 also states that a prefix is a word element that comes at the beginning of a word. Note that the word prefix itself contains a prefix, namely, pre-. The second part of the word prefix is "fix," which gives us a perfect definition of prefix: something af<u>fix</u>ed to (attached) to the front of or before (pre-) something else. Most of the prefixes occurring in medical terms are also found in everyday English. Although we have all used many of the prefixes contained in this chapter, we may have done so without realizing that they are prefixes. For example, when we are admitted to an anteroom, we may not stop to think that the prefix **ante-** means "before" and that an anteroom is so called because it is a room we enter before entering another room.

ROOTS TO COMBINE WITH THE SUFFIXES INTRODUCED IN THIS CHAPTER

Table 2-1 lists some roots to get you started on your journey of learning hundreds of medical terms. You may wish to memorize the roots given in the table now, given that there are not many. Or if you prefer, just give them a quick glance now and, as you go through the chapter, refer back to this table whenever you run across a term with a root you don't recognize.

CATEGORIES OF SUFFIXES

Dividing suffixes into functional categories makes them easier to learn than they would be otherwise. A medical term suffix adds to or changes a root in one of four different ways, as indicated in the following list:

- Signifies a medical condition
- Signifies a diagnostic term, test information, or surgical procedure
- Indicates a medical specialty or specialist
- Converts a noun to an adjective

TABLE 2-1 SOME COMMON WORD ROOTS TO BEGIN BUILDING TERMS	
arter/i/o	artery
arthr/o	joint
card/i/o	heart
derm/at/o	skin
gen/i/o	origin, cause, formation
ger/o/onto	old age
hem/a/t/o	blood
iatr/o	physician
muscul/o	muscle
neur/o	nerve
ost/e/o	bone
path/o	disease
ped/i/o	child
phren/o	mind
psych/o	mind
skelet/o	skeleton
spin/o	spine
tend/i/n/o	tendon

The suffix stenosis, for example, indicates a narrowing or blockage in a body part, which is a condition. Consider, then, the term **arteriostenosis**. Because the root arter/i/o means artery, we may conclude that arteriostenosis is a narrowing of an artery. Observe how this term is divided into word elements:

TERM	ELEMENTS	MEANING
arteriostenosis	root: arter/i/o = artery	narrowing of an artery
	suffix: -stenosis = narrowing	

Suffixes Signifying Medical Conditions

The suffix **-porosis**, which means porous, is added to the root **oste/o**, to form the term *osteoporosis*, which means "a porous condition of bone." See Table 2-2 for more examples.

Suffixes Signifying Diagnostic Terms, Test Information, or Surgical Procedures

Suffixes that form terms related to test information, diagnoses, and procedures are often attached to a root that signifies a body part. The term **appendectomy** is an example. The suffix **-ectomy** means "removal of," and **append** is the root for appendix. Thus, the term means "removal of the appendix." Table 2-3 lists common suffixes that signify diagnostic terms, test information, or procedures.

Suffixes That Name a Medical Specialty or Specialist

Some suffixes relating to medical specialties and specialists are derived from the Greek word *iatros*, which means "physician" or "medical treatment." This Greek word is the source of the root iatr/o. For practical purposes, you may consider the root iatr as an integral part of the suffixes **-iatric**, and **-iatry**, and so on (e.g., in the terms *geriatrics, psychiatric, psychiatry, psychiatrist, pediatrics*, and *pediatrician*). Although both -ician and -ist are used in referring to a specialist, the suffix -ist is perhaps the more common one. An example is the **gerontologist**, a physician who diagnoses and treats disorders brought on by aging.

TABLE 2-2 SUFFIXES THAT SIGNIFY MEDICAL CONDITIONS

Suffix	Meaning of the Suffix	Example	Definition of the Example
-algia	pain	arthralgia	pain in a joint
-dynia	pain	arthrodynia	pain in a joint
-ectasis, -ectasia	expansion or dilation	angiectasis	dilation of a vessel
-iasis	presence of; formation of	cholelithiasis; sometimes also spelled chololithiasis	stones in the gallbladder or bile ducts
-itis	inflammation	appendicitis	inflammation of the appendix
-malacia	softening	osteomalacia	softening of the bones
-megaly	enlargement	gastromegaly	enlargement of the stomach
-oma	tumor	gastroma	tumor of the stomach
-osis	abnormal condition	osteoporosis	condition of porous bones
-penia	reduction of size or quantity	leukopenia	low number of white blood cells
-plegia	paralysis	hemiplegia	paralysis on one side of the body
-pnea	breathing	tachypnea	rapid breathing
-porosis	porous condition	osteoporosis	porous
-ptosis	downward displacement	nephroptosis	downward displacement of a kidney
-rrhage	flowing forth	hemorrhage	significant discharge of blood from blood vessels
-rrhexis	rupture	hysterorrhexis	rupture of the uterus
-spasm	muscular contraction	angiospasm	muscular contraction of a vessel

TABLE 2-3 SUFFIXES THAT SIGNIFY DIAGNOSTIC TERMS, TEST INFORMATION, OR SURGICAL PROCEDURES

Suffix	Refers to	Examples
-centesis	surgical puncture	thoracentesis
-desis	surgical binding	arthrodesis
-ectomy	surgical removal	appendectomy
-gen, -genic, -genesis	origin, producing	osteogenic
-gram	written or pictorial record	electrocardiogram
-graph	device for graphic or pictorial recording	electrocardiograph
-graphy	act of graphic or pictorial recording	electrocardiography
-meter	device for measuring	audiometer
-metry	act of measuring	audiometry
-pexy	surgical fixation	hysteropexy
-plasty	surgical repair	rhinoplasty
-rrhaphy	suture	herniorrhaphy
-scope	device for viewing	arthroscope
-scopy	act of viewing	arthroscopy
-tomy	incision	colotomy
-tripsy	crushing	lithotripsy

TABLE 2-4	SUFFIXES THAT SIGNIFY MEDICAL SPECIALTIES AND SPECIALISTS	
Suffix	**Refers to**	**Examples**
-ian	specialist	pediatrician
-iatrics	medical specialty	pediatrics
-iatry	medical specialty	psychiatry
-ics	medical specialty	orthopedics
-ist	specialist in a field of study	orthopedist
-logy	study of	gynecology

Terms denoting a field or medical specialty may also end with the suffix **-logy**. Table 2-4 lists the suffixes for medical specialties and specialists.

Root or suffix? The element **gen** can act as a suffix or a root, but as is the case with iatr, it combines nicely with several suffixes and may be considered as a part of them. Terms formed with **-genic** are adjectives, owing to the **-ic** ending. As will become evident later, -ic can act as a suffix by itself, too.

Suffixes That Denote Adjectives

As with suffixes that signify medical specialties and specialists, suffixes used to create adjective forms are not governed by a clear set of rules. Nevertheless, there are some rules that come into play (i.e., the rules of English pronunciation). For example, we replace the final letter, *x*, in the word appendix with a *c* to form the adjective appendicitis because "appendixitis" does not sound much like an English word.

In creating adjectives, we also sometimes change noun terms that name specialties. For example, psychiatry and pediatrics are the names of specialties. Dropping the *y* from psychiatry and adding the adjective suffix -ic converts the specialty name to an adjective:

psychiat**ric** medicine   psychiat**ric** hospital

With pediatrics, on the other hand, all we need to do to form the adjective is drop the *s*:

pediat**ric** medicine   pediat**ric** hospital

Examples of adjective suffixes are listed in Table 2-5.

CATEGORIES OF PREFIXES

Not all medical terms include a prefix, but when one is present, it is critical to the term's meaning. For example, **hyper**glycemia (high blood sugar) and **hypo**glycemia (low blood sugar) name conditions that are exact opposites. Confusing those two prefixes create a malaprop, a language error, as explained in Chapter 1. In fact, two other similar-sounding prefix pairs are prone to malaprop formation as well. They are ante- and anti- (ante- means "before" and anti- means "against.")

TERM	ELEMENTS	MEANING
hypoglycemia	prefix: hypo = low	low blood sugar
	root: glyc/o = sugar	
	suffix: -emia = condition	

TABLE 2-5	SUFFIXES THAT DENOTE ADJECTIVES	
Suffix	**Meaning**	**Examples**
-ac, -al, -an, -aneous, -ar, -ary, -eous, -iac, -iatric, -ic, -ical, -oid, -otic, -ous, -ular	converts a root or noun to an adjective	geriatric, orthopedic, ocular

Dividing prefixes into functional categories, just as we did with suffixes, makes them easier to learn. There are four logical divisions:

- Prefixes of time or speed
- Prefixes of direction
- Prefixes of position
- Prefixes of size or number

Seeing prefixes in words we already know helps us assimilate their meanings quickly and enables us to understand medical terms we encounter later on. For that reason, common English words are included as examples in some of the following paragraphs and tables.

Prefixes of Time or Speed

Prefixes denoting time or speed are used in everyday English. **Pre**historic and **post**graduate are common words with a prefix relating to time. Table 2-6 lists examples of this category of prefix.

TABLE 2-6	PREFIXES DENOTING TIME OR SPEED		
Prefix	**Refers to**	**Examples**	**Definition**
ante-, pre-	before	antepartum, premature	before birth, before full development
brady-	abnormally slow rate of speed	bradycardia	abnormally slow heartbeat
neo-	new	neonatal	newborn (adjective)
post-	after	postscript	a written thought added after the main message
tachy-	rapid, abnormally high rate of speed	tachycardia	abnormally fast heartbeat

Prefixes of Direction

The word **ab**normal is an example of a word containing a prefix that signifies direction.

We use prefixes in everyday life without bothering to analyze them. For example, we normally would not take the time to think about the prefix **contra-** (against) in the word contradiction, yet we understand its meaning. Prefixes relating to direction are listed in Table 2-7.

Prefixes of Position

Infrastructure (infra- means "inside" or "below"), **inter**state (inter- means "between"), and **para**legal (para- means "alongside") are all words we frequently use that include prefixes of position. Having these prefix meanings already in our vocabularies makes it easier to learn their medical uses. Prefixes of position are commonly used during diagnostic and treatment procedures. Table 2-8 lists the prefixes related to position.

TABLE 2-7	PREFIXES OF DIRECTION		
Prefix	**Refers to**	**Examples**	**Definition**
ab-	away from, outside of, beyond	abnormal	not normal
ad-	toward, near to	adjective	toward a noun
con-, sym-, syn-	with; within	congenital, sympathetic, synthetic	with (or at) birth, with feeling toward, with the same idea or purpose
contra-	against	contraband	substance against the law
dia-	across, through	diameter	a line through the middle

TABLE 2-8   PREFIXES OF POSITION

Prefix	Refers to	Examples	Definition
ec-, ecto-, ex-, exo-	outside	extraction	removal to the outside
en-	inside	encephalopathy	disease inside the head; brain disease
endo-	within	endoscopy	visual examination of the inside of some part of the body
epi-	upon, subsequent to	epigastric	adjective referring to something above the stomach
extra-	beyond	extracellular	adjective referring to something outside a cell or cells
hyper-	above, beyond normal	hyperglycemia	high blood sugar
hypo-	low, below, below normal	hypogastric	region beneath the stomach
infra-	inside or below	infrarenal	adjective referring to something below the kidneys
inter-	between	interosseous	between bones
intra-	inside, within	intracerebral	inside the cerebrum
meso-	middle	mesothelioma	tumor arising from the mesothelium
meta-	beyond	metacarpal	the bone beyond the carpus; one of five bones in either hand
pan-	all or everywhere	pancarditis	general inflammation of the heart
para-	alongside, like	paraplegia	paralysis of the lower half of the body
peri-	around	perivascular	in the tissues surrounding a vessel
retro-	backward, behind	retrosternal	adjective referring to something behind the sternum

Prefixes of Size and Number

A **semi**annual (semi- means "half"; annual means "yearly") sale is one that occurs every 6 months. The **uni**corn (uni- means "one") is a fictitious creature that has one horn. Prefixes of size and number are very common. Table 2-9 lists prefixes of size and number; many are easily recognizable.

Suffixes and prefixes as presented in this chapter will become familiar as you progress through the chapters on body systems. Review the study tables and perform the exercises for self-testing.

TABLE 2-9   PREFIXES OF SIZE AND NUMBER

Prefix	Refers to	Examples
bi-	two	biannual
di-, dipl-	two, twice	diplopia
hemi-, semi-	half	hemiplegia
macro-	big	macrocyte
micro-	small	microscope
mono-	one	monocyte
olig-, oligo-	a few	oliguria
pan-	all or everywhere	pancarditis
poly-	many	polydactyly
quadri-	four	quadriplegia
semi-	half, partial	semiannual
tetra-	four	tetradactyl
tri-	three	triceps
uni-	one	unicellular

Study Table — COMMON SUFFIXES

SUFFIX	MEANING	EXAMPLES
-ac, -al, -an, -aneous, -ar, -ary, -eal, -eous, -iac, -iatric, -ic, -ical, -oid, -otic, -ous, -tic, -ular	converts a root or a noun term to an adjective	geriatric, orthopedic, ocular, dental, cutaneous, cyanotic, atrial, cardiac, ureteral
-cele	protrusion, hernia	rectocele
-centesis	surgical puncture	thoracentesis
-cyte	cell	leukocyte
-desis	surgical binding	arthrodesis
-dynia, -algia	pain	arthrodynia
-ectasis, -ectasia	expansion or dilation	angiectasis
-ectomy	surgical removal	appendectomy
-edema	excessive fluid in intracellular tissues	angioedema
-emesis	vomiting	hematemesis
-emia	blood	uremia
-genic	origin, producing	osteogenic
-gram	written or pictorial record	electrocardiogram
-graph	device for graphic or pictorial recording	electrocardiograph
-graphy	act of graphic or pictorial recording	electrocardiography
-ian, -iatrist, -ist, -logist, -logy, -ics, -iatry, -iatrics	specialty of, study of, practice of	geriatrist, pediatrician, gynecology
-iasis	a suffix used to convert a verb to a noun indicating a condition	cholelithiasis
-ism	a condition of; a process; or a state of	dwarfism, gigantism
-itis	inflammation	appendicitis
-lith	stone, calculus, calcification	pneumolith
-lysis	disintegration	hemolysis
-malacia	softening	osteomalacia
-megaly	enlargement	gastromegaly
-meter	device for measuring	audiometer
-metry	act of measuring	audiometry
-oid	resembling or like	android
-oma	tumor	gastroma
-opsy	visual examination	biopsy
-osis	abnormal condition	osteoporosis, arthrosis
-pathy	disease	cardiopathy

(continued)

SUFFIX	MEANING	EXAMPLES
-penia	reduction of size or quantity	leukopenia
-pexy	surgical fixation	hysteropexy
-phobia	fear, appears mainly as a suffix	claustrophobia
-plasia	abnormal formation	chondroplasia
-plasty	surgical repair	rhinoplasty
-plegia	paralysis	hemiplegia
-pnea	breath, respiration	tachypnea
-poiesis	producing	erythropoiesis
-porosis	porous condition	osteoporosis
-ptosis	downward displacement	nephroptosis
-rrhage	flowing forth	hemorrhage
-rrhaphy	suture	herniorrhaphy
-rrhea	discharge	diarrhea
-rrhexis	rupture	hysterorrhexis
-sclerosis	hardness	arteriosclerosis
-scope	device for viewing	arthroscope
-scopy	act of viewing	arthroscopy
-spasm	muscular contraction	arteriospasm
-stasis	level; unchanging	hemostasis
-stenosis	narrowed; blocked	arteriostenosis
-stomy	permanent opening	colostomy
-tome	instrument for cutting	osteotome
-tomy	incision	osteotomy
-tripsy	crushing	lithotripsy

Study Table   COMMON PREFIXES

PREFIX	MEANING	EXAMPLES
ab-	away from, outside of, beyond	abnormal
ad-	toward, near to	addiction
ante-, pre-	before	antepartum, premature
anti-	against, opposed	antibiotic
bi-	two	biannual
brady-	abnormally slow rate of speed	bradycardia
con-, sym-, syn-	with	congenital, sympathetic, synarthrosis
contra-	against	contralateral
dia-	across, through	diagnosis

PREFIX	MEANING	EXAMPLES
dys-	painful, bad, difficult	dyspnea
ec-, ecto-	outside, away from	ectopy
en-, endo-	inside	endoscopy
epi-	upon, subsequent to	epigastric
ex-, exo-	outside	exoskeleton
extra-	beyond	extrasystole
hemi-, semi-	half	hemiplegia
hyper-	above, beyond normal	hypergastric
hypo-	below, below normal	hypogastric
infra-	inside or below	infrastructure
inter-	between	intercostal
intra-	inside	intracerebral
macro-	big	macrocyte
meso-	middle	mesothelium
meta-	beyond	metacarpal
micro-	small	microscope
mono-, uni-	one	monocyte
neo-	new	neoplasm
olig-, oligo-	a few	oliguria
pan-	everywhere	pancarditis
para-	alongside, like	paraplegia
post-	after	postsynaptic
quadri-	four	quadriceps
retro-	backward, behind	retroperitoneal
tachy-	abnormally high rate of speed	tachycardia
tri-	three	tricep

EXERCISES

EXERCISE 2-1 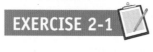 COMBINING ROOTS AND SUFFIXES THAT
SIGNIFY MEDICAL CONDITIONS

NOTE: As the object of this chapter section is to introduce suffixes, not whole terms, these
particular roots were selected for use only because they combine easily with more than one
suffix. Additional roots will be introduced within the various anatomical system chapters.

**Build terms by combining the correct form of each of the roots with the suffixes appearing
next to it. Suffixes and their definitions may be found in the Study Table on suffixes for this
chapter. Write a definition for each term in the space to the right. Use a medical dictionary
for definitions if needed.**

ROOT	SUFFIX	WORD	MEANING
1. card/i/o	-cele	_____	_____
	-dynia	_____	_____
	-ectasia	_____	_____
	-itis	_____	_____
	-malacia	_____	_____
	-megaly	_____	_____
	-ptosis	_____	_____
	-plegia	_____	_____
	-rrhexis	_____	_____
	-spasm	_____	_____
2. dermat/o	-itis	_____	_____
	-oma	_____	_____
	-megaly	_____	_____
	-osis	_____	_____
3. hem/o, hemat/o	-lysis	_____	_____
	-genesis	_____	_____
	-oma	_____	_____
	-osis	_____	_____

4. neur/o   -algia   _____   _____

-ectasis   _____   _____

-itis   _____   _____

-oma   _____   _____

5. oste/o   -dynia   _____   _____

-oma   _____   _____

-malacia   _____   _____

-penia   _____   _____

-porosis   _____   _____

-itis   _____   _____

6. psych/o   -osis   _____   _____

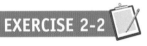

EXERCISE 2-2 COMBINING ROOTS AND SUFFIXES THAT SIGNIFY DIAGNOSTIC TERMS, TEST INFORMATION, OR SURGICAL PROCEDURES

Build terms by combining the correct form of each of the roots with the suffixes appearing next to it. Suffixes and their definitions may be found in the Study Table on suffixes for this chapter. Write a definition for each term in the space to the right. Use a medical dictionary for definitions if needed.

ROOT	SUFFIX	WORD	MEANING
1. card/i/o	-genic	_____	_____
	-gram	_____	_____
	-graph	_____	_____
	-graphy	_____	_____
	-pathy	_____	_____
	-rrhaphy	_____	_____
2. dermat/o	-plasty	_____	_____
3. hemat/o	-genesis	_____	_____
	-metry	_____	_____

4. neur/o   -ectomy   _____   _____

             -genic   _____   _____

             -genesis   _____   _____

5. oste/o   -rrhaphy   _____   _____

             -plasty   _____   _____

             -genesis   _____   _____

             -ectomy   _____   _____

             -tomy   _____   _____

6. path/o   -gen   _____   _____

             -genic   _____   _____

             -genesis   _____   _____

7. psych/o   -genic   _____   _____

             -genesis   _____   _____

             -metry   _____   _____

             -pathy   _____   _____

EXERCISE 2-3 COMBINING ROOTS AND SUFFIXES ASSOCIATED WITH A MEDICAL SPECIALIST OR SPECIALTY

Build terms by combining the correct form of each of the roots with the suffixes appearing next to it. Suffixes and their definitions may be found in the Study Table on suffixes for this chapter. Write a definition for each term in the space to the right. Use a medical dictionary for definitions if needed.

ROOT	SUFFIX	WORD	MEANING
1. card/i/o	-logy	_____	_____
	-logist	_____	_____
2. derm/o, dermat/o	-logy	_____	_____
	-logist	_____	_____
3. ger/o/nt/o	-iatrics	_____	_____
	-logy	_____	_____
	-logist	_____	_____

4. hem/o, hemat/o   -logy   _____   _____

   -logist   _____   _____

5. neur/o   -logy   _____   _____

   -logist   _____   _____

6. oste/o   -logy   _____   _____

   -logist   _____   _____

7. path/o   -logy   _____   _____

   -logist   _____   _____

8. psych/o   -logy   _____   _____

   -iatry   _____   _____

   -iatrist   _____   _____

EXERCISE 2-4 COMBINING ROOTS AND SUFFIXES THAT DENOTE ADJECTIVES

Build terms by combining the correct form of each of the roots with the suffixes appearing next to it. Suffixes and their definitions may be found in the Study Table on suffixes for this chapter. Write a definition for each term in the space to the right. Use a medical dictionary for definitions if needed.

ROOT	SUFFIX	WORD	MEANING
1. card/i/o	-ac	_____	_____
2. hem/o, hemat/o	-toxic	_____	_____
3. derm/o, dermat/o	-al	_____	_____
	-ic	_____	_____
4. ger/o, geront/o	-iatric	_____	_____
	-al	_____	_____
5. neur/o	-al	_____	_____
	-ic	_____	_____
6. spin/o	-al	_____	_____
	-ous	_____	_____
7. oste/o	-al	_____	_____
	-oid	_____	_____

EXERCISE 2-5 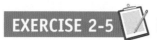 MATCHING SUFFIXES WITH MEANINGS

Choose the letter next to the Column 2 definition corresponding to each suffix in Column 1 and write it in the space provided. Suffixes and their definitions may be found in the Study Table on suffixes for this chapter.

COLUMN 1	COLUMN 2
1. ___G___ -cyte	A. a morbid impulse toward a specific object or thought
2. ___I___ -edema	B. vomiting
3. ___B___ -emesis	C. a stone, calculus, calcification
4. ___M___ -sclerosis	D. a condition, a process or state of
5. ___J___ -tome	E. disease
6. ___D___ -ism	F. visual examination
7. ___C___ -lith	G. cell
8. ___H___ -lysis	H. disintegration
9. ___F___ -opsy	I. excessive fluid in intracellular tissues
10. ___E___ -pathy	J. instrument for cutting
11. ___A___ -phobia	K. level; unchanging
12. ___O___ -poiesis	L. narrowed; blocked
13. ___N___ -stomy	M. hardness
14. ___K___ -stasis	N. permanent opening
15. ___L___ -stenosis	O. producing

EXERCISE 2-6 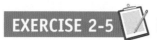 ADDING PREFIXES OF TIME OR SPEED

Add each prefix in the list to the word or word part appearing next to it, and write the definition of the word thus formed in the space to the right. Refer to a standard English dictionary as needed.

PREFIX	WORD	WORD FORMED	MEANING
1. ante-	room	_____	_____
2. neo-	classic	_____	_____
3. post-	glacial	_____	_____
4. pre-	dominant	_____	_____
5. tacho-	meter	_____	_____

EXERCISE 2-7 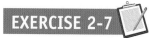 ADDING PREFIXES OF DIRECTION

Add each prefix in the list to the word or word part appearing next to it, and write the definition of the word thus formed in the space to the right. Refer to a standard English dictionary as needed.

PREFIX	WORD	WORD FORMED	MEANING
1. ab-	normal		
2. ad-	joining		
3. con-	centric		
4. contra-	lateral		
5. dia-	gram		
6. sym-	pathetic		
7. syn-	thesis		

EXERCISE 2-8 ADDING PREFIXES OF POSITION

Add each prefix in the list to the word or word part appearing next to it, and write the definition of the word thus formed in the space to the right. Refer to a standard English dictionary as needed.

PREFIX	WORD	WORD FORMED	MEANING
1. ec-	centric		
2. ecto-	morph		
3. en-	slave		
4. endo-	cardial		
5. epi-	demic		
6. ex-	change		
7. exo-	sphere		
8. extra-	terrestrial		
9. hyper-	sensitive		
10. hypo-	thesis		
11. infra-	structure		

12. inter-   collegiate   _____   _____

13. intra-   mural   _____   _____

14. meso-   sphere   _____   _____

15. meta-   physics   _____   _____

16. pan-   orama   _____   _____

17. para-   legal   _____   _____

18. retro-   rocket   _____   _____

EXERCISE 2-9 ADDING PREFIXES OF SIZE OR NUMBER

Add each prefix in the list to the word or word part appearing next to it, and write the definition of the word thus formed in the space to the right. Refer to a standard English dictionary as needed. The prefixes may all be found in the Study Table on prefixes or in the text.

PREFIX	WORD	WORD FORMED	MEANING
1. bi-	annual	_____	_____
2. hemi-	sphere	_____	_____
3. macro-	cosm	_____	_____
4. micro-	scope	_____	_____
5. mono-	rail	_____	_____
6. olig-	archy	_____	_____
7. quadri-	lateral	_____	_____
8. semi-	annual	_____	_____
9. tri-	angle	_____	_____
10. uni-	cycle	_____	_____

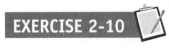

EXERCISE 2-10   CROSSWORD PUZZLE: COMMON SUFFIXES AND PREFIXES

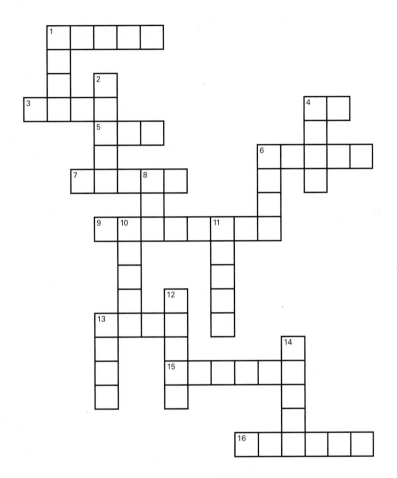

ACROSS

1. prefix, big
3. suffix, study of
4. prefix, away from
5. prefix, total or everywhere
6. prefix, between or across
7. suffix, pictorial recording device
9. suffix, narrowing
13. suffix, cell
15. suffix, removal of
16. prefix, four

DOWN

1. prefix, one
2. prefix, above or beyond normal
4. prefix, against
6. suffix, inflammation
8. prefix, before
10. prefix, abnormally fast
11. suffix, act of viewing
12. suffix, device for measuring
13. suffix, protrusion
14. suffix, pain

◀ CHAPTER 2 QUIZ

Suffixes

For each of the following questions or statements, write the answer in the space to the right.

1. What two suffixes mean "pain"?

    1. _____

2. *Ang/i/o* is a root meaning "blood vessel." What term means "dilation of a blood vessel"?

    2. _____

3. Angioid means "resembling blood vessels." What part of speech is angioid?

    3. _____

4. Define *angiorrhaphy*.

    4. _____
    _____

5. What suffix would you add to the root *ang/i/o* to form a term meaning "the act of making a pictorial record of blood vessels"?

    5. _____

6. What is an angioma?

    6. _____

7. What does *-plasty* mean?

    7. _____
    _____
    _____
    _____

8. What term denotes a skin specialist?

    8. _____

9. A gerontologist treats what age of patients, young or old?

    9. _____

10. What is the difference in meaning between *gerontology* and *geriatrics*?

    10. _____
    _____
    _____
    _____

Prefixes

For each of the following questions or statements, write the answer in the space to the right.

1. The prefixes *ab-* and *ad-* are opposites; which one means "toward"?

   1. _____

2. The prefix *pre-* means "before"; what other prefix means the same thing?

   2. _____

3. Write a brief definition of bradycardia.

   3. _____
      _____
      _____

4. What does the prefix *extra-* mean in the word extrasensory?

   4. _____

5. What prefix would you use in a term that means "high blood pressure"?

   5. _____

6. Given the meaning of *anti-*, what would be the purpose of an anticollision radar?

   6. _____
      _____

7. Given the meaning of the prefix *tri-*, how many engines does a trijet have?

   7. _____

8. Does the prefix *micro-* refer to the physical size of a microscope? If not, what does its presence in the word tell us?

   8. _____
      _____
      _____
      _____

9. Write a medical term by combining the prefix *endo-* with the root *card/i/o*, meaning "heart," and the suffix that means "inflammation." Using only your knowledge of these three word elements, write the best definition you can for the term.

   9. _____
      _____
      _____
      _____
      _____

10. The suffix *-pnea*, meaning "breathing" or "respiration," can follow both *tachy-* and *dys-*. Define the terms *tachypnea* and *dyspnea*.

  10. _____
      _____
      _____
      _____
      _____

3 *The Body's Organization*

LEARNING OBJECTIVES

Upon completion of this chapter, you should be able to:

- Discuss the levels of body organization.
- Describe the anatomical position and cite the directional terms used in relation to the body.
- Name the planes of the body.
- Name the body cavities.
- Name the divisions of the abdomen and back.
- Analyze, define, and pronounce the new terms introduced in this chapter.

INTRODUCTION

Learning about human body construction will help you retain the medical terms you are learning by creating a mental picture of where things are. It is also useful to know the distinction between the terms *anatomy* and *physiology*. Anatomy comes to us from the Greek word *anatome*, which means "dissection." You may have recognized the element -tome, which indicates that anatomy has something to do with cutting. Physiology, on the other hand, is one of the many "ology" words; in this case, it means study of how the body's parts work together. In short, anatomy reveals the "what it is" and physiology the "how it works."

The "what it is" begins with chemicals that act together to form cells. The cells process the food we eat and the air we breathe. Cells also reproduce themselves, each cell according to the DNA code it contains.

WORD ELEMENTS OFTEN USED IN TERMS RELATED TO BODY ORGANIZATION

Table 3-1 lists many of the elements making up terms related to the body as a whole. Not surprisingly, many of them have to do with what constitutes a major category or where things are located.

LEVELS OF ORGANIZATION

The body has four levels of organization: cells, tissues, organs, and systems; each level is defined subsequently under its own heading (Fig. 3-1).

TABLE 3-1	COMMON WORD ELEMENTS RELATED TO BODY ORGANIZATION
Element	**Meaning**
anter/o (root)	front, anterior
cerv/o (root)	neck
chondr/o (root)	cartilage
cyt/o, -cyte (root, suffix)	cell
dors/o (root)	back
inguin/o (root)	groin
my/o (root)	muscle
myel/o (root)	spinal cord
neur/o (root)	nerve, neuron
poster/o (root)	posterior, back
proxim/o (root)	near
super/o (root)	superior
trans- (prefix)	across

Cells

A human body is said to have 10 trillion to 100 trillion cells, depending on whom you ask. Of course, no one has ever actually counted the number of cells in a body, but as all the estimates are in the trillions, it's easy to appreciate the body's complexity as a functioning whole. Cells work both individually and together (Fig. 3-2). Although cells differ from one another and consist of different components, they do have some common elements:

- A cell membrane that allows certain substances in and out
- A nucleus that directs activities within the cell (Exception: red blood cells do not have nuclei.)
- Cytoplasm, a watery fluid that fills the spaces outside the nucleus

Tissue

Cells make up tissue, which is composed of similar cells working together to perform common tasks. The four types of body tissues are muscular, connective, nervous, and epithelial.

Organs

Tissues with common functions come together to form the body's organs, which perform specialized functions. Examples are the brain, stomach, and heart.

Systems

A group of organs forms a system, and each system has its own special purpose. Therefore, this book discusses each system in a chapter of its own.

NAVIGATING THE BODY

Health care professionals need to be familiar with directional and positioning terms, which are frequently used during examinations, diagnostic procedures, and treatments of patients.

Anatomical Position and Directional and Positional Terms

Standard **anatomical terms of location** are designations employed in science to deal with the anatomy of animals and thus avoid confusion. They are not language-specific and thus require no translation. They are universal terms that may be readily understood by zoologists who speak any language.

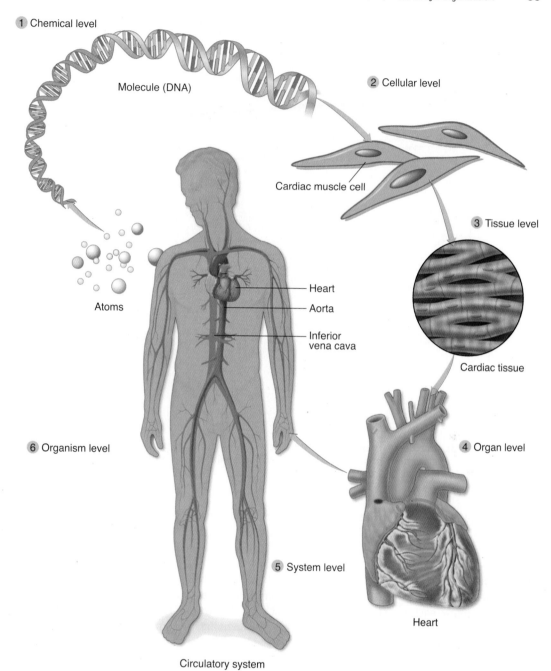

FIGURE 3-1 Body organization. The six levels of the body's organization can be seen here: 1. chemical level, 2. cellular level, 3. tissue level, 4. organ level, 5. system level, and finally 6. organism level, the human body. *From Premkumar K. The Massage Connection: Anatomy and Physiology. Baltimore, MD: Lippincott Williams & Wilkins; 2004.*

However, while standardized anatomical terms exist within specific fields of biology, they differ dramatically from one discipline to another, particularly between zoological anatomy (zootomy) and human anatomy.

Directional terms in the field of human anatomy differ in two ways: first, unlike terms of location in zoology, **they are language-specific**; second, they are specified relative to the **anatomical**

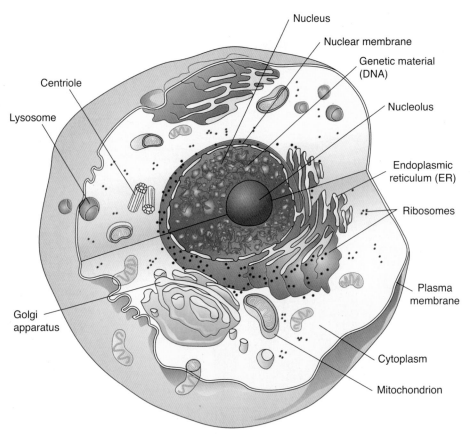

FIGURE 3-2   Basic structure of a cell. The basic structure of a cell includes the cell membrane, the nucleus, and the cytoplasm. *Modified from Cohen BJ, Wood DL.* Memmler's The Human Body in Health and Disease. *9th ed. Philadelphia, PA: Lippincott Williams & Wilkins; 2000.*

position. In the anatomical position, the body is erect and facing forward, and the arms are at the sides with the palms of the hands facing forward (Fig. 3-3). Left and right are from the subject's perspective, not the observer's.

> The inhabitants of Pormpuraaw, a remote Aboriginal community in Australia, have no words for "left" or "right." Instead, they speak of everything in terms of absolute cardinal directions (north, south, east, west). They say things such as, "There's an ant on your southwest leg." To say hello in Pormpuraaw, one asks, "Where are you going?" An appropriate response might be, "A long way to the south-southwest. How about you?" The Pormpuraawans not only know instinctively which direction they are facing, they also spontaneously use their spatial orientation to represent both position and time.[1]

Directional terms are adjectives that help describe a complaint, symptom, body part, or process. **Superior** means above or nearer to the head. One might use this term when describing an observation (e.g., "The bruise is superior to the eyebrow"). **Inferior** means below or toward the feet. **Anterior** is a directional term that relates to the front of the body. An example of the use of anterior would be, "The rash covered the entire anterior of the left thigh." **Ventral** is an adjective that refers to the front of the body.

---

[1] Paraphrased from a story in the *Wall Street Journal*, July 23, 2010.

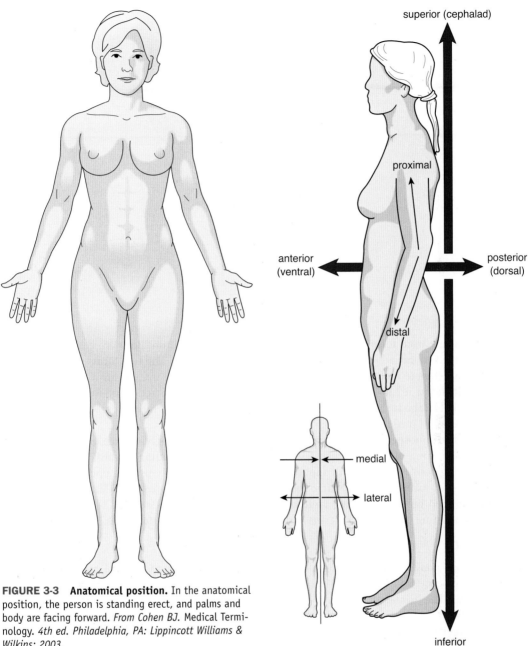

FIGURE 3-3   Anatomical position. In the anatomical position, the person is standing erect, and palms and body are facing forward. *From Cohen BJ. Medical Terminology. 4th ed. Philadelphia, PA: Lippincott Williams & Wilkins; 2003.*

FIGURE 3-4   Directional terms. Directional terms are frequently used to describe a symptom, a body part, or how one part is related to another. For example, the shoulder is proximal to the elbow. *Modified from Cohen BJ, Wood DL. Memmler's The Human Body in Health and Disease. 9th ed. Philadelphia, PA: Lippincott Williams & Wilkins; 2000.*

Posterior and **dorsal** are terms that specify the back or toward the back of the body. **Medial** means toward the midline of the body, and **lateral** means away from the midline or toward the side. You may see the adjective lateral used for descriptive purposes as in, "The tumor is located on the lateral wall of the left lung." The final two directional terms are **proximal** and **distal**. Proximal refers to something nearer to the point of attachment to the body or origin. An example of this is as follows: the shoulder is proximal to the elbow. Distal means further from the origin or point of attachment: the wrist is distal to the shoulder and the elbow. See Figure 3-4 for an illustration showing directional terms.

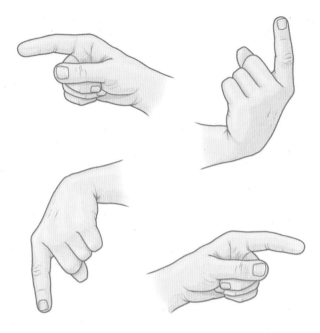

Two terms are used for placing patients in a lying down position. Both are common English words that have become adopted children of medical terminology. The two terms are **supine** and **prone**. Supine refers to a position in which the patient is lying face up. (It means the same thing in plain English, but it can also mean lazy or simply disinclined to act.) Noticing that the word "up" is included in the first syllable of the word "supine" will help you remember its meaning of "face up" in medical prose.

Prone is the opposite of supine, which means that the patient is lying face down. Prone, too, means the same thing in plain English with another meaning: "tending toward," as in "Smith is prone to making poor choices." Both supine and prone are frequently used in operating room and X-ray reports. For example, "The patient was placed in the supine position." This means that the patient was placed on the operating table on his or her back, lying face up. See Figure 3-4 and Table 3-2 for a listing of directional terms and additional examples of the terms.

Body Planes

Body planes are imaginary surfaces within the body (Fig. 3-5). The anatomical position is always their reference point. Four planes are frequently used to locate structural arrangements:

- **Frontal**: The frontal plane separates the front of the body from the back.
- **Sagittal**: The sagittal plane divides the body or organ into unequal left and right sides.
- **Midsaggittal**: The midsagittal plane divides the body or organ into equal left and right sides.
- **Transverse** or **horizontal**: This plane separates the body into upper and lower planes, cutting "across" the body.

 Aren't some of these terms just plain English? Yes. Alert readers will have noticed that at least some of the adjectives identifying body planes are also present in contexts outside of medicine.

THE BODY CAVITIES AND DIVISIONS

A body cavity is defined as a hollow space that contains body organs. The body has two major cavities: one in the front of the body and one in the back. The front body cavity is called the **ventral cavity**. The adjective ventral comes from the Latin word *venter*, meaning "belly." The cavity in the

TABLE 3-2 BODY POSITION AND DIRECTIONAL TERMS

Term	Direction	Example
anterior or ventral	toward the front; away from the back of the body	The nose is on the anterior side of the face; the toes are anterior to the ankle.
posterior or dorsal	near the back; toward the back of the body	The spine is on the posterior side of the body.
superior or cephalad	above; toward the head	The neck is superior to the chest.
inferior or caudal	below; toward the soles of the feet	The knee is inferior to the hip; the stomach is inferior to the chest.
proximal	near the point of attachment to the trunk	The elbow is proximal to the wrist.
distal	farther from the point of attachment to the trunk	The fingers are distal to the wrist.
lateral	pertaining to the side; away from the middle	The eyes are lateral to the nose.
medial	toward the middle of the body	The nose is medial to the eyes.
prone	lying horizontal and face down (or turned to the side)	The patient was placed on the operating table in a prone position.
supine	lying horizontal and face up	The patient was placed on the operating table in a supine position.

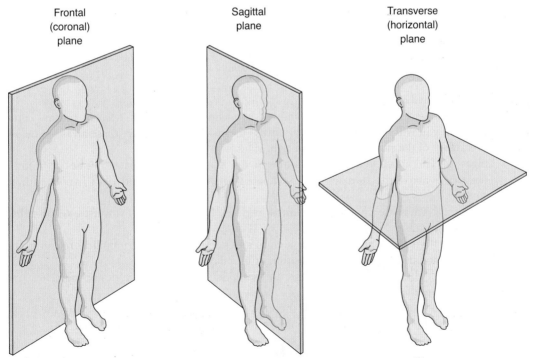

Frontal (coronal) plane   Sagittal plane   Transverse (horizontal) plane

FIGURE 3-5 Body planes. The three body planes are frequently used to locate structures or may be used for diagnostic testing. For example, planes are used to describe positioning or views in X-rays and other special radiographic tests. *From Cohen BJ, Wood DL. Memmler's The Human Body in Health and Disease. 9th ed. Philadelphia, PA: Lippincott Williams & Wilkins; 2000.*

back of the body is called the **dorsal cavity**, from the Latin word *dorsum*, which means "back." The dorsal cavity is subdivided into the **cranial** and **spinal cavities**, which house the brain and spinal cord, respectively (Fig. 3-6).

The ventral cavity extends from the neck to the pelvis and is subdivided into the **thoracic** and **abdominopelvic cavities**. The diaphragm, which is the muscle that initiates respiration, physically divides the thoracic and abdominopelvic cavities.

Divisions of the Abdominopelvic Cavity

A person documenting a physical examination or a surgical procedure needs to describe incisions, procedures, location of organs, etc. In order to do this effectively, he or she may need to know that the abdomen is divided into sections, which consist of either nine regions or four quadrants (Fig. 3-7A, B; Tables 3-3 and 3-4).

Nine Regions

Region designation is primarily for describing the location of underlying organs. Note that in the following list, the number in parentheses refers to two sides within the region, a left and a right, and counts as two regions (see Fig. 3-7A). The regions are named as follows:

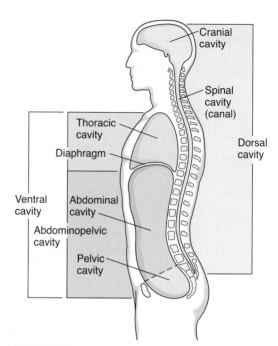

FIGURE 3-6   Body cavities. The body is divided into two major cavities—ventral and dorsal. There are five cavities within the ventral and dorsal cavities: The ventral cavity includes the thoracic, abdominal, and pelvic cavities; the dorsal cavity includes the cranial and spinal cavities. Reprinted with permission from *Cohen BJ, Wood DL.* Memmler's The Human Body in Health and Disease. *9th ed. Philadelphia, PA: Lippincott Williams & Wilkins; 2000.*

- Hypochondriac (2): There are right and left hypochondriac regions. *Chondr-* means "cartilage," and you will recall that the prefix *hypo-* means "below." Hence, these areas are below the cartilage of the ribs on the left and right sides.
- Epigastric: This area is just above the stomach. *Epi-* is a prefix that means "beside" or "upon." This area is above the stomach and is situated between the left and right hypochondriac regions.
- Lumbar (2): There are right and left lumbar regions. They are located at waist level on either side of the navel.
- Umbilical: If you look at the nine regions as a tic-tac-toe chart, the umbilical region is the middle section. It contains the belly button or umbilicus.
- Hypogastric: This is the bottom square in the middle column of the tic-tac-toe chart, just below the umbilical section.
- Inguinal (2): There are right and left inguinal sections. They lie on either side of the hypogastric section. Inguinal also refers to the "groin" area (see Fig. 3-7A and Table 3-3).

Doesn't the word hypochondriac have another definition? Yes, someone with imaginary pains is called a hypochondriac, and the reason for this usage came about because the left side hypochondriac region is roughly where a hypersensitive person might interpret any discomfort as a heart attack.

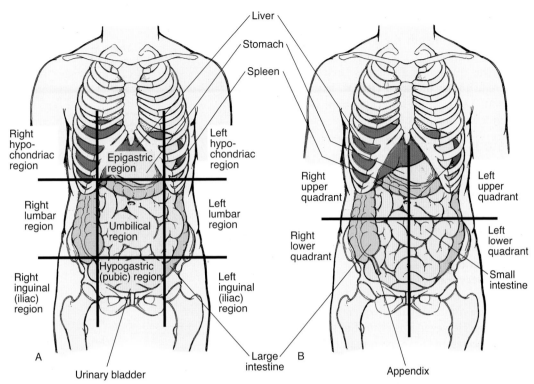

FIGURE 3-7 **Abdominopelvic cavity. A.** The nine regions of the abdomen. **B.** The four quadrants of the abdomen. *From* Stedman's Medical Dictionary. *27th ed. Baltimore, MD: Lippincott Williams & Wilkins; 2000.*

TABLE 3-3   NINE REGIONS OF THE ABDOMEN

left hypochondriac region	left lateral region just below the ribs
left lumbar region	left lateral region in the middle row
left inguinal region	left lower region of the lower row by the groin
epigastric region	middle region in the upper row
umbilicus	middle region in the middle row
hypogastric region	middle section in the lower row
right hypochondriac region	right lateral region just below the ribs
right lumbar region	right lateral region in the middle row
right inguinal region	right lower region of the lower row by the groin

TABLE 3-4   FOUR QUADRANTS OF THE ABDOMEN

Term	Organs in Quadrant
left upper quadrant (LUQ)	left lobe of liver, spleen, stomach, portions of the pancreas, small intestines, and colon
right upper quadrant (RUQ)	right lobe of liver, gallbladder, portions of the pancreas, small intestines, and colon
right lower quadrant (RLQ)	contains portions of small intestines and colon, right ovary and fallopian tube, appendix, and right ureter
left lower quadrant (LLQ)	contains portions of small intestines and colon, left ovary and fallopian tube, and left ureter

Four Quadrants

Four quadrants identify the abdomen (see Fig. 3-7B and Table 3-4). The center point is the navel. The quadrants are abbreviated as follows: right upper quadrant (**RUQ**), left upper quadrant (**LUQ**), right lower quadrant (**RLQ**), and left lower quadrant (**LLQ**).

Divisions of the Back

The back is divided into five sections that correspond to the sections of the spinal column (Fig. 3-8; Table 3-5):

1. **Cervical**
2. **Thoracic**
3. **Lumbar**
4. **Sacral**
5. **Coccygeal**

Some terms get to be quite lengthy, and health care professionals frequently use abbreviations. However, it is critical to know that some abbreviations have more than one meaning. For example, CRF may mean chronic renal failure, case report form, or any one of another 29 meanings listed in Wikipedia (which in all probability omits still more possible meanings). Abbreviations related to each chapter topic are presented in subsequent chapters.

TABLE 3-5	DIVISIONS OF THE BACK
Term	**Area of the Back**
cervical	neck
thoracic	chest
lumbar	lower back below waist
sacral	lower back
coccyx	tailbone

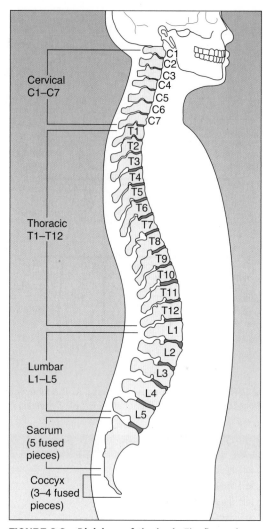

FIGURE 3-8 Divisions of the back. The five main divisions of the back include the cervical vertebra, the thoracic vertebra, the lumbar vertebra, the sacrum, and the coccyx. The sections are frequently named by the capital letter of the section (e.g., the second cervical vertebra is C2). *From Willis MC. Medical Terminology: A Programmed Learning Approach to the Language of Health Care. Baltimore, MD: Lippincott Williams & Wilkins; 2002.*

Abbreviation Table — BODY ORGANIZATION

ABBREVIATION	MEANING
LUQ	left upper quadrant
RUQ	right upper quadrant
LLQ	left lower quadrant
RLQ	right lower quadrant

Study Table — BODY ORGANIZATION

TERM	PRONUNCIATION	MEANING
hypochondriac	hy-poh-KON-dree-ak	below the ribs; also used as a noun to refer to a person whose illnesses are imaginary
hypogastric	hy-poh-GAS-tric	below the stomach
inferior	ihn-FEER-ee-ohr	below or in the direction away from the cranium
inguinal	IN-gwin-uhl	groin
lateral	LAT-eh-rahl	away from the middle of and toward the side of the body
medial	MEE-dee-ahl	toward the midline of the body
myalgia	my-AL-jee-ah	muscle pain
posterior	poss-TEE-ree-ohr	toward the back of the body
proximal	PROX-ih-mahl	toward the point of fixation to the body
sacrum	SAY-krum	five fused bones of the lower back
superior	soo-PEER-ee-ohr	above; toward the cranium
thoracic	tho-RASS-ik	adjective for chest
thorax	THOR-ax	chest
umbilicus	um-BILL-ih-kuhs	navel, belly button
ventral	VEHN-trahl	toward the front of the body and away from the back of the body

EXERCISES

EXERCISE 3-1 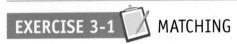 MATCHING

Insert the letter from the right-hand column that matches each numbered item in the left-hand column.

A. PLANES OF THE BODY

1. _____ frontal plane

2. _____ sagittal plane

3. _____ transverse plane

A. divides the body into upper and lower

B. divides the body into left and right

C. divides the body into anterior and posterior

B. DIRECTIONAL TERMS

1. _____ superior

2. _____ lateral

3. _____ posterior

4. _____ medial

5. _____ distal

6. _____ prone

7. _____ supine

8. _____ inferior

9. _____ anterior

10. _____ proximal

A. lying horizontal and face up

B. near the point of attachment to the trunk

C. toward the front; away from the back of the body

D. below; toward the soles of the feet

E. lying horizontal and face down

F. above; toward the head

G. toward the side; away from the middle

H. near the back; toward the back of the body

I. farther from the point of attachment to the trunk

J. toward the middle of the body

EXERCISE 3-2 FILL IN THE BLANK

Select the correct word from the following list and complete the sentence.

anterior	dorsal	lateral	posterior	superior
distal	inferior	medial	proximal	ventral

1. The wrist is _____ to the elbow.

2. The _____ end of the lower leg communicates with the ankle.

3. The sternum is _____ to the spinal cord.

4. The knee cap is on the _____ side of the body.

5. The head is _____ to the neck.

6. The ears are located on the _____ of the head.

7. The shoulder blades are on the _____ side of the body.

8. The chin is _____ to the forehead.

EXERCISE 3-3 WORD BUILDING

Add the correct prefix or suffix to the word root to make a new term. Select from the following word elements: *-itis, -ic, -al, hypo-, hyper-, epi-, and trans-*. The first exercise is an example.

WORD ROOT OR "COMBINING FORM"	ADD PREFIX OR SUFFIX	MEANING	TERM
1. gastr/o	*hypo-* *-ic*	below the stomach	*hypogastric*
2. dors/o	_____	pertaining to the back	_____
3. chondr/o	_____	inflammation of the cartilage	_____
4. thorac/o	_____	across the chest or thorax	_____
5. neur/o	_____	inflammation of a nerve	_____
6. cardi/o	_____	pertaining to the region above or upon the heart	_____

EXERCISE 3-4 CROSSWORD PUZZLE: THE BODY'S ORGANIZATION

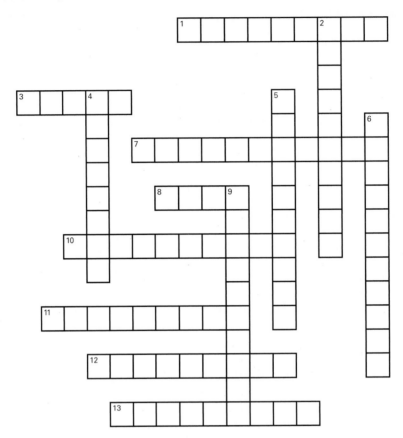

ACROSS

1. Belly button
3. Groups of these make a body system
7. Lungs are part of this system
8. Number of body cavities
10. Type of supportive tissue
11. Stomach is in this system
12. Toward the back
13. Watery fluid in the cells

DOWN

2. Contains the genetic code
4. Toward the front
5. Separates the body into upper and lower parts
6. Region below the umbilicus
9. Type of tissue that lines the body cavities

◀ CHAPTER 3 QUIZ

Write the answers to the following six questions using the spaces provided to the right of each question.

1. What word describes the position of the ear in relation to the nose? _____
   _____

2. What does posterior mean? _____

3. What word describes the position of the elbow in relation to the wrist? _____
   _____

4. When the body is in the anatomical position, which direction are the palms of the hands facing? _____

5. What does myalgia refer to? _____

True or false? Circle the correct answer.

6. Prone is lying face up.   TRUE   FALSE

7. The left hypochondriac region is above the left lumbar region.   TRUE   FALSE

8. The little toe is medial to the big toe.   TRUE   FALSE

9. The diaphragm is a muscle.   TRUE   FALSE

10. There are five divisions to the back.   TRUE   FALSE

11. The sacrum is also called the tailbone.   TRUE   FALSE

12. The sagittal plane divides the body into right and left portions.   TRUE   FALSE

13. In the anatomical position, the body is horizontal.   TRUE   FALSE

14. The opposite of lateral is proximal.   TRUE   FALSE

15. The terms *ventral* and *anterior* both mean front.   TRUE   FALSE

4 The Integumentary System

LEARNING OBJECTIVES

Upon completion of this chapter, you should be able to:

- Name the two primary layers of the skin.
- Name the accessory structures of the integumentary system.
- Pronounce and define terms related to the integumentary system.
- Interpret abbreviations associated with the integumentary system.

INTRODUCTION

The largest organ of the body is the skin, which covers the entire body—more than 20 square feet on average—and weighs about 24 pounds. It is the main part of the integumentary system, which also includes hair, nails, and **sebaceous** (oil) and **sudoriferous** (sweat) glands.

Integumentum is Latin for "covering" or "shelter," and thus the skin, nails, and hair that cover our bodies are called, collectively, the integumentary system. One might think that this Latin word would provide us with a valuable root for forming terms related to the skin, nails, and hair. But one would be wrong. In fact, naming the system is its only job.

WORD ELEMENTS OFTEN USED IN INTEGUMENTARY SYSTEM TERMS

Each body covering—skin, hair, and nails—has one or more roots of its own, as shown in Table 4-1. It's a good idea to study those word elements, along with the others given in the table, before you go any further. That way, as you go through the text, you can practice deciphering terms using context *and* etymology.

The physician who specializes in the diagnosis and treatment of skin disorders is called a **dermatologist** (dermato + log + ist). The field is called **dermatology** (dermato + logy). As you go through the following paragraphs, note the new terms introduced (they are in boldface type) and chart each element, as was just done for you for the terms dermatologist and dermatology. All word elements not learned in previous chapters are to be found in Table 4-1. After making these charts, study them and then complete the unnumbered exercise at the end of the "Structure" heading.

STRUCTURE OF THE SKIN, HAIR, AND NAILS

The skin consists of two layers: the **epidermis** and **dermis**. A layer of connective tissue called the **subcutaneous** layer lies beneath the dermis. Although the subcutaneous layer is not, technically speaking, part of the integumentary system, it is mentioned in this chapter because it connects the dermis to the muscles and organs beneath it (Fig. 4-1).

The epidermis is the outside layer of skin. It is made up of epithelial tissue, which is, incidentally, also found in other parts of the body. The epidermis protects the body from the outside world, a pretty big job for something only 3 one-thousandths of an inch thick. It does not contain blood vessels and is therefore said to be **avascular**, also a characteristic of epithelial tissue found elsewhere in the body. The epidermis on the palms of our hands and the soles of our feet is somewhat thicker than that on the rest of our skin, but only about 2 one-hundredths of an inch thick even there. **Melanocytes** produce a pigment called melanin, which provides color and protection against sunlight.

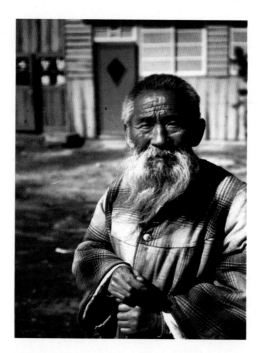

TABLE 4-1	COMMON WORD ELEMENTS RELATED TO THE INTEGUMENTARY SYSTEM	
Anatomical Element	**Function**	**Refers to**
cutane/o	root	skin
-cyte, cyt/o	suffix; root	cell
derm/o, dermat/o	root	skin
onych/o	root	nail
pil/o	root	hair
seb/o	root	sebum (oil; fat)
sudor/i/	root	sweat
Element Naming a Color, Position, or other Feature	**Function**	**Meaning**
albin/o	root	white
cirrh/o, jaund/o, xanth/o	root	yellow
cyan/o	root	blue
epi-	prefix	upon
erythr/o	root	red
fero	root	Latin word meaning "to carry"
ichthy/o	root	dry, scaly (fishlike)
kerat/o	root	hornlike
melan/o	root	black
myc/o	root	fungus
scler/o	root	hardening
sub-	prefix	below
xer/o	root	dry

Word Elements Exercise FILL IN THE BLANKS

Study Table 4-1 before attempting to complete this exercise. When you are confident that you know the meanings of each of the elements introduced in the table, fill in the blanks. Compare your answers to the answer key in Appendix A and make corrections as needed.

1. derm/o/at/ato   root   _____

2. myc/o   root   _____

3. -cyte, cyt/o   suffix; root _____

4. sudor/i/   root   _____

5. erythr/o   root   _____

6. xer/o   root   _____

7. fero   root   _____

8. sub-   prefix   _____

9. seb/o   root   _____

10. epi-   prefix   _____

11. albin/o   root   _____

12. cyan/o   root   _____

13. ichthy/o   root   _____

14. cutane/o   root   _____

15. kerat/o   root   _____

16. derm/o, dermat/o   root   _____

17. onych/o   root   _____

18. melan/o   root   _____

19. pil/o   root   _____

20. scler/o   root   _____

21. cirrh/o, jaund/o, xanth/o root   _____

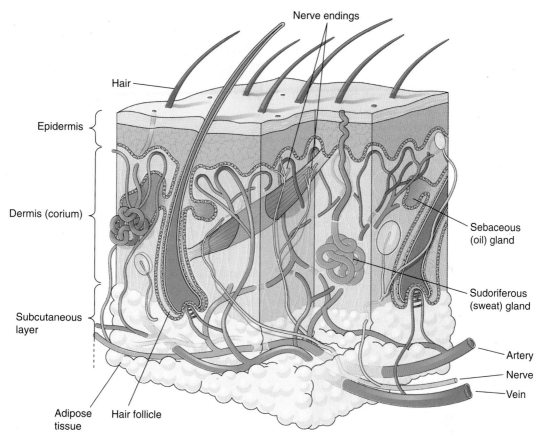

FIGURE 4-1   Cross-section of the skin. The layers of the skin: epidermis (epi- is a prefix meaning "upon" or "on top"; dermis is a root for skin) and dermis, or corium. The subcutaneous tissue is not part of the skin but is normally considered in the study of the skin (sub- is a prefix meaning "under"; cutane is a root meaning "skin"). *Modified from Cohen BJ, Taylor J. Memmler's Structure and Function of the Human Body. 8th ed. Baltimore, MD: Lippincott Williams & Wilkins; 2005.*

 Quick Check: Structure of the Skin, Hair, and Nails

Fill in the suffixes, and write the resulting word in the TERM column. The word that appears in boldface type in the MEANING column is a clue.

PREFIX	ROOT	SUFFIX	TERM	MEANING
sub-	cutane/o	_____	_____	**adjective** meaning "below the skin"
no prefix	melano	_____	_____	a pigment-producing cell
no prefix	seb/o	_____	_____	**adjective** referring to sebum, which may be described as an **oil or fat**

Unlike the epidermis, the dermis (sometimes also called the **corium**) contains blood vessels and nerves. So if you get a scratch that hurts and/or bleeds, you will know that you have injured the dermis. The dermis also contains **sebaceous** glands (oil producing) and **sudoriferous** glands (sweat producing).

Hair follicles produce the hair distributed over much of the body. Hair fibers are composed of a hard protein called **keratin**. Like skin, hair color is determined by the pigment melanin, which is produced from special cells called melanocytes. These melanocytes surround the hair shaft. When a small quantity of melanin is present, the hair color will be light or blonde, and as the quantity of melanin increases, the hair darkens. Gray hair occurs as melanin production decreases with age or injury.

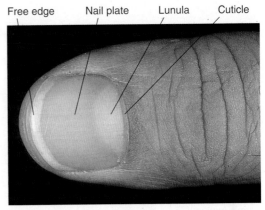

FIGURE 4-2 **Superior view of a nail.** The cuticle is the thin band of tissue that seals the nail plate to the skin. *From Cohen BJ, Taylor J. Memmler's Structure and Function of the Human Body. 8th ed. Baltimore, MD: Lippincott Williams & Wilkins; 2005.*

The sebaceous glands, which are situated close to hair follicles, secrete **sebum**, an oily fluid, onto the hair shaft. Sebum moves along the hair shaft toward the surface of the epidermis and provides lubrication to both skin and hair.

The sudoriferous glands are found over most of the body but are most numerous in the palms of the hands, soles of the feet, forehead, and armpits. These glands secrete a watery fluid that evaporates to help cool the body. The nails, the final accessory structures of the integumentary system, are composed of the protein keratin. The **lunula** (a Latin word meaning "little moon") is the whitish crescent region of the nail. The **cuticle** (cutane/o is the root) is the thin band of tissue that seals the nail plate to the skin (Fig. 4-2).

DISORDERS AND TREATMENTS

The skin, being visible in its entirety, makes diagnosis of some of its abnormalities uncomplicated. Moreover, the skin can sometimes provide clues to underlying bodily disorders, which may be signaled by changes in color or by the development of **lesions** and other eruptions.

Skin Lesions

A lesion may have many different causes. They may be flat, elevated, or depressed, (Fig. 4-3) and each variation has its own medical term, as shown in the following list:

Flat lesions:
- **Macule**: Flat, colored spot less than 1 cm in diameter (e.g., freckle)
- **Plaque**: Flat or lightly raised lesion more than 1 cm in diameter

Elevated lesions:
- **Bulla**: Raised, fluid-filled lesion or blister greater than 1 cm in diameter
- **Nodule**: Solid, raised lesion larger than a papule, 0.6 to 2 cm in diameter
- **Papule**: Small, circular, solid elevation of the skin less than 1 cm in diameter (e.g., wart, pimple)
- **Pustule**: Small, circular, pus-filled elevation of the skin, usually less than 1 cm in diameter
- **Vesicle**: Small, circular, fluid-filled elevation of the skin less than 1 cm in diameter
- **Wheal**: Smooth, rounded, slightly raised area often associated with itching

Depressed lesions:
- **Fissure**: Crack or break in the skin; a slit of any size
- **Ulcer**: An open sore or crater that extends to the dermis resulting from destruction of the skin

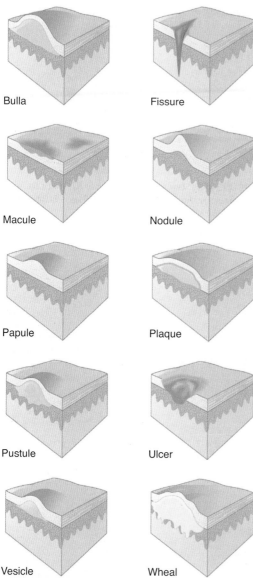

FIGURE 4-3   Skin lesions. Illustrations of some of the more common skin lesions. *From Cohen BJ. Medical Terminology: An Illustrated Guide. 5th ed. Philadelphia, PA: Lippincott Williams & Wilkins; 2007.*

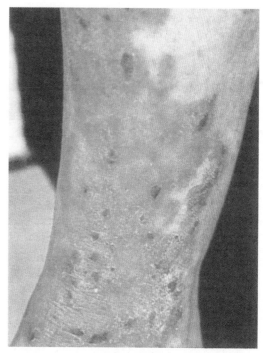

FIGURE 4-4   Eczema (dermatitis). *From Cohen BJ. Memmler's The Human Body in Health and Disease. 10th ed. Philadelphia, PA: Lippincott Williams & Wilkins; 2005.*

Inflammatory Disorders

Many skin disorders are characterized by inflammation. Contact **dermatitis** can be caused by exposure to an allergen or by direct contact with a chemical or plant. Poison ivy, for example, may be the diagnosis if the skin is red (**erythematous**), is covered with tiny vesicles, and is itchy. The word **pruritic** is sometimes used instead of itchy to indicate the presence of an itch. It comes from the Latin verb *prurio*, which means to itch. There is no corresponding root, although two other terms come from this same verb. They are **pruritus** and **prurigo**, which refer to a number of chronic skin disorders that involve itch.

Eczema is the generic term for inflammation of the skin (Fig. 4-4). **Psoriasis** names an inherited inflammatory condition of the skin (Fig. 4-5). Neither of these terms is derived from actual roots, although the suffix -iasis is a common one that, as you may recall from Chapter 2, means condition.

Scleroderma, as its etymology indicates, is taut, thick, leatherlike skin.

Skin Infections

Skin is our protective barrier; when it breaks down, bacteria, viruses, fungi, and parasites have an opportunity to invade our bodies. Many infections, however, can be more annoying than they are serious.

- **Impetigo**: caused by bacteria (*Staphylococcus aureus*) (Fig. 4-6)
- **Scabies**: caused by an egg-laying mite (Fig. 4-7)
- **Tinea**: caused by a fungus (Fig. 4-8)

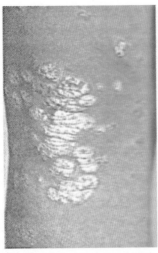

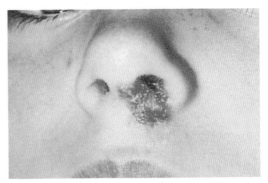

FIGURE 4-6 **Impetigo.** *From Cohen BJ. Medical Terminology: An Illustrated Guide. 5th ed. Philadelphia, PA: Lippincott Williams & Wilkins; 2007.*

FIGURE 4-5 **Psoriasis.** *From Cohen BJ. Memmler's The Human Body in Health and Disease. 10th ed. Philadelphia, PA: Lippincott Williams & Wilkins; 2005.*

- **Shingles** (**herpes zoster**): caused by a virus; symptoms include pain and a vesicular rash that develops along the path of a nerve

Burns

A burn is an injury to the skin caused by heat from any source. The severity of a burn is categorized by the depth of the layers of skin involved. See Table 4-2.

FIGURE 4-7 **Scabies.** *From Fleisher GR, Ludwig S, Baskin MN. Atlas of Pediatric Emergency Medicine. Philadelphia, PA: Lippincott Williams & Wilkins; 2004.*

Other Skin Disorders

Melanoma is a serious form of skin cancer. Some other skin and nail disorders also fail to fit previously mentioned categories. They include **decubitus** (from a Latin verb that means "to lie down") **ulcers**, also known as bedsores; **acne**, a disease of the sebaceous glands common in teens and young adults; **vitiligo**, depigmented blotches or macules that appear on the skin (Fig. 4-9); and **paronychia**, an infection of the skin around the nails (Fig. 4-10).

Alopecia is the technical term for baldness. It is not formed from a standard root, although the -ia suffix is standard. Other skin conditions include **erythema** and **ichthyosis**, both of which are formed from standard roots and suffixes. **Edema** comes from a Greek word that means swelling. It is a standard medical term referring to swelling that occurs anywhere in the body.

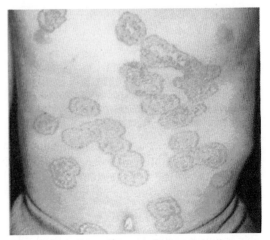

FIGURE 4-8 **Tinea (ringworm).** *From Cohen BJ. Memmler's The Human Body in Health and Disease. 10th ed. Philadelphia, PA: Lippincott Williams & Wilkins; 2005.*

TABLE 4-2	CLASSIFICATION OF BURNS
Type of Burn	**Layers of Skin Involved**
first degree	erythema (redness); superficial damage to epidermis; no blisters
second degree	blisters; erythema
third degree	charring; damage to the epidermis, dermis, subcutaneous layers, muscle, and bone

TREATMENTS

Surgical procedures may be performed on the integumentary system for diagnosis or treatment of abnormal conditions. These procedures may include a **biopsy**, which involves the surgical removal of a small piece of skin for examination, or **cryogenic surgery**, also called **cryosurgery** or **cryotherapy**. The root cry/o- comes from the Greek word *kryos* meaning "cold." This root is found in many terms, both within medicine and physics. In medicine, cryogenic techniques are commonly used to destroy abnormal tissues such as warts, moles, and tumors. Cryogenic surgery often involves the use of liquid nitrogen, which evaporates, or "boils," at $-321°$ F.

In the case of burns and some ulcerated areas, dead tissue prevents new, healthy tissue from growing. In such cases, a surgical procedure known as **debridement** may be used to remove dead tissue. Once again, the standard word elements you learned are absent from this term, which comes from a French adverb meaning "unbridled." That French word does indeed describe the purpose of debridement, which is to "unbridle" the body of dead tissue so that new, healthy tissue will be free to replace it.

Nonsurgical treatments include medications applied to the surface of the skin. The term often used to identify this type of treatment is "topical" (i.e., on top of the skin).

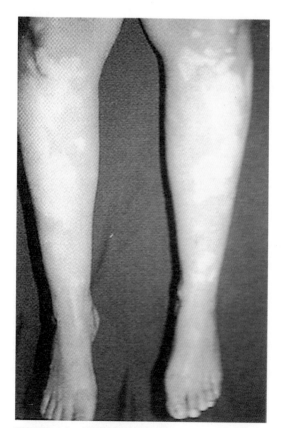

FIGURE 4-9 Vitiligo. *From Cohen BJ. Medical Terminology: An Illustrated Guide. 5th ed. Philadelphia, PA: Lippincott Williams & Wilkins; 2007.*

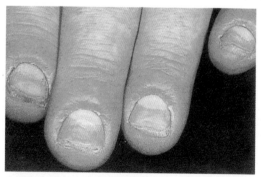

FIGURE 4-10 Paronychia. *From Cohen BJ. Medical Terminology: An Illustrated Guide. 5th ed. Philadelphia, PA: Lippincott Williams & Wilkins; 2007.*

Doesn't topical mean "relating to a particular topic," such as a topic in the news? Occasionally, the meaning of an English word changes when a segment of the population begins using it to mean something other than its traditional meaning. The word *topical* is such a word. However, its "medical" meaning most likely came first, given that its medical use dates back to the 17th century. Still, dictionaries include the notation *medical* alongside it, probably because English speakers may do a mental double take when encountering its medical use for the first time. Medical terms that fall into this category are identified throughout this book so that, as a medical professional, you will be aware of the possible confusion their use may cause, especially among patients.

Other treatments may include oral or injected medication. Classifications of topical medications are listed in the following:

- **Antipruritics** to relieve discomfort and itching caused by rashes or dermatitis
- **Antifungals** to treat minor infections
- **Antiseptics** and **bacteriostatics** to kill or inhibit bacteria
- **Scabicides** to treat scabies
- **Antibiotics** to prevent infection in burn cases

Abbreviation Table THE INTEGUMENTARY SYSTEM	
ABBREVIATION	**MEANING**
BSA	body surface area (used in describing skin damage assessment caused by burns)
LE	lupus erythematosus
SLE	systemic lupus erythematosus
SPF	sun protection factor
STSG	split-thickness skin graft
UV	ultraviolet

Study Table	THE INTEGUMENTARY SYSTEM	
TERM AND PRONUNCIATION	**ANALYSIS**	**MEANING**
adipose (AD-ih-pohs)	from the Latin word *adeps* (fat)	fatty tissue
corium (KO-ree-uhm)	Latin word *corium* (skin)	synonym for dermis
cutaneous (cue-TAYN-ee-uhs)	from another Latin word *cutis* (skin)	adjective referring to the skin
cuticle (CUE-tih-kuhl)	from the Latin word *cutis* (skin)	the thin band of tissue that seals the nail plate to the skin
dermatologist (dur-muh-TAHL-uh-jist)	*dermat/o* (skin); *-logist* (practitioner)	a specialist who diagnoses and treats skin diseases
dermatology (dur-muh-TAHL-uh-jee)	*dermat/o* (skin); *-logy* (study)	study of the integumentary system
dermis (DUR-mis)	from the Greek word *derma* (skin)	inner layer of skin
epidermis (epp-ih-DUR-mis)	*epi-* (upon); *dermis* (skin)	outer layer of the skin
follicle (FAWL-ik-uhl)	from the Latin word *folliculus* (a small sac)	small sac in the skin from which a hair grows
keratin (KERR-uh-tin)	from the Greek word *keras* (horn)	protein that forms hair, nails, and the tough outer layer of skin
lunula (LOO-new-luh)	from the Latin word *luna* (moon)	white, crescent-shaped area of a nail
melanin (MELL-uh-nihn)	from the Greek word *melas* (black)	dark pigment present in skin and other parts of the body
melanocyte (MEL-uh-no-site)	from the Greek word *melas* (black); *-cyte* (cell)	cell that produces melanin
sebaceous (se-BAY-shus)	from the Latin word *sebum* (tallow and by extension, grease, oil, fat)	oil-producing gland
subcutaneous (sub-ku-TAY-nee-us)	*sub-* (beneath); *cutane* (skin); *-ous* (adjective suffix)	beneath the skin
sudoriferous (soo-doe-RIFF-uh-russ)	from two Latin words: *sudor* (sweat) and *fero* (to carry)	sweat-producing glands
Disorders and Symptoms		
abscess (AB-sehs)	from the Latin word *abscessus* (a going away)	localized collection of pus in any body part; frequently associated with swelling and inflammation
acne (ak-nee)	a common English word	inflammatory papular and pustular eruption of the skin
albinism (al-BY-nih-zm)	from a Latin word *albus* (white) and *-ism* (condition)	partial or total absence of pigment of the skin, hair, and eyes

(continued)

TERM AND PRONUNCIATION	ANALYSIS	MEANING
alopecia (al-oh-PEE-shee-uh)	from a Greek word *alopekia* (fox mange)	partial or complete loss of hair; baldness
comedo (KOM-eh-do)	a Latin word (glutton)	blackhead; dilated hair follicle filled with bacteria; primary lesion in acne
cyanosis (SY-uh-no-siss)	*cyan/o* (blue); *-osis* (abnormal condition)	abnormal condition signaled by bluish discoloration of tissue
cyst (sih-st)	from the Greek word *kystis* (bladder)	closed sac or pouch in or under the skin that contains fluid or solid material
dermatitis (dur-muh-TY-tiss)	*dermat/o* (skin); *-itis* (inflammation)	inflammation of the skin
dermatomycosis (DUR-matt-oh-MI-ko-sis)	*dermat/o* (skin); *myc/o* (fungus); *-osis* (abnormal condition)	fungal infection of the skin
diaphoresis (dy-ah-for-EE-sis)	a Greek word (perspiration)	synonym for perspiration
ecchymosis (ek-ee-MOH-sis)	*ec-* (out); from *chymos* (Greek word for juice); *-osis* (abnormal condition)	a purple patch more than 3 mm in diameter caused by blood under the skin; see also petechiae
eczema (EK-zee-ma)	from the Greek word *eczeo* (boil over)	inflammatory condition of the skin characterized by erythema, vesicles, and crusting with scales
epidermitis (epp-ih-dur-MY-tiss)	*epi-* (upon); *-dermis* (skin); *-itis* (inflammation)	inflammation of the epidermis
erythema (ehr-ih-THEE-ma)	Greek word (flush)	abnormal redness of the skin
excoriation (ex-COR-ee-at-shun)	from the Latin verb *excorio* (to skin)	scratch mark; linear break (caused most often from scratching) in the skin surface
hemangioma (hee-man-jee-OH-ma)	*hem/o* (blood); *angi/o* (vessel); *-oma* (tumor)	benign tumor of blood vessels; birthmark
hyperhidrosis (hyper-HY-droh-sis)	*hyper-* (above normal); *hidr* (sweat); *-osis* (condition)	profuse sweating; increased or excessive perspiration; may be caused by heat, menopause, or infection
ichthyosis (ik-thee-OH-sis)	*ichthy/o* (fishlike); *-osis* (abnormal condition)	abnormally dry skin; scaly; resembling fish skin
impetigo (im-peh-TYE-goh)	from the Latin verb *impeto* (attack)	inflammatory skin disease with pustules that rupture and become crusted
keloid (KEE-loid)	from the Greek word *kelis* (tumor); and *-oid* (like)	overgrowth of scar tissue
lesion (LEE-shun)	from the Latin verb *laedo* (to injure)	wound, injury, or pathologic change in body tissue
macule (MAK-yul)	from the Latin word *macula* (spot)	flat, discolored area that is flush with the skin; birthmark or freckle

TERM AND PRONUNCIATION	ANALYSIS	MEANING
melanoma (mel-uh-NO-muh)	*melan/o* (black); *-oma* (tumor)	tumor of the melanocytes; skin cancer characterized by dark-pigmented, irregular-shaped lesion
nevus (NEE-vuhs)	Latin word for birthmark	mole; pigmented skin blemish that is usually benign but may become cancerous
nodule (NOD-yul)	from the Latin word *nodus* (knot)	a small node or circumscribed swelling
onychomalacia (ON-ih-ko-muh-LAY-shee-uh)	*onych/o* (nail); *-malacia* (softening)	softening of the nails
onychopathy (on-ih-KOP-uh-thee)	*onych/o* (nail); *-pathy* (disease)	any disease of the nails
papule (pap-yul)	from the Latin word *papula* (pimple)	small, circumscribed solid elevation of the skin
paronychia (pahr-oh-NIK-ee-ah)	*para-* (adjacent); *onych/o* (nail); *-ia* (condition)	infection around a nail
petechia (peh-TEEK-ia); petechiae (plural)	from the Italian word *peticchie* (small hemorrhagic spots)	tiny hemorrhagic spot(s) on the skin less than 3 mm in diameter; see also ecchymosis
polyp (PAHL-ip)	from the Latin word *polypus* (a growth on a stem)	a mass of tissue that bulges outward from the skin's surface on a stem or stalk of mucous membrane
pruritus (pru-RY-tis)	from the Latin verb prurio (to itch)	itching
psoriasis (soh-RY-ih-sis)	Greek word for itch	chronic skin disease characterized by itchy, red, silvery-scaled patches
pustule (PUHST-yul)	from the Latin word *pustula* (pimple)	small (up to 1 cm in diameter) circumscribed elevation of the skin containing pus
scabies (SKAY-bees)	from the Latin verb scabo (to scratch)	contagious infection caused by a mite
scleroderma (sklehr-oh-DER-ma)	*scler/o* (hardness); *-derma* (skin)	chronic disease characterized by thickening and hardening of the skin
shingles; herpes zoster (HER-peez ZAHS-tuhr)	from the Greek word *herpo* (to creep)	viral infection producing the eruption of highly painful vesicles that may follow a nerve path
tinea (TIN-ee-uh)	Latin word for worm	any fungal infection of the skin (tinea barbae = beard; tinea capitis = head; tinea pedis = athlete's foot)
ulcer (UL-ser)	from the Latin word *ulcus* (a sore)	an open sore or lesion of the skin; a lesion through the skin or a mucous membrane resulting from loss of tissue

(continued)

TERM AND PRONUNCIATION	ANALYSIS	MEANING
urticaria (ur-tih-KAR-ee-uh)	from the Latin word *uro* (to burn)	hives; allergic reaction of the skin characterized by eruption of pale red elevated patches
verruca (ve-ROO-kah)	Latin word for wart	wart; caused by a virus
vesicle (VES-ih-kal)	from the Latin word *vesicula* (blister)	small, fluid-filled, raised lesion; a blister
vitiligo (vit-il-IH-go)	from the Latin word *vitium* (blemish)	localized loss of skin pigmentation characterized by milk-white patches

Diagnoses, Procedures, and Treatments

analgesic (an-uhl-GEE-sik)	*ana-* (without); *gesic* (pain)	agent that relieves pain
antibiotic (an-ty-BYE-ah-tik)	*anti-* (against); *biotic* (organism)	agent that kills bacteria
antifungal (an-ty-FUNG-ul)	*anti-* (against); *fungal* (fungus)	agent that kills fungus
anti-inflammatory (an-ty-ihn-FLAM-ah-tor-ee)	*anti-* (against); *inflammatory* (inflammation)	agent to reduce inflammation
antipruritic (an-ty-pryu-RIH-tik)	*anti-* (against); *pruritic* (itching)	agent that reduces itching
antipyretic (an-ty-PEYE-reh-tik)	*anti-* (against); *pyretic* (burning)	agent that reduces fever
antiseptic (an-tih-sehp-tik)	*anti-* (against); *septic* (poison)	agent that inhibits the growth of infectious agents
antiviral (an-ty-VY-rahl)	*anti-* (against); *viral* (virus)	agent that destroys viruses
debridement (deh-BREED-ment)	*de-* (removal); *bridement* (from the word *bridle*, the part of the riding harness by which a rider controls the horse)	removal of necrotic or dead tissue from a wound or burn
dermatoplasty (dur-MAT-oh-plass-tee)	*dermat/o* (skin); *-plasty* (surgical repair)	plastic surgery repair performed on the skin
incision and drainage (I&D)	common English words	cutting open of a wound or lesion, such as an abscess, and letting out or draining the contents, such as pus
onychectomy (ON-ihk-EHK-toh-mee)	*onych/o* (nail); *-ectomy* (excision)	surgical removal of a nail
onychotomy (on-ih-KOT-oh-mee)	*onych/o* (nail); *-tomy* (incision)	incision into a nail
scabicide (SKA-bih-seyed)	*scabies* (see above); *-cide* (destruction)	agent lethal to mites
transdermal (trans-DUR-mahl)	*trans-* (across); *derm/o* (skin); *-al* (adjective suffix)	a method of administering medication through the unbroken skin via patch or ointment

EXERCISES

| EXERCISE 4-1 | CASE STUDY |

Read the case and write a definition for each underlined term in the appropriate space. Then read it a second time and write down any questions you think it fails to answer. For example, who diagnosed what? What do pets and children have to do with a diagnosis? And so on. Complete item 10, making sure you answer all your own questions. Compare your rewritten version with the one given in the answer key. They won't be identical, but the questions addressed should be similar. If your version is better than the one in the answer key, don't be alarmed. It means either that you are already an accomplished communicator or that you learned something from the exercise—maybe both.

CHIEF COMPLAINT: Rash on the face

PRESENT ILLNESS: A 29-year-old white female states that last week, she started having some itching on her forehead. She went to the doctor who prescribed erythromycin, an (1) antibiotic. Two days later, the rash covered her entire face. The patient was diagnosed with (2) impetigo and was admitted to the hospital for treatment.

CONSULTATION: Dr. Smith, a (3) dermatologist, saw the patient. The chart was reviewed, and the patient was examined. She is married and has no children and no pets. She developed (4) dermatitis on her forehead 2 weeks ago that has spread to her entire face. The rash has become more (5) erythematous, and she now has (6) pustules on her forehead, nose, and cheeks. Facial (7) edema persists, and she is almost unable to open her eyes. She has been given additional antibiotics and an (8) antipruritic medication. She developed (9) pruritus on her feet, which was thought to be a reaction to the antibiotic, so the medication was changed to another antibiotic.

IMPRESSION: Impetigo; allergic response to erythromycin. Patient responding to change in antibiotic. Continue with current antibiotic regimen and continue to monitor patient. Thank you for allowing me to participate in this interesting case. I will follow patient and provide additional suggestions if warranted.

Dr. Smith

TERM	DEFINITION
1. _____	_____
2. _____	_____
3. _____	_____
4. _____	_____
5. _____	_____
6. _____	_____
7. _____	_____
8. _____	_____
9. _____	_____

10. Rewrite this report to improve its readability and effectiveness

_____

_____

_____

_____

_____

_____

EXERCISE 4-2 LABELING THE SKIN

Using the following list, choose the correct terms to label the diagram correctly.

adipose tissue	epidermis	nerve	subcutaneous layer
artery	hair	nerve endings	sudoriferous gland
dermis	hair follicle	sebaceous gland	vein

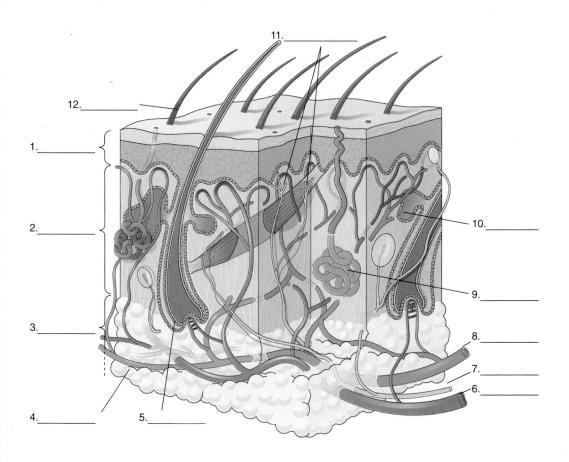

EXERCISE 4-3 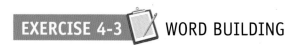 WORD BUILDING

Add the correct prefix or suffix to each word root to satisfy the corresponding definition. Select from the following word elements: *-pathy, -osis, -logy, -oma, -itis,* and *epi-*. Remember to avoid double vowels and double consonants between elements and remember also to omit hyphens.

WORD ROOT	ADD PREFIX OR SUFFIX	MEANING	TERM
1. dermat/o	_____	inflammation of the skin	_____
2. melan/o	_____	malignant black tumor	_____
3. dermis	_____	outer layer of skin	_____
4. onych/o	_____	disease of the nail	_____
5. dermat/o	_____	study of the skin	_____
6. ichthy/o	_____	dry, scaly, fishlike skin	_____

Use the following prefixes and suffixes to write terms for the following definitions.

epi- on, upon, over; *per-* through; *intra-* within; *sub-* under; *-al, -ous,* adjective suffix

7. under the skin   _____

8. through the cutaneous layer   _____

9. within the skin   _____

10. on the surface of the skin   _____

EXERCISE 4-4 MATCHING

Match the terms in Column 1 with the best definitions in Column 2.

TERM	DEFINITION
1. _____ nevus	A. birthmark
2. _____ verruca	B. thickened scar
3. _____ macule	C. blackhead
4. _____ alopecia	D. mole
5. _____ keloid	E. wart
6. _____ comedo	F. baldness
7. _____ diaphoresis	G. profuse sweating; increased perspiration
8. _____ erythema	H. abrasion of upper skin layers
9. _____ excoriation	I. flat, discolored spot
10. _____ hemangioma	J. redness of the skin

EXERCISE 4-5 WORD ANALYSIS

Write the prefix, root(s), and suffix of each of the following terms as they apply, and then write a definition in the final column.

TERM	PREFIX	ROOT(S)	SUFFIX	DEFINITION
1. dermatitis	_____	_____	_____	_____
2. hematoma	_____	_____	_____	_____
3. dermatomycosis	_____	_____	_____	_____
4. onychia	_____	_____	_____	_____
5. pachyderma	_____	_____	_____	_____
6. onychomalacia	_____	_____	_____	_____
7. paronychia	_____	_____	_____	_____
8. piloid	_____	_____	_____	_____
9. pyoderma	_____	_____	_____	_____
10. seborrhea	_____	_____	_____	_____

EXERCISE 4-6 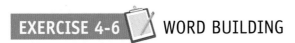 WORD BUILDING

Read the following clues beneath the spaces to build the terms for the provided definitions.

1. fungus infection of a nail

   _____   _____   _____   _____
   (nail)   (fungus)   (condition)   term

2. study of the integumentary system

   _____   _____   _____
   (skin)   (study)   term

3. inflammation of the epidermis

   _____   _____   _____   _____
   (upon)   (skin)   (inflammation)   term

4. thickening or hardening of the skin

   _____   _____   _____
   (hardening)   (skin)   term

5. surgical removal of a nail

   _____   _____   _____
   (nail)   (excision)   term

6. surgical repair or replacement of skin

   _____   _____   _____
   (skin)   (surgical repair)   term

7. nail biting

   _____   _____   _____
   (nail)   (eating)   term

8. adjective form of epidermis

   _____   _____   _____   _____
   (upon)   (skin)   (adjective suffix) term

9. any medical condition of the skin

   _____   _____   _____
   (skin)   (condition)   term

10. thin, transparent layer of skin located at the nail root

   _____   _____   _____   _____
   (upon)   (nail)   (structure)   term

EXERCISE 4-7 ✎ SENTENCE COMPLETION

Complete the following sentences.

1. Alopecia is a term meaning _____.

2. Loss of all hair on the scalp is called _____.

3. The medical term for a bruise is _____.

4. Any skin disease marked by scaling and shedding of the skin is called _____.

5. The now-common English word laser was originally an acronym, its letters standing for
   _____.

6. The Latin word *adiposus* means _____ giving us the term
   _____ tissue.

7. An adjective used to refer to sweat-producing glands is _____.

8. The epidermis is _____, which means without veins.

9. Sebum is a natural oil produced in the body that provides lubrication and bacterial control of
   _____.

10. The outermost sublayer of the epidermis is called the _____.

EXERCISE 4-8 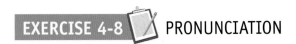 PRONUNCIATION

In the online student resources, go to the Audio Glossary and select Chapter 4, The Integumentary System. Select a term that you are unfamiliar with and "listen" to the pronunciation. Write the term and definition of the term in the following list. Repeat for a total of 20 terms. Be prepared to pronounce these terms in class.

AUDIO PRONUNCIATION GLOSSARY: THE INTEGUMENTARY SYSTEM

TERM	DEFINITION
1. _____	_____
2. _____	_____
3. _____	_____
4. _____	_____
5. _____	_____
6. _____	_____
7. _____	_____
8. _____	_____
9. _____	_____
10. _____	_____
11. _____	_____
12. _____	_____
13. _____	_____
14. _____	_____
15. _____	_____
16. _____	_____
17. _____	_____
18. _____	_____
19. _____	_____
20. _____	_____

EXERCISE 4-9 CROSSWORD PUZZLE: THE INTEGUMENTARY SYSTEM

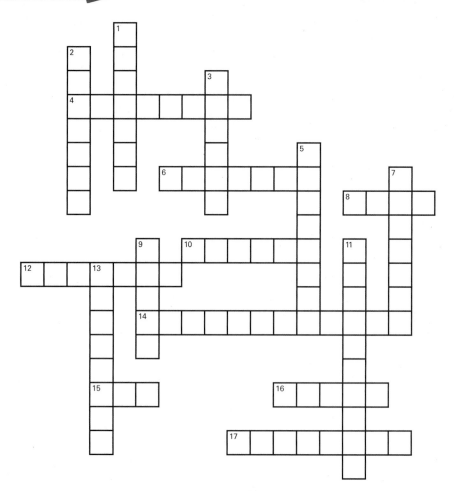

ACROSS

4. vesicular rash that develops along the path of a nerve
6. fatty tissue
8. root word that means "dead"
10. wound or injury
12. pigment that determines hair and skin color
14. term for "redness"
15. root word for "freezing"
16. root word for "nail"
17. depigmented blotches that appear on the skin

DOWN

1. thin band of tissue that seals the nail plate to the skin
2. small, circular, pus-filled elevation of the skin
3. thick layer of tissue just below the epidermis
5. a very common type of skin cancer with irregular borders and a variance in color that progresses to a dark or almost black shade
7. infection caused by an egg-laying mite
9. fungal infection
11. an infection of the skin around the nails
13. baldness

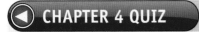

CHAPTER 4 QUIZ

Choose the correct answer for the following multiple choice questions.

1. If **myc/o** is the root for fungus, what is the term that means "condition of the nail caused by fungus"?
   a. mycosis
   b. onychomycosis
   c. trichomycosis
   d. onychomalacia

2. If **ichthy** is the root word for dry, fishlike, what is the term for a condition of being extremely dry?
   a. ichthyioma
   b. ichthyosis
   c. ichthyema
   d. ichthiitis

3. The term to describe a lesion of the skin containing pus is:
   a. verruca
   b. pustule
   c. bulla
   d. macule

4. A large blister filled with fluid is called:
   a. hemangioma
   b. furuncle
   c. cutis
   d. bulla

5. **Tinea** means a fungal infection. Which term best describes a fungal infection of the skin and/or accessory structures?
   a. tinea pedis
   b. tinea cruris
   c. tinea capitis
   d. all of the above

6. The term for natural or abnormal baldness that may be total or partial is:
   a. amastiac
   b. alopecia
   c. urticaria
   d. desquamation

7. The term used for a condition of profuse sweating is:
   a. diaphoresis
   b. sebaceous
   c. halitosis
   d. peristalsis

8. The term that best describes the thin band of tissue that seals the nail plate to the skin is:
   a. corium
   b. follicle
   c. cuticle
   d. epidermis

9. The term that best describes the cell that produces the pigment that provides color to the skin and hair is:
   a. keratocyte
   b. melanocyte
   c. erythrocyte
   d. leukocyte

10. Which term describes a fungal infection of the skin?
    a. dehiscence
    b. dermatomycosis
    c. dermatitis
    d. evisceration

Match each term listed here with the definitions that follow.

albinism	cyanosis	keloid	scleroderma
alopecia	ecchymosis	petechia	urticaria
biopsy	fissure	polyp	vitiligo

11. A firm scar that forms in the healing of a sore or wound is a _____.

12. _____ is a small slit or cracklike lesion.

13. _____ is a condition with a bluish discoloration of tissue.

14. A chronic disease characterized by thickening and hardening of the skin is called _____.

15. Absence or loss of hair is a condition called _____.

16. Partial or complete absence of pigment of the skin, hair, and eyes is termed _____.

17. A loss of skin pigmentation with milk-white skin patches is a condition known as _____.

18. _____, or hives, is an allergic reaction of the skin characterized by pale red eruptions.

19. The removal of a small piece of living tissue for examination under a microscope is called a(n) _____.

20. A(n) _____ is a mass of tissue that bulges outward and grows on a stem or stalk.

5 *The Skeletal System*

LEARNING OBJECTIVES

Upon completion of this chapter, you should be able to:

- Name the major structures and functions of the skeletal system.
- Name the medical specialists and health care professionals who treat disorders of the skeletal system.
- Define skeletal medical terms from your understanding of word elements.
- Differentiate between the axial and appendicular skeletons.
- State the medical terms that name the three types of joints.
- Interpret abbreviations used in connection with the skeletal system.
- Define the new terms introduced in this chapter.

INTRODUCTION

Our skeletons form the basic structures of our bodies, much like the framework of concrete and steel does in a tall building. Buildings constructed in earthquake zones are designed to move and sway so they won't fall down when the earth moves beneath them. We look upon such buildings as marvels of modern engineering, perhaps without giving a thought to the human skeleton, which allows us to walk, run, talk, gesture, throw things, and even draw up plans for tall buildings.

WORD ELEMENTS OFTEN USED IN REFERRING TO THE SKELETAL SYSTEM

Many terms having to do with the skeletal system are made up of the elements listed in Table 5-1. Other elements already learned are also used to make up some terms in this chapter. Prefixes you learned in Chapter 2, such as dia- (through), epi- (outside), endo- (inside), and peri- (around), for example, will be evident in terms introduced under the "Structure and Function" heading.

Study Table 5-1 carefully before attempting to complete Exercise 5-1. After completing the exercise, compare your answers with those in Appendix A and correct any mistakes you made.

AN OVERVIEW OF THE SKELETAL SYSTEM

The human skeleton begins to form about 6 weeks after fertilization and continues to grow and develop until the person is 25 years old. Its approximately 206 bones perform many duties.

> Isn't it true that some people have more than 206 bones? The response 206 was deemed correct on a Jeopardy television program. It must be true! All joking aside, the exact number of bones can vary slightly from one person to another, but the number 206 satisfies those who avoid arcane discussions of extra ribs, vertebrae, etc.

TABLE 5-1	WORD ELEMENTS COMMON WITHIN SKELETAL SYSTEM TERMS	
Element	Type	Meaning
-algia	suffix	pain
amphi-	prefix	both sides
ankyl/o	root	stiff, fused, closed
arthr/o	root	joint
brachi/o	root	arm
calcane/o	root	calcaneus, heel bone
carp/o	root	wrist
cervic/o	root	neck
cheir/o	root	hand
chondr/o	root	cartilage
cost/o	root	rib
crani/o	root	cranium
dactyl/o	root	finger, toe
-desis	suffix	stabilize or fuse
-ectomy	suffix	removal of, excision of
electr/o	root	electricity
femur/o	root	femur, thighbone
-gram	suffix	written record of
humer/o	root	humerus, upper arm bone
-itis	suffix	inflammation
kinesi/o	root	movement
-kinesia	suffix	movement
kyph/o	root	hump
-logy	suffix	study of
lord/o	root	swayback, curve
lumb/o	root	lower back
-malacia	suffix	softening
my/o, muscul/o	root	muscle
myel/o	root	bone marrow
-oma	suffix	tumor
orth/o	root	correct, straight
os/te/o	root	bone
ped/o	root	foot, child
pelv/o	root	pelvis
phalang/o	root	bones of fingers and toes
-physis	suffix	to grow
-plasty	suffix	surgical repair
-porosis	suffix	porous
-scopy	suffix	to visually examine
spondyl/o, vertebr/o	root	vertebrae
syn-	prefix	joined together
thorac/o	root	thorax, chest
zygo-	prefix	joined (yoked) together

Word Elements Exercise FILL IN THE BLANKS

Study Table 5-1 before attempting to complete this exercise. When you are confident that you know the meanings of each of the elements introduced in the table, fill in the blanks.

ELEMENT	MEANING
1. lord/o	_____
2. zygo-	_____
3. carp/o	_____
4. ped/o	_____
5. os/te/o	_____
6. phalang/o	_____
7. -algia	_____
8. crani/o	_____
9. syn-	_____
10. -itis	_____
11. my/o, muscul/o	_____
12. -scopy	_____
13. kinesi/o	_____
14. orth/o	_____
15. femur/o	_____
16. -malacia	_____
17. -plasty	_____
18. arthr/o	_____
19. pelv/o	_____
20. -physis	_____
21. brachi/o	_____
22. dactyl/o	_____

(continued)

23. cost/o _____

24. myel/o _____

25. electr/o _____

26. thorac/o _____

27. humer/o _____

28. -desis _____

29. -porosis _____

30. ankyl/o _____

31. spondyl/o, vertebr/o _____

32. -gram _____

33. -kinesia _____

34. amphi- _____

35. calcane/o _____

36. kyph/o _____

37. cervic/o _____

38. cheir/o _____

39. -logy _____

40. chondr/o _____

41. lumb/o _____

42. -ectomy _____

43. -oma _____

The skeleton serves as a rigid but articulating (articulating means movable) framework for muscles and other tissues. It also protects our vital organs by forming a shield against bumps and such. Its less obvious jobs are to produce and store essential minerals and to make blood cells.

The skeleton may be divided into two parts: the **axial** and **appendicular** skeletons (Fig. 5-1). The words axial and appendicular are adjective forms of the words axis and appendix. Axis is a common English word sometimes used metaphorically to describe political alliances but most often denoting an imaginary straight line, such as the one between the north and south poles of the earth. The axial skeleton has an axis running from the middle of the top of your head to the bottom of your spine. The axial skeleton therefore includes the bones of the skull, chest, and spinal column.

The appendicular skeleton comprises the arms and legs, along with the shoulder and pelvic bones. While the appendicular skeleton has nothing to do with the body's "appendix," those two body parts do have a common classical word origin: the Latin word *appendix* refers to something attached to something else. Thus, the appendicular skeleton is attached to the axial skeleton, the main hub of the body, and, as you probably already know, the appendix is attached to the large intestine.

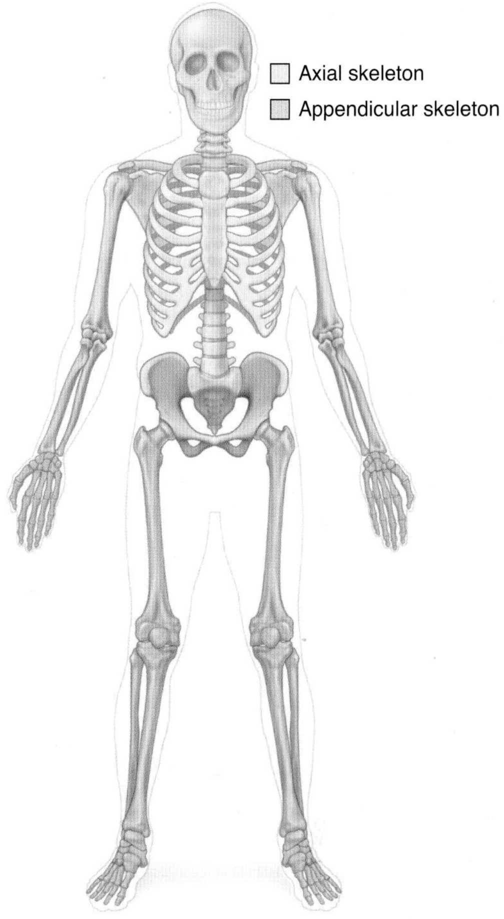

The skeletal system depends on **ligaments**, **tendons**, and **joints** to allow for movement. Ligament comes from the Latin word *ligamentum*, meaning "a tie" or "binding," which is what ligaments do (i.e., "tie" bones together). Tendon, on the other hand, comes from another Latin word, the verb *tendere*, which means to stretch, which is what tendons do. Strictly speaking, of course, these two terms belong to the muscular system, but they are mentioned here because their function is essential to the skeleton.

Joints are simply the places where bones come together. The word joint also has classical language roots, but we may simply relate the word joint to junction, a common English word referring to where roads, rail lines, or any other kind of lines meet. In other words, a joint is a junction, or a place at which two or more things come together.

☐ Axial skeleton
☐ Appendicular skeleton

FIGURE 5-1   Axial and appendicular skeletons.
The axial and appendicular skeletons differentiated. The axial skeleton is shown in *yellow;* the appendicular (consisting of the arms and legs) is in *gray*.

STRUCTURE AND FUNCTION

Bone formation begins early in fetal development when the skeleton is composed mostly of cartilage. **Ossification**—ossify means "to form bone"–occurs during the second and third month of fetal development as cartilage hardens and turns into bone. Bone is made up of **osseous** tissue, which consists of special mature bone cells called **osteocytes**.

The bones of the skeleton are of different shapes and sizes. They may be essentially flat, such as those found in the cranium and ribs. They also may be short, such as those in the wrist and ankles, or long, such as those found in the arms, legs, hands, and feet.

Long bones have subparts that are named. The term **diaphysis** is the shaft of a long bone, and the term **epiphysis** is the name given to each end of a long bone. The term for the inside of the diaphysis is **medullary cavity**. Because it's a cavity, it is hollow, of course, and medullary means that the cavity contains marrow. The Latin word *medius*, meaning "middle," is also the basis for the word **medulla** (marrow).

Most bones are covered with a membrane called the **periosteum**. The inner surface of the medullary cavity is lined with a thin layer of cells called the **endosteum** (Fig. 5-2).

By now, you are probably familiar with the prefixes peri- and endo-. But if you didn't automatically identify those prefixes, as meaning around and inside, you may benefit from a review of Chapter 2, Table 2-8.

As indicated in the foregoing discussion, not every term has a root. The reason is simple: we borrow freely from Greek and Latin, and if you stop to think about that practice, you will realize that every word or word fragment we use is—in a narrow sense at least—a potential root. In other words, prefixes and suffixes can sometimes form the central idea of a term.

The Axial Skeleton

The axial skeleton is composed of the **cranial**, **facial**, **thoracic**, and **spinal** bones. The six main cranial bones are the **frontal** bone; two **parietal** bones, one on each side; two **temporal** bones, on the sides of the head; and the **occipital** bone. The cranial bones are joined by **sutures**, which are fibrous membranes that join them (Fig. 5-3). Cranial bones enclose and protect the brain.

The main facial bones are the **nasal** bone, **zygomatic** bones (two), and the **maxilla** and **mandible**. The nasal bone forms the bridge of the nose, and the two zygomatic bones form the cheeks. The maxilla is the upper jawbone, and the mandible is the lower jawbone.

Isn't *maxilla* Latin for jawbone? Although the mandible is regarded as "the jawbone," *maxilla* is the Latin word for jawbone. The Latin verb *mandere*, from which "mandible" is derived, means "to chew or devour."

The **thoracic** bones, which include the **sternum**, **ribs**, and associated cartilage, are known collectively as the **thoracic cage** (Fig. 5-4). The adjective thoracic is formed from the word thorax, which is Latin for "breastplate" (chest armor). The two major organs inside the thoracic cage are the heart and lungs.

The posterior (back) rib pairs are attached to their correspondingly numbered **vertebrae**. All but the last two anterior (front) ribs are attached to the **sternum** (flat bone in the chest). The last

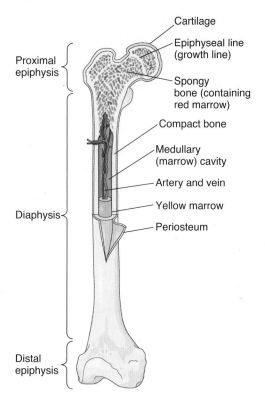

FIGURE 5-2 Structure of a long bone. The epiphyses, or ends of the bone, are shown in relation to the diaphysis or shaft of the bone. The periosteum covers the bone's outer surface. The medullary is the middle of the bone and houses the blood vessels and marrow. *From Cohen BJ. Medical Terminology: An Illustrated Guide. 5th ed. Philadelphia, PA: Lippincott Williams & Wilkins; 2007.*

Bones of the skull:

- Frontal
- Parietal
- Sphenoid
- Temporal
- Nasal
- Maxilla
- Occipital
- Zygomatic
- Mandible

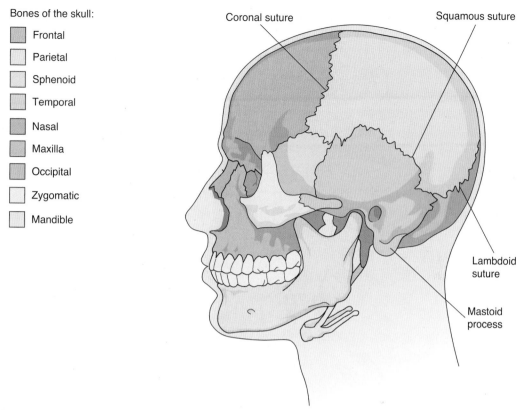

Coronal suture · Squamous suture · Lambdoid suture · Mastoid process

FIGURE 5-3 **The skull.** View from the left side. The bones of the skull are indicated by different colors. The sutures, also known as suture joints, are the lines of junction between the two bones. These joints are usually immovable. *Modified from Cohen BJ*. Medical Terminology: An Illustrated Guide. *5th ed. Philadelphia, PA: Lippincott Williams & Wilkins; 2007.*

two rib pairs "float," which means that they are attached only to the vertebrae. The lower end of the sternum is a bony daggerlike projection called the **xiphoid process**. This term comes from the Greek word, *xiphos*, which means "sword."

Why can't we use the words floating, false, and true instead of fluctuantes, spuriae, and verae when talking about ribs? We can, and we do. However, the medical phrase for floating ribs is **costae fluctuantes**. Rib pairs 8, 9, and 10, together with the "floating ribs" 11 and 12, are sometimes collectively called **costae spuriae**, which means (false ribs). The first seven pairs of ribs are called **costae verae** (true ribs). If you know the English words fluctuate, spurious, and verify, you can associate them with these terms as a help in remembering them. If you are unfamiliar with those English words, look them up in a good dictionary and make them part of your general vocabulary.

The spinal column includes five sections of vertebrae (singular: vertebra). The naming of a vertebra consists of a prefix letter (C for cervical, T for thoracic, and L for lumbar), followed by a number indicating the placement on the column. A couple of examples would be C1 for the first cervical vertebra and L5 for the fifth lumbar vertebra in the lower back region. The distribution of the vertebrae of the cervical, thoracic, and lumbar regions is shown in Figure 5-5. The illustration shows the **sacrum** and **coccyx** at the base of the spine.

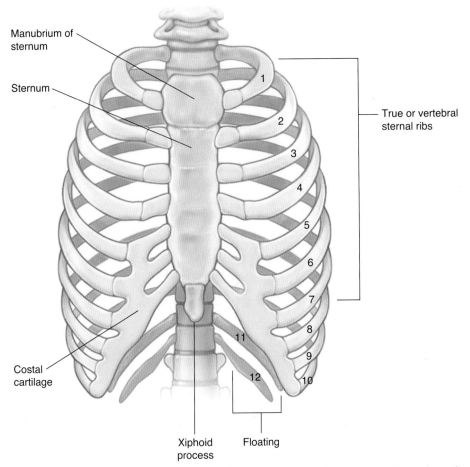

Manubrium of
sternum

Sternum

Costal
cartilage

True or vertebral
sternal ribs

Xiphoid
process

Floating

FIGURE 5-4   Thoracic cage. The thorax comprises the sternum, manubrium of the sternum, ribs, and costal cartilage. The first seven ribs articulate or join the sternum or breastbone by means of the costal cartilage. The last five ribs are not directly joined to the sternum, and the last two ribs are attached posteriorly to the thoracic vertebrae.

 Isn't the cervix part of the womb? The words cervix and cervical also refer to the "neck" of the uterus, part of the female reproductive system (see Chapter 14).

The sacrum is joined to the hip bones and, therefore, is part of the pelvic girdle, which is in turn part of the appendicular skeleton. Although the sacrum is not part of the axial skeleton, it is mentioned here because of its association with the spinal column.

The Appendicular Skeleton

As mentioned previously, the appendicular skeleton consists of the body's appendages (arms and legs) and the areas to which these appendages are attached: the shoulder and pelvic girdles. Shoulder bones, although associated with the chest, are part of the appendicular skeleton. The main bones of the shoulder girdle are the **clavicle** (collarbone) and the **scapula** (shoulder blade) (Fig. 5-6).

The long bone extending from the shoulder and ending at the elbow is called the **humerus**, not because it is the "funny bone" but because *humerus* is the Latin word for "shoulder." However, there is a connection with the word "humorous." The phrase "funny bone" was most probably coined as a joke because the ulnar nerve, which causes the pins-and-needles sensation when it is

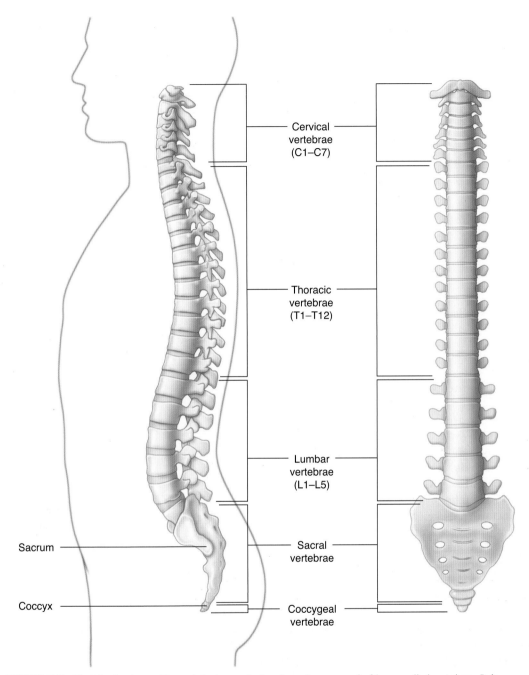

Cervical
vertebrae
(C1–C7)

Thoracic
vertebrae
(T1–T12)

Lumbar
vertebrae
(L1–L5)

Sacrum

Sacral
vertebrae

Coccyx

Coccygeal
vertebrae

FIGURE 5-5 **Vertebral column.** The vertebral, or spinal, column is composed of bones called vertebrae. It is divided into five regions: cervical, thoracic, lumbar, sacral, and coccygeal. These are often abbreviated by their first letter. For example, C7 is the seventh cervical vertebra.

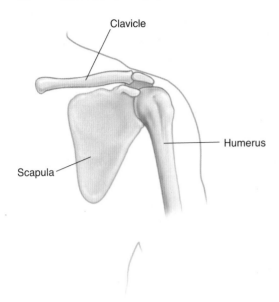

FIGURE 5-6   **The bones of the shoulder.** The bones of the shoulder include the clavicle, humerus, and scapula.

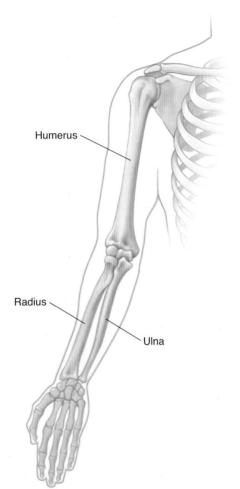

FIGURE 5-7   **The bones of the arm.** The bones of the arm include the humerus, radius, and ulna. The humerus, or upper arm bone, articulates with the scapula at the shoulder and the radius and ulna at the elbow. The radius and ulna, or lower arm bones, articulate with the humerus at the elbow and the carpals at the wrist.

struck, is located where the humerus joins the elbow.

The forearm consists of the **ulna** and **radius**, which extend from the elbow down to the wrist (Fig. 5-7). The wrist includes eight bones called **carpals**, from the Greek word *karpos*, meaning "wrist." As we learned in Chapter 2, meta- is a prefix meaning "beyond"; therefore, the **metacarpals** lie "beyond" the carpals, connecting the wrist to the fingers. The **phalanges** are the bones that make up the fingers. The term phalanges is the plural form of *phalanx*, which is Greek for "line of soldiers." The bones of the wrist and hand are shown in Figure 5-8.

The pelvic girdle, so named because it surrounds and protects the pelvic organs, consists of the two hip bones, right and left, along with the sacrum, noted previously in connection with the spinal column. The hip bone, also called the **os coxae**, is a fusion of three bones: the **ilium**, the **ischium**, and the **pubis**.

The **femur**, Latin for "thigh," is a long bone that extends from the hip to the knee, and the **tibia** and **fibula** are long bones that extend from the knee to the ankle (Fig. 5-9). The tibia, Latin for "shin," is the shin bone or heavy bone of the lower leg; the fibula, from the Latin word *figibula*, meaning "fastener," does not bear the body's weight, but together with the tibia, it is connected to the **talus** (ankle bone). The **patella** (kneecap) is a "floating" bone that is imbedded in the tendon of the thigh muscle. It offers protection to the knee joint.

Tarsus (from the Greek *tarsos*, meaning "a flat surface") is sometimes used as a technical name for the ankle. The **tarsals** and **metatarsals** of the ankle and foot correspond with the carpal and metacarpal bones of the wrist and hand. The bones making up the fingers and toes are both called **phalanges**. The bony protrusions at the distal end of the fibula are called, respectively, the **medial** and

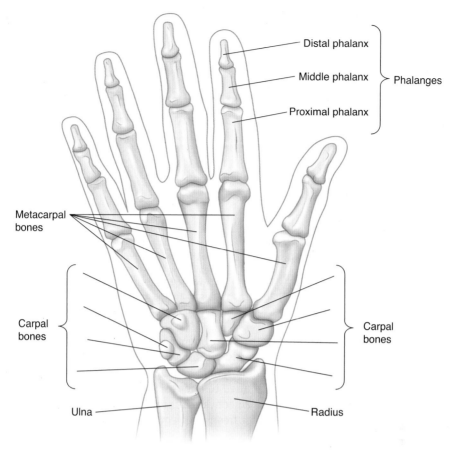

FIGURE 5-8 **Hand and wrist bones.** The wrist is made up of eight carpal bones. They join the metacarpals, which extend out to the phalanges or fingers. Meta- means "beyond," so the metacarpals, or bones of the palm of the hand, are beyond the wrist bones.

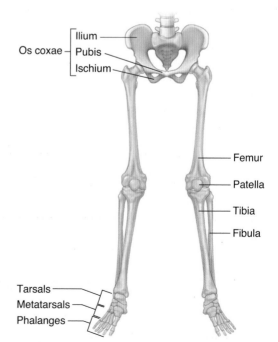

FIGURE 5-9 **Bones of the pelvic girdle and legs.**
The pelvis is formed from three fused bones, the ilium, ischium, and pubis, which are collectively termed the os coxae. The femur is the longest bone in the body and is located in the thigh. The tibia and fibula are the lower leg bones. The tarsals or ankle bones join the metatarsal bones in the foot, which are connected to the phalanges or toes. (Note: Phalanges are both finger and toe bones.)

lateral malleolus. These may be referred to as the "ankle bones," but they are really part of the tibia and fibula. The heel bone, or **calcaneus**, is one of the larger bones in the foot. Figure 5-10 shows the bones of the ankle and foot.

Joints

As noted previously, a **joint** is the place where bones come together. Some joints, such as the knee and elbow joints, are highly movable, and some are capable of little or no movement. A joint with no movement is called a **synarthrosis**. A joint with little movement is called an **amphiarthrosis**. Any of the suture joints in the cranium would be a good example of a synarthrosis, and the vertebral bodies within the spinal column are examples of amphiarthroses.

A joint that has free movement is called a **diarthrosis** or a **synovial joint**.

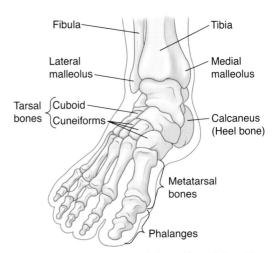

FIGURE 5-10   The bones of the ankle and foot. The medial and lateral malleolus are protrusions from the lower leg bones that we know as "ankle" bones. The tarsals are the ankle bones, and the metatarsals (meta- means "beyond") are the bones just beyond the tarsals.

Why was my definition of diarthrosis wrong when I depended on word elements for the answer? The word elements within the term diarthrosis fail to reveal a clear definition. The prefix dia- (through) and *arthroun*, a Greek word for joint, would give us "through a joint." Maybe that is why the term synovial joint is also used to refer to a free-moving joint: syn (with), ovi (egg white), and -al combine to make an adjective that provides a hint that fluid (something resembling the white of an egg?) allows for free movement.

The spaces within each synovial joint are filled with a viscous liquid called **synovial fluid**. Although the spaces in even a large joint are so tiny that less than 1/100th of an ounce of synovial fluid is needed to fill it, the fluid is needed to lubricate the joint as it moves and to cushion it against shock. Synovial joints permit a variety of movements. The knee and elbow joints, for example, are "hinge joints" that provide for **flexion** and **extension**. The ball and socket joint of the shoulder, also a synovial joint, provides a range of motions including rotation. Figure 5-11 shows the various movements of the synovial joints, and Table 5-2 describes their various movements.

Cartilage, a precursor of bone tissue, is classified as connective tissue, but it is mentioned here because cartilage enables movement in the synovial joints.

Bursae (singular: **bursa**) are found wherever tendons or ligaments impinge on other tissues. Bursae are spaces within connective tissue filled with synovial fluid.

PRACTICE AND PRACTITIONERS

A number of specialists work in the branch of **orthopedic** medicine, all of them engaged in the diagnosis and treatment of patients with musculoskeletal disorders. **Orthopedic physicians** coordinate patient care with **physical therapists**, **occupational therapists**, **kinesiologists**, or other practitioners in sports medicine. The **rheumatologist** is a physician who specializes in the treatment of joint disorders and arthritic conditions.

DISORDERS AND TREATMENTS

A **sprain** is a tear in a ligament or the fibrous tissue that connects bones. A **fracture** is a broken bone. However, all fractures are not the same. Some are simple breaks, and some are not. If the fracture is a **closed fracture**, there is no wound or open skin. If the broken bone protrudes through the skin, it is called an **open** or **compound fracture**. Table 5-3 names and illustrates these and the other kinds of fractures.

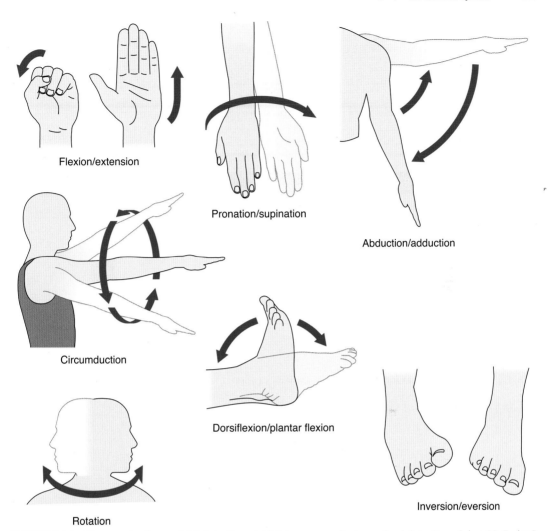

FIGURE 5-11 **Movements at synovial joints.** Synovial joints are more freely moving joints. *From Cohen BJ, Taylor J. Memmler's Structure and Function of the Human Body. 8th ed. Baltimore, MD: Lippincott Williams & Wilkins; 2005.*

TABLE 5-2	MOVEMENTS OF SYNOVIAL JOINTS
Movement	**Description**
abduction	movement away from the midline of the body
adduction	movement toward the midline of the body
circumduction	movement in a circular direction from a central point
dorsiflexion	backward bending as of the hand or foot
eversion	turning outward
extension	movement that brings the limb into a straight position
flexion	bending or being bent
inversion	turning inward
plantar flexion	bending the sole of the foot or pointing the toes downward
pronation	to turn downward or backward as with the hand or foot
rotation	moving around a central axis
supination	turning the palm or foot upward

Quick Check: Structure of the Skeletal System

Fill in the blanks.

1. Osseous tissue consists of special mature bone cells called _____.

2. A diarthrosis is a joint that has free movement. It is also called a _____ joint.

3. The facial bones include the nasal bone, the two zygomatic bones, the maxilla, and the _____.

TABLE 5-3	COMMON FRACTURES	
Fracture	**Description**	**Example**
hairline closed	break without separation simple fracture with no open wound	
Colles	break in the distal end of the radius (wrist)	
comminuted	break in which the bone is crushed or splintered	
compression	fracture or break caused by a squeezing or opposing force; loss of height in a vertebra due to disease or trauma	
greenstick	incomplete break; one side of the bone is broken and the other is bent	

TABLE 5-3	COMMON FRACTURES *(continued)*	
Fracture	**Description**	**Example**
impacted	break where one bone fragment is pushed or driven into another	
oblique	break is at an angle to the bone	
open	skin is broken through the fracture; bone protrudes through the skin	
Pott	fracture of the distal end of the fibula	
spiral	break is S-shaped, usually caused by twisting injury	
transverse	break is straight across the bone, at a right angle to the long axis of the bone	

Treatment of a fracture consists of **reduction** (realignment) of the broken bone. In some cases, **traction** (using elastics or pulley and weights to maintain alignment) may be needed. Casts and splints are used to immobilize a broken bone during the healing process.

Bone disorders arising from disease include conditions such as **osteomyelitis**, an inflammation caused by bacteria.

Osteoporosis is a bone disorder characterized by a decrease in bone density and mass. Two other bone disorders are **rickets** and **osteomalacia**. These two conditions result from vitamin deficiency and lack of calcium absorption. **Neoplasms** or tumors of the bone may be primary or secondary (from other sites in the body). **Osteosarcoma** is a tumor of the bone. **Chondrosarcoma** is a tumor that arises in cartilage.

Joint disorders include **arthritis**, a general term used to denote joint inflammation. General wear and tear on joints results in **osteoarthritis**. Treatment may include medication for pain and inflammation and/or physical therapy. **Arthrocentesis** may be used to drain the fluid and relieve the pressure in the joint.

Rheumatoid arthritis is attributed to an immunologic abnormality that causes an inflammatory response with subsequent tissue destruction. Treatments consist of medication, rest, and physical therapy (Fig. 5-12).

A disc that protrudes into the spinal canal and puts pressure on the spinal nerve is called a **herniated disc**. It can be discovered in a number of ways, including by means of a **myelogram**.

Compression fractures of the vertebrae may produce **kyphosis** (humpback) and loss of height. **Lordosis** (swayback) involves the lumbar region. **Scoliosis** is a sideways curvature of the spine that may occur in any region of the spine (Fig. 5-13).

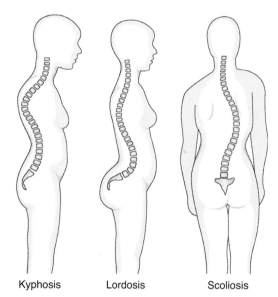

Kyphosis   Lordosis   Scoliosis

FIGURE 5-13 Curvatures of the spine. Kyphosis is an exaggerated thoracic curve; lordosis is an exaggerated lumbar curve; scoliosis is a sideways curve in any region. *From Cohen BJ. Medical Terminology: An Illustrated Guide. 5th ed. Philadelphia, PA: Lippincott Williams & Wilkins; 2007.*

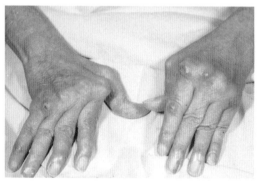

FIGURE 5-12 Advanced rheumatoid arthritis. The hands show swelling of the joints and deviation of the fingers. *From Cohen BJ. Medical Terminology: An Illustrated Guide. 5th ed. Philadelphia, PA: Lippincott Williams & Wilkins; 2007.*

Abbreviation Table 🔵 THE SKELETAL SYSTEM

ABBREVIATION	MEANING
ACL	anterior cruciate ligament
C (C1, C2, etc.)	cervical
CT	computed tomography
CTS	carpal tunnel syndrome
Fx	fracture
L (L1, L2, etc.)	lumbar
LE	lower extremity
RA	rheumatoid arthritis
ROM	range of motion
S	sacral
T	thoracic
THR	total hip replacement
TKA	total knee arthroplasty
TKR	total knee replacement
Tx	traction

Study Table THE SKELETAL SYSTEM

TERM AND PRONUNCIATION	ANALYSIS	MEANING
Structure and Function		
amphiarthrosis (AM-fee-ar-THRO-sihs)	*amphi-* (both sides); *arthr/o* (joint); *-osis* (abnormal condition)	joint with little movement
appendicular (APP-ehn-DIHK-yu-lahr)	adjective referring to something that is added or attached	having to do with something attached
axial (AX-ee-uhl)	adjective form of axis, a common English word	straight line through a physical body
brachial (BRAY-kee-uhl)	*brachi/o* (arm); *-al* (adjective suffix)	having to do with an arm
bursa (BUR-sah)	a Latin word meaning "purse"	saclike connective structure found in some joints; protects moving parts from friction
calcaneus (kal-KAY-nee-uhs)	Latin word for heel	the heel bone
carpal (KAR-pahl)	adjective form of carpus (wrist)	a wrist bone
cartilage (CAR-tih-lij)	from the Latin word *cartilagin* (gristle)	dense, flexible connective tissue

(continued)

TERM AND PRONUNCIATION	ANALYSIS	MEANING
cervical (SUR-vih-kuhl)	*cervic/o* (neck); *-al* (adjective suffix)	adjective describing the vertebrae (C1–C7) in the neck region; also used in connection with the uterus, which is part of the female reproductive system
cervix (SUR-vix); the adjective is cervical	Latin word for neck	neck (also the neck of the uterus)
chondrogenesis (konn-droh-JENN-uh-sihs)	*chondr/o* (cartilage); *-genesis* (origin)	formation of cartilage
chondroid (KONN-droyd)	*chondr/o* (cartilage); *-oid* (similar to)	resembling cartilage
clavicle (KLAV-ih-cuhl); the adjective is clavicular (kla-VIK-yu-luhr)	from the Latin word *clavicula* (a small key)	the collarbone
coccyx (KOK-six); the adjective is coccygeal (kok-SIH-jee-uhl)	from the Greek word *kokkyx* (cuckoo)	the tailbone, made up of the four fused vertebrae at the base of the spinal column
cranial bones (KRAY-nee-uhl)	*crani/o* from the Greek word *kranion* (skull); *-al* (adjective form)	collectively, and along with other minor bones, the frontal bone, two parietal bones, two temporal bones, and the occipital bone
diaphysis (dye-AFF-ih-sihs)	a Greek word (growing between)	shaft of the long bone
diarthrosis (dy-ar-THRO-sihs)	a Greek word (articulation)	synonym for synovial joint
endosteum (ehn-DOST-ee-um)	*endo-* (inside); *oste/o* (Greek word for bone)	inner membrane layer of the bone
epiphysis (eh-PIFF-ih-sihs)	*epi-* (upon); *-physis* (growth)	end of the long bone (distal, proximal)
extension (ehx-TEN-shun)	a common English word	to straighten a joint
femur (FEE-muhr)	a Latin word (thigh)	thighbone
fibula (FIHB-yu-lah)	a Latin word (clasp)	the lateral leg bone
flexion (FLEHX-shun)	from the Latin verb *flecto* (bend)	bending a joint
frontal bone (FRUN-tuhl)	frontal (adjective form of English noun: front)	one of the six main cranial bones
humerus (HUE-muh-ruhs)	a Latin word (shoulder)	the long bone extending from the shoulder to the elbow
ilium (IL-ee-uhm)	a Latin word (flank)	one of the three bones fused together to form the hip bone
ischium (IS-kee-uhm)	a Latin word (hip)	one of the three bones fused together to form the hip bone

TERM AND PRONUNCIATION	ANALYSIS	MEANING
lumbar (LUM-bar)	from *lumbus* (Latin for loin); *-ar* (adjective suffix)	adjective describing the vertebrae (L1–L5) in the lower spinal column
malleolus (mahl-ee-OHL-us)	from the Latin word *malleus* (hammer)	bony protrusion on either side of the ankle (medial and lateral)
mandible (MAN-dih-buhl); the adjective is mandibular (man-DIB-yu-luhr)	a Latin word (jaw)	the lower jawbone
maxilla (MAX-ih-luh); the adjective is maxillary (MAX-ih-lahr-ee)	a Latin word (jawbone)	the bone above the upper teeth
medullary cavity (MED-yul-her-ee)	an adjective form of *medulla* (Latin for marrow)	bone marrow cavity
metacarpal (MEHT-uh-KAR-puhl)	*meta-* (beyond); carp from *carpus* (wrist); *-al* (adjective suffix)	short for metacarpal bone; one of the five bones extending from the wrist to the first knuckle in each hand
metatarsals (MEH-tah-TAHR-sahlz)	*meta-* (beyond); tarsal from *tarsos* (flat surface); *-al* (adjective suffix)	short for metatarsal bones; the bones between the tarsals and the phalanges (toes) of the foot
nasal bone (NAY-zuhl)	*nas/o* (nose); *-al* (adjective suffix)	a facial bone (nose)
occipital bone (ox-SIP-it-uhl)	*occiput* (Latin for back of the head); *-al* (adjective suffix)	one of the six main cranial bones
os coxae (OSS COX-ay)	*os* (Latin for bone); *coxae* (Latin: genitive case for hip)	hip bone
osseous (OSS-ee-us)	from the Latin word *osseus* (bony); *-ous* (adjective suffix)	bone tissue
ossification (OSS-ihf-ih-KAY-shun)	*os* (bone); *facio* (Latin verb for make)	bone formation
osteocytes (OSS-tee-oh-syt)	*oste/o* (bone); *-cyte* (cell)	mature bone cells
osteogenesis (oss-tee-oh-JENN-uh-suhs)	*oste/o* (bone); *-genesis* (origin)	formation of bone
parietal bones (puh-RY-uh-tuhl)	from a Latin word *paries* (wall) and *-al* (adjective suffix)	two of the six main cranial bones
patella (pah-TELL-ah)	a Latin word (small plate)	kneecap
pectoral girdle (pek-TOR-uhl)	from *pectus*, a Latin word (chest); *-al* (adjective suffix)	the shoulder girdle
periosteum (pair-ee-OST-ee-um)	*peri-* (around); *oste/o* (bone)	membrane that surrounds the outside of the bone
phalanges (FAY-lanj-es)	plural of the Greek word *phalanx* (a column of soldiers)	fingers (singular form is phalanx)

(continued)

TERM AND PRONUNCIATION	ANALYSIS	MEANING
pubis (PYU-bihs)	short for "os pubis"; from the Latin word *pubertas* (grown up)	one of the three bones fused together to form the hip bone
radius (RAY-dee-uhs); the adjective is radial (RAY-dee-uhl)	a Latin word (a rod or a spoke of a wheel)	one of the two bones (the other is the ulna) extending from the elbow to the wrist
sacrum (SAK-rum); the adjective is sacral (SAK-ruhl)	short for "os sacrum," a Latin word meaning "sacred"	bone formed from five vertebrae fused together near the base of the spinal column
scapula (SKAP-yu-luh); plural is scapulae (SKAP-yu-lay); the adjectival form is scapular (SKAP-yu-luhr)	a Latin word for shoulder blade	the shoulder blade
sternum (STUR-nuhm)	from a Greek word *sternon* (chest)	the breastbone
suture (SOO-chur)	from the Latin word *sutura* (seam)	in the skeletal system, a fibrous membrane joining bones, especially the cranial bones
synarthrosis (syn-AR-thr-oh-sihs)	*syn-* (together); *arthr/o* (joint); *-osis* (condition)	joint with no movement
synovial (sy-NOH-vee-ahl)	*syn-* (together); Latin *ovum* (egg); *-al* (adjective suffix)	adjective form of synovia, a synonym for synovial fluid
talus (TAY-luhs)	a Latin word (ankle)	the bone in the ankle that articulates with the tibia and fibula
tarsals (TAR-sahlz)	from Greek *tarsos* (a flat surface, sole of the foot)	the bones of the sole of the foot
tarsus (TAR-suhs)	from Greek *tarsos* (a flat surface)	instep or sole of the foot; collectively, the seven bones making up the bottom of the foot
temporal bones (TEMP-uh-ruhl)	from the Latin *tempus* (time, temple)	two of the six main cranial bones; located on the side of the head near the ears
thoracic (tho-RASS-ik)	from the Greek *thorax* (breastplate, the chest)	adjective form of thorax
thorax (THOR-ax)	from Greek *thorax* (breastplate, the chest)	chest
tibia (TIH-bee-ah); the adjective form is tibial (TIH-bee-al)	a Latin word (flute)	shin bone
ulna (ULL-nah); the adjective is ulnar (ULL-nahr)	a Latin word (elbow; forearm)	one of the two bones (the other is the radius) extending from the elbow to the wrist

TERM AND PRONUNCIATION	ANALYSIS	MEANING
vertebra (VUR-tuh-bruh); plural is vertebrae (VUR-tuh-bray)	from the Latin *verto* (to turn)	one of the thirty-three segments making up the spinal column
xiphoid process (ZEYE-foyd)	from the Greek *xipho* (sword), *-oid* (resemblance to)	bony, daggerlike structure at the lower end of the sternum
zygomatic bones (ZI-go-MAT-ik)	from Greek *zygoma* (bolt or bar); *-tic* (adjective suffix)	a facial bone (cheek, one of two)
Common Disorders		
arthralgia (ar-THRAL-jee-uh)	*arthr/o* (joint); *-algia* (pain)	pain in a joint
arthritis (ar-THRY-tuhs)	*arthr/o* (joint); *-itis* (inflammation)	inflammation of a joint
arthrocele (ARTH-roh-seel)	*arthr/o* (joint); *-cele* (hernia)	swelling of a joint
arthrochondritis (ARTH-roh-konn-DRY-tihs)	*arthr/o* (joint); *chondr/o* (cartilage); *-itis* (inflammation)	inflammation of cartilage in a joint
arthrodynia (arth-roh-DINN-ee-uh)	*arthr/o* (joint); *-dynia* (pain)	pain in a joint
arthropathy (ar-THROP-ah- thee)	*arthr/o* (joint); *-pathy* (disease or disorder)	any disorder of a joint
arthrosis (ar-THROW-sihs)	*arthr/o* (joint); *-osis* (abnormal condition of)	disintegration of a joint
brachialgia (BRAY-kee-AL-jee-uh)	*brachi/o* (arm); *-algia* (pain)	pain in the arm
bursitis (burr-SY-tihs)	*burs/o* (bursa); *-itis* (inflammation)	inflammation of a bursa
carpal tunnel syndrome (KAR-puhl TUN-uhl SINN-druhm)	*carp/o* (wrist); *-al* (adjective suffix); *syn-* (together); from the Greek *dromos* (a running)	condition characterized by wrist pain, often occurring during sleep
chondrodynia (konn-droh-DINN-ee-uh)	*chondr/o* (cartilage); *-dynia* (pain)	pain originating in cartilage
chondromalacia (konn-droh-muh-LAY-she-uh)	*chondr/o* (cartilage); *-malacia* (softening)	softening of cartilage
chondropathy (kon-DROP-ah-thee)	*chondr/o* (cartilage); *-pathy* (disease or disorder)	disease of cartilage
chondrosarcoma (KONN-droh-sar-KOH-ma)	*chondr/o* (cartilage); *sarc/o* (flesh); *-oma* (tumor)	malignant tumor arising from the cartilage
compound fracture (KOM-pound FRAK-chur)	from the Latin *fractura* (a break)	break in the bone where the bone comes through the skin; open fracture
costalgia (koss-TAL-jee-uh)	*cost/o* (rib); *-algia* (pain)	pain in a rib(s)
costochondritis (KOSS-toh-kon-DRY-tihs)	*cost/o* (rib); *chondr/o* (cartilage); *-itis* (inflammation)	inflammation of rib cartilage
dactylalgia (DAKK-tihl-AL-jee-uh)	*dactyl/o* (finger, toe); *-algia* (pain)	pain in a finger (or toe)
dactylodynia (DAKK-tihl-oh-DINN-ee-uh)	*dactyl/o* (finger, toe); *-dynia* (pain)	pain in a finger (or toe)

(continued)

TERM AND PRONUNCIATION	ANALYSIS	MEANING
dactylomegaly (DAKK-tih-lo-MEG-uh-lee); more often called megadactyly (meg-uh-DAKK-tuh-lee), probably because "mega" has so many common uses as an English prefix	*dactyl/o* (finger, toe); *-megaly* (enlargement)	enlargement of one or more fingers or toes
fracture (FRAK-chur)	from Latin word *fractura* (break)	break in a bone
herniated disc (HER-nee-ay-ted disk)	from Latin word *hernia* (rupture); *disc/o* (disk)	protrusion of a fragmented intervertebral disc in the intervertebral foramen with potential compression of a nerve
kyphosis (ky-FOH-sihs)	*kyph/o* (humped); *-sis* (condition)	humpback; anteriorly concave curvature of the thoracic and sacral region of the spine
lordosis (lohr-DOH-sihs)	from the Greek word *lordosis* (a bending backwards)	swayback; abnormal anteriorly convex curvature of the lumbar part of the spine
ostealgia (oss-tee-AL-jee-uh)	*oste/o* (bone); *-algia* (pain)	pain in a bone
osteitis (oss-tee-EYE-tihs)	*oste/o* (bone); *-itis* (inflammation)	inflammation of bone
osteochondritis (OSS-tee-oh-konn-DRY-tihs)	*oste/o* (bone); *chondr/o* (cartilage); *-itis* (inflammation)	inflammation of bone and associated cartilage
osteodynia (oss-tee-oh-DINN-ee-uh)	*oste/o* (bone); *-dynia* (pain)	pain in a bone
osteomalacia (OSS-tee-oh-muh-LAY-she-uh)	*oste/o* (bone); *-malacia* (softening)	softening of bone
osteomyelitis (OSS-tee-oh-my-eh-LY-tihs)	*oste/o* (bone); *myel/o* (marrow); *-itis* (inflammation)	inflammation of bone marrow
osteopenia (oss-tee-oh-PEEN-ee-uh)	*oste/o* (bone); *-penia* (deficiency)	abnormally low bone density
osteoporosis (OSS-tee-oh-puh-RO-sihs)	*oste/o* (bone); *por/o* (porous); *-sis* (condition)	atrophy and thinning of bone tissue
osteosarcoma (OSS-tee-oh-sar-KOH-ma)	*oste/o* (bone); *sarc/o* (fleshlike); *-oma* (tumor)	highly malignant tumor of the bone
rheumatoid arthritis (ROO-mah-toid ar-THRY-tuhs)	from the Greek word *rheuma* (flux); *-oid* (resemblance of)	systemic disease occurring more often in women that affects the connective tissue; involves many joints, especially those of the hands and feet
rickets (RIH-kehts)	common English word	disease due to vitamin D deficiency characterized by deficient calcification and soft bones associated with skeletal deformities

TERM AND PRONUNCIATION	ANALYSIS	MEANING
scoliosis (skohl-ee-OH-sihs)	*scoli/o* (twisted); *-sis* (condition)	lateral curvature of the spine; S-shaped curvature
sprain (SPRAYN)	common English word	injury to a ligament
syndrome (SIN-drum)	*syn-* (together); from the Greek *dromos* (running)	collection of signs and symptoms occurring together and characterizing a medical condition

Practice and Practitioners

orthopedics (or-thoh-PEE-diks)	*orth/o* (straight or correct); *ped-* (child); *-ic* (adjective suffix)	the medical specialty concerned with the development, preservation, restoration, and function of the musculoskeletal system
orthopedic surgeon (or-thoh-PEE-dik)	*orth/o* (straight or correct); *ped-* (child); *-ic* (adjective suffix)	a physician in the field of orthopedics (can be MD or DO)
rheumatologist (ROO-mah-tah-lo-gist)	*rheumat/o* (flux); *-logist* (one who studies a certain field)	physician who treats joint and connective tissue disorders such as arthritis
rheumatology (ROO-mah-tah-lo-gee)	*rheumat/o* (flux); *-logy* (the study of)	field of specialty that deals with joints and connective tissue disorders

Diagnosis and Treatment

analgesics (an-al-GEE-ziks)	*an-* (absence); from the Greek word *gesis* (sensation)	medication used to relieve pain
anti-inflammatory (AN-ty-in-FLAMM-ah-tohr-ee)	*anti-* (against); inflammatory (common English word)	medication used to reduce inflammation (example: used to reduce joint inflammation in arthritis)
arthrocentesis (arth-roh-senn-TEE-sihs)	*arthr/o* (joint); *-centesis* (surgical puncture for aspiration)	removing fluid from a joint
arthrogram (ARTH-roh-gram)	*arthr/o* (joint); *-gram* (record or picture)	radiograph of a joint
arthrometry (arth-ROM-uh-tree)	*arthr/o* (joint); *-metry* (process of measuring)	measurement of the amount of movement in a joint
arthroscope (ARTH-roh-skope)	*arthr/o* (joint); *-scope* (instrument for viewing)	device used in arthroscopy
arthroscopy (ahr-THRAW-skoh-pee)	*arthr/o* (joint); *-scopy* (use of instrument for viewing)	examination of the interior of a joint
CT scan	abbreviation for computed tomography	noninvasive imaging test; imaging anatomical information from a cross-sectional plane of the body

(continued)

TERM AND PRONUNCIATION	ANALYSIS	MEANING
MRI	abbreviation for magnetic resonance imaging	a diagnostic radiograph in which the magnetic nuclei of a patient are aligned in a magnetic field; these signals are converted into tomographic images
myelogram (MY-el-loh-gram)	*myel/o* (bone marrow); *-gram* (record or picture)	X-ray of the spinal column using contrast medium
narcotic (nahr-KAH-tik)	*narc/o* (sleep)	drug derived from opium with potent analgesic effects; potential effects of dependency through prolonged use
NSAIDs	abbreviation for nonsteroidal anti-inflammatory drugs	medication that exerts analgesic and anti-inflammatory actions
reduction (ree-DUK-shun)	common English word	correcting a fracture by realigning the bone pieces
traction (TRAK-shun)	common English word	using elastics or pulley and weights to maintain alignment; a pulling or dragging force exerted on a limb in a distal direction
Surgical Procedures		
arthrectomy (ar-THREK-tuh-mee)	*arthr/o* (joint); *-ectomy* (surgical removal)	excision of a joint
arthroplasty (ARTH-roh-plass-tee)	*arthr/o* (joint); *-plasty* (surgical repair)	surgical repair of a joint
arthrotomy (ar-THRAWT-uh-mee)	*arthr/o* (joint); *-tomy* (cutting operation)	surgical incision into a joint
carpectomy (kar-PEK-tuh-me)	*carp/o* (wrist); *-ectomy* (surgical removal)	excision of part of the wrist
chondroplasty (KONN-droh-plass-tee)	*chondr/o* (cartilage); *-plasty* (surgical repair)	surgical repair of cartilage
costectomy (koss-TEK-tuh-mee)	*cost/o* (rib); *-ectomy* (surgical removal)	excision of a rib
ostectomy (oss-TECK-tuh-mee)	*oste/o* (bone); *-ectomy* (surgical removal)	surgical removal of bone
osteoplasty (OSS-tee-oh-plass-tee)	*oste/o* (bone); *-plasty* (surgical repair)	surgical repair of bone
osteorrhaphy (OSS-tee-oh-raff-ee)	*oste/o* (bone); *-rrhaphy* (surgical suturing)	suturing together the parts of a broken bone
osteotomy (oss-tee-AW-tuh-mee)	*oste/o* (bone); *-tomy* (cutting operation)	surgical cutting of bone
vertebrectomy (ver-tuh-BREKK-tuh-mee)	from the Latin word *verto* (to turn); *-ectomy* (surgical removal)	excision (resectioning) of a vertebra

EXERCISES

EXERCISE 5-1 FIGURE LABELING: SKELETON

Write the name of each numbered part in the corresponding line.

calcaneus	facial bones	mandible	phalanges	sternum
carpals	femur	metacarpals	radius	tarsals
clavicle	fibula	metatarsals	ribs	tibia
costal cartilage	humerus	patella	sacrum	ulna
cranium	ilium	pelvis	scapula	vertebral column

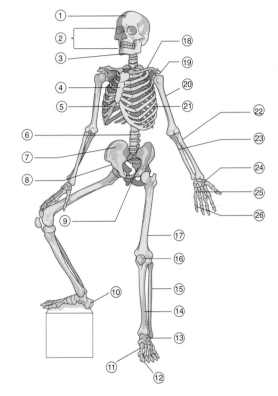

1. _____

2. _____

3. _____

4. _____

5. _____

6. _____

7. _____

8. _____

9. _____

10. _____

11. _____

12. _____

13. _____

14. _____

15. _____

16. _____

17. _____

18. _____

19. _____

20. _____

21. _____

22. _____

23. _____

24. _____

25. _____

26. _____

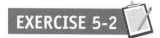

EXERCISE 5-2 FIGURE LABELING: LONG BONE

Write the name of each numbered part in the corresponding line below.

cartilage	diaphysis	epiphyseal line	periosteum	spongy bone
compact bone	distal epiphysis	medullary cavity	proximal epiphysis	yellow marrow

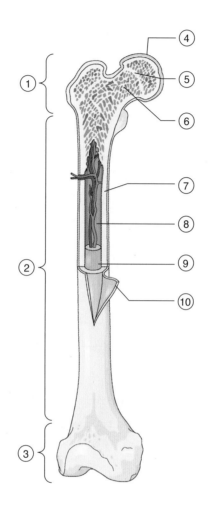

1. _____ 6. _____

2. _____ 7. _____

3. _____ 8. _____

4. _____ 9. _____

5. _____ 10. _____

EXERCISE 5-3   WORD BUILDING

Use the word elements listed to build the terms defined.

-algia = pain
arthr/o = joint
cardi/o = heart
chondr/o = cartilage
cost/o = rib
-desis = fusion/ fixation

-ectomy = removal
electr/o = electricity
-gram = record
inter- = between
-itis = inflammation
kinesi/o = movement

-logy = study
-malacia = softening
my/o = muscle
myel/o = marrow/ spine
-oma = tumor
oste/o = bone

-plasty = plastic repair
-porosis = porous
sarc/o = flesh
-scopy = visual exam

1. _____ inflammation of the bone and bone marrow

2. _____ visual examination of a joint

3. _____ abnormal softening of cartilage

4. _____ a radiograph of a joint

5. _____ the fusion or fixation of a joint

6. _____ the study of movement of body parts

7. _____ surgical repair of cartilage

8. _____ pertaining to the area between the ribs

9. _____ inflammation of the bone

10. _____ a highly malignant tumor of the bone

11. _____ surgical repair of a joint

12. _____ X-ray of the spine

13. _____ inflammation of the cartilage

14. _____ bones with diminished density; porous

15. _____ pain in the ribs

EXERCISE 5-4 🖊 MATCHING: TERMS OF JOINT MOVEMENT

Match each term in Column 1 with its best definition in Column 2.

TERM	DEFINITION
1. _____ abduction	A. backward bending of hand or foot
2. _____ rotation	B. bending the foot toward the ground
3. _____ plantar flexion	C. straightening or stretching
4. _____ extension	D. motion around a central axis
5. _____ dorsiflexion	E. motion away from the body
6. _____ flexion	F. bending motion
7. _____ adduction	G. motion toward the body

EXERCISE 5-5 🖊 MATCHING: TYPES OF FRACTURES

Match each term in Column 1 with its best definition in Column 2.

TERM	DEFINITION
1. _____ comminuted	A. break at an angle
2. _____ greenstick	B. S-shaped break
3. _____ compound	C. bone splintered or crushed
4. _____ simple	D. bone pressed into itself
5. _____ impacted	E. broken straight across bone
6. _____ transverse	F. skin has been broken along with the bone
7. _____ oblique	G. no open wound, broken bone
8. _____ spiral	H. bone only partially broken

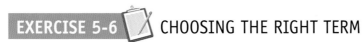

EXERCISE 5-6   CHOOSING THE RIGHT TERM

Circle the term defined.

1. A cartilaginous growth or tumor
   a. osteochondroma
   b. chondroma
   c. chondroid
   d. osteoma

2. Inflammation of the bone marrow and adjacent bone
   a. arthritis
   b. bursitis
   c. osteomyelitis
   d. periostitis

3. The surgical loosening of an ankylosed joint
   a. arthrolysis
   b. arthrodesis
   c. arthrocentesis
   d. rachiolysis

4. The formation of a bone
   a. osteoporosis
   b. osteology
   c. orthogenesis
   d. osteogenesis

5. The bony structure that forms the upper part of the sternum
   a. manubrium
   b. mandible
   c. temporomadibular joint
   d. maxilla

6. An abnormal increase in the outward curvature of the spine
   a. spondylosis
   b. lumbago
   c. lordosis
   d. kyphosis

7. Correction of a fracture or dislocation without opening the skin
   a. osteoclasis
   b. spinal fusion
   c. closed reduction
   d. magnetic resonance

8. A fracture in which the bone is splintered or crushed
   a. spiral fracture
   b. stress fracture
   c. transverse fracture
   d. comminuted fracture

9. The cartilaginous lower portion of the sternum
   a. xiphoid process
   b. sacroiliac
   c. olecranon process
   d. pelvic girdle

EXERCISE 5-7 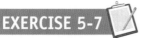 WRITING DESCRIPTIONS TO FIT MEDICAL TERMS

The underlined medical terms refer to a physician, a condition, or a treatment. Replace the underlined terms with a description.

Mrs. Smith, an 82-year-old woman, was out walking her dog on a cold day. She slipped on a patch of ice, fell, and incurred painful injuries. In the emergency room, Dr. Farley Burrows, an <u>orthopedic surgeon</u> (1), examined her. Mrs. Smith had limited <u>ROM</u> (2) in her right wrist and was experiencing pain in her left hip. Dr. Burrows ordered X-rays, which revealed a <u>comminuted fracture</u> (3) in the wrist and an <u>impacted fracture</u> (4) in the hip. He then performed a <u>reduction</u> (5) of the wrist bone and ordered that Mrs. Smith be admitted to the hospital and placed in <u>traction</u> (6) to maintain realignment of her hip.

Write your descriptions of each of the underlined terms or phrases in the spaces.

1. _____

2. _____

3. _____

4. _____

5. _____

6. _____

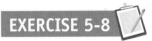 EXERCISE 5-8   CROSSWORD PUZZLE: THE SKELETAL SYSTEM

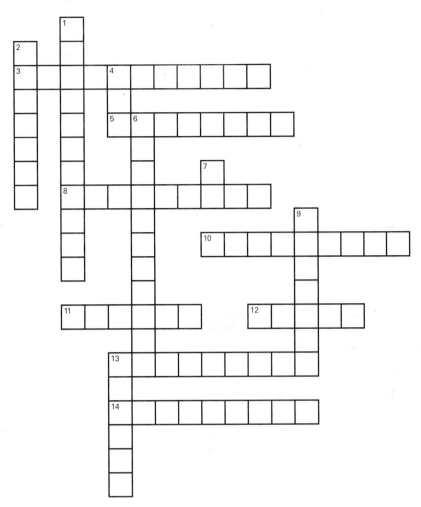

ACROSS

3. instrument used to view inside a joint
5. lower jawbone
8. inflammation of a joint
10. fingers and toes
11. root for cartilage
12. root for cranium
13. heel bone
14. pain in a rib

DOWN

1. surgical repair of a bone
2. upper jawbone
4. abbreviation for range of motion
6. joint pain
7. abbreviation for computed tomography
9. wrist bones
13. tailbone

◀ **CHAPTER 5 QUIZ**

Identify the proper medical term.

1. Collar bone
   a. ischium
   b. ulna
   c. clavicle
   d. zygomatic

2. Bones of the hands
   a. tarsals
   b. metacarpals
   c. metatarsals
   d. calcaneus

3. Bones of the fingers and toes
   a. metatarsals
   b. carpals
   c. phalanges
   d. fibulas

4. Heel bone
   a. ilium
   b. zygomatic
   c. ulna
   d. calcaneus

5. Back bone/spine
   a. vertebrae
   b. temporals
   c. maxilla
   d. scapula

6. Shoulder blade
   a. scapula
   b. sternum
   c. maxilla
   d. scoliosis

Each of the following groups of words has a word that does not belong. Identify this term.

7. a. scoliosis   b. rickets   c. RA   d. diaphysis

8. a. humerus   b. fibula   c. radius   d. ulna

9. a. tibia   b. fibula   c. femur   d. ulna

10. a. deltoid   b. patella   c. sternum   d. carpal

11. a. sclerosis   b. kyphosis   c. scoliosis   d. lordosis

12. a. cervical   b. parietal   c. thoracic   d. lumbar

13. a. patella   b. sternum   c. phalanges   d. diaphragm

14. a. comminuted   b. insertion   c. compound   d. greenstick

Fill in the blank with the correct term.

15. An incision into the chest is termed _____.

16. The word that means "inflammation of a joint" is _____.

17. Aspiration of fluid from a joint by a needle puncture is a(n) _____.

18. The study and treatment of disorders of the musculoskeletal system is

   _____.

19. To "reduce" a fracture is to _____.

20. The specialist who treats disorders of the skeletal system is called a(n) _____.

6 The Muscular System

INTRODUCTION

In the preceding chapter, you may recall having read that there are approximately 206 bones in the human body. The total number of muscles is harder to calculate because of the various ways to distinguish them. But it is safe to say that there are approximately three times as many muscles as there are bones. Moreover, muscles make up about half of our total body weight.

We normally think of muscles as necessary for lifting objects, running, jumping, throwing a ball, or swinging a golf club. Even though that assumption is accurate, muscles are also needed for seeing, talking, eating, digesting, breathing, smiling, frowning, blinking, and so on. And let's not forget the muscle that pumps blood through our bodies, even though the heart is included in another chapter.

WORD ROOTS SPECIFIC TO THE MUSCULAR SYSTEM

The roots shown in Table 6-1 are often found in terms related to the muscular system. You will recognize them in many of the terms you will learn in this chapter.

STRUCTURE AND FUNCTION

Muscles can be characterized by their location, control action (voluntary or involuntary), and cell appearance (striated or nonstriated). There are three types of muscles: skeletal, smooth, and cardiac (Fig. 6-1).

Of the three types, skeletal muscle is the largest group, comprising more than 600 separate muscles. These muscles are made up of fibers enclosed in a fibrous sheath of **fascia** attached to bones by **tendons** made up of connective tissue (Figs. 6-2 and 6-3). **Ligaments** connect bones to bones and offer support to muscles.

Skeletal muscles do their jobs by contracting and relaxing. These two actions make all movement possible. Skeletal muscles are attached to bones, of course, and these contractions and relaxations change the position angles of bones to effect skeletal movement. The terms defined in Table 6-2, therefore, name each kind of movement involved in contraction and relaxation.

Skeletal muscle is also known as striated muscle because the dark and light bands in the muscle fibers create a striated (striped) appearance. Skeletal muscle is responsible not only for voluntary

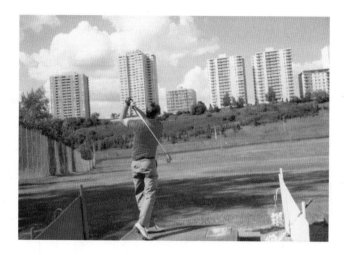

movement but also for heat, which is generated by rapid, small contractions (shivering), and for maintenance of posture.

Smooth Muscle

Smooth muscle, which acts involuntarily, is located in the blood vessels, respiratory passageways, digestive tract, and walls of hollow internal organs. The functions of smooth muscle are to control and move substances through passageways with wavelike motions and to regulate the diameter of the openings of vessels and hollow organs.

Cardiac Muscle

Cardiac muscle, also known as the heart or **myocardial muscle**, forms the wall of the heart. It acts involuntarily and has a lightly striated appearance. The contraction and relaxation of the cardiac muscle is responsible for the heart's pumping action. This subject is discussed in detail in Chapter 9.

TABLE 6-1	WORD ELEMENTS COMMON WITHIN THE MUSCULAR SYSTEM	
Element	**Type**	**Meaning**
fasci/o	root	fibrous membrane
fibr/o	root	fiber
hemi-	prefix	half
kine-, kinesi/o	root	movement
ligament/o	root	ligament
muscul/o	root	muscle
my/o	root	muscle
para-	prefix	beside, beyond, near
-paresis	suffix	partial or incomplete paralysis
-plegia	suffix	paralysis
quadri-	prefix	four
sthen/o	root	strength
tend/o, tendin/o	root	tendon
ton/o	root	tone

Comparison of the different types of muscle			
	Smooth	Cardiac	Skeletal
Location	Wall of hollow organs, vessels, respiratory passageways	Wall of heart	Attached to bones
Cell characteristics	Tapered at each end, single nucleus, non-striated	Branching networks, single nucleus, lightly striated	Long and cylindrical, multi-nucleated, heavily striated
Control	Involuntary	Involuntary	Voluntary

FIGURE 6-1   Comparison of muscle types. A comparison of the types of muscles, their location, cell characteristics, and type of control. *From Cohen BJ, Wood DL*. Memmler's The Human Body in Health and Disease. *9th ed. Philadelphia, PA: Lippincott Williams & Wilkins; 2000.*

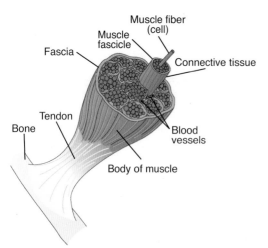

FIGURE 6-2   Structure of a skeletal muscle.
Muscle cells are referred to as fibers that are held in bundles by connective tissue. A sheet of fascia covers the muscle. *From Cohen BJ*. Medical Terminology: An Illustrated Guide. *5th ed. Philadelphia, PA: Lippincott Williams & Wilkins; 2007.*

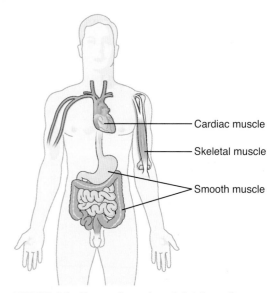

FIGURE 6-3   Types of muscles: skeletal, cardiac, and smooth. Smooth muscle makes up the wall of ducts and hollow organs, such as the stomach and intestine; cardiac muscle makes up the wall of the heart; skeletal muscle is attached to bones. *From Cohen BJ*. Medical Terminology: An Illustrated Guide. *5th ed. Philadelphia, PA: Lippincott Williams & Wilkins; 2007.*

TABLE 6-2 TERMS THAT NAME MUSCLE MOVEMENTS

Movement	Definition	Example
abduction	movement away from midline	moving the arms outward from the body
adduction	movement toward midline	return of the lifted arms to sides
eversion	turning outward	turning the sole of the foot outward
inversion	turning inward	turning the sole of the foot inward
extension	opening the angle of a joint	straightening of the knee
flexion	closing the angle of a joint	bending the knee
pronation	turning downward	turning the palm of the hand downward
supination	turning upward	turning the palm of the hand upward
dorsiflexion	bending backward	pointing the toes backward toward your nose
plantar flexion	bending the sole of the foot	pointing the toes downward
rotation	turning a body part on its own axis	turning the head

Word Elements Exercise IDENTIFYING WORD ELEMENTS AND THEIR MEANINGS

Thoroughly familiarize yourself with Table 6-1 before attempting to complete this exercise. Without referring to the table again, write the element type (prefix, root, or suffix) in the column marked Type. Write the meaning of each element in the column marked Meaning.

ELEMENT	TYPE	MEANING
1. ligament/o		
2. tend/o, tendin/o		
3. ton/o		
4. -plegia		
5. muscul/o		
6. kine-, kinesi/o		
7. -paresis		
8. sthen/o		
9. my/o		
10. quadri-		
11. fasci/o		
12. fibr/o		
13. hemi-		
14. para-		

✔ *Quick Check: The Three Types of Muscles*

What are the three types of muscles? Give an example of where each is found.

TYPE	WHERE LOCATED
1. _____	_____
2. _____	_____
3. _____	_____

PRACTICE AND PRACTITIONERS

The medical specialists who treat disorders of the muscular system include **neurologists** and **orthopedic surgeons**, who also treat skeletal and neurologic disorders, as noted in Chapter 5. A neurologist is a physician who specializes in the diagnosis and treatment of both the muscular and nervous systems. The area of study is called **neurology**. Many conditions involve joints as well as muscles, and orthopedic physicians diagnose and treat patients with joint disorders. Other health care professionals who work with patients who have muscular system disorders include **occupational therapists** and **physical therapists**.

DISORDERS AND TREATMENTS

Disorders of the muscular system often involve other systems. However, the terms introduced in the following discussion are specific to the muscular system only.

Most muscle disorders are caused by physical trauma, such as those occurring in sports or accidents. Others are chronic and are listed first.

Chronic Disorders

Muscular dystrophy causes weakness without affecting the nervous system. Its most common form, which affects only male children, is called **Duchenne's muscular dystrophy**.

Myasthenia gravis is an immunologic disorder characterized by fluctuating weakness, especially of the facial and external eye muscles. Symptoms can include **dysphagia**.

Fibromyalgia is a disorder characterized by widespread aching and stiffness of muscles and soft tissues, fatigue, tenderness, and sleep disorders. The cause of fibromyalgia is unknown, and it may coexist with other chronic diseases.

Amyotrophic lateral sclerosis (also called **Lou Gehrig's Disease**), also noted as a neurologic disease, is a fatal, progressive degeneration of the nerve tracts of the spinal cord leading to muscular **atrophy**.

Cumulative Trauma and Sports Injuries

Cumulative trauma disorders are often caused by repetitive, work-related motions that damage muscles, tendons, joints, or nerves. A common one is **carpal tunnel syndrome**, which is a skeletal disorder involving the carpal bones. It is also considered a cumulative trauma disorder of the muscular system because it affects the tendons of the wrist (Fig. 6-4).

A **rotator cuff injury**, which affects the shoulder, occurs to people who perform repeated activities such as swimming or throwing. The rotator cuff is formed by four muscles that may become inflamed and swollen when overused.

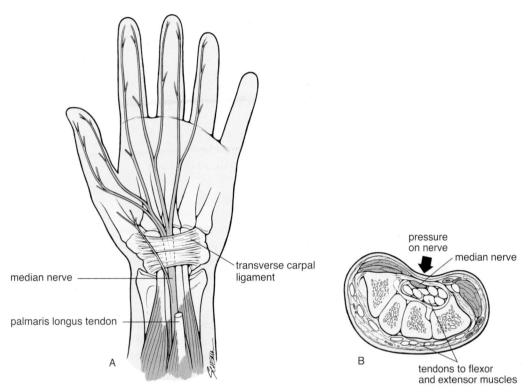

median nerve

palmaris longus tendon

transverse carpal ligament

A

pressure on nerve

median nerve

B

tendons to flexor and extensor muscles

FIGURE 6-4   Carpal tunnel syndrome. A. Pressure on the median nerve as it passes through the carpal (wrist) bone causes numbness and weakness in the areas of the hand supplied by the nerve. **B.** Cross-section of the wrist showing compression of the median nerve. *From Cohen BJ.* Medical Terminology: An Illustrated Guide. *5th ed. Philadelphia, PA: Lippincott Williams & Wilkins; 2007.*

Epicondylitis, also commonly called tennis elbow, is an inflammation of the medial and lateral epicondyles, bony projections of the distal portion of the humerus (Fig. 6-5).

Plantar fasciitis is an inflammation of the plantar fascia (connective tissue in the arch of the foot) that can cause intense pain when walking or running. It may be caused by long periods of weight bearing, sudden changes in activity, or obesity.

Sports injuries often occur to overstressed or poorly conditioned muscles. However, injuries occur even to professional athletes in good physical condition. Two examples are the **hamstring injury** and **shin splints**. A **hamstring injury** is a strain or tear in one of the hamstring muscles (group of four posterior thigh muscles). This injury is common among sprinters, track hurdlers, and baseball or football players. Treatment consists of rest, ice, compression (bandaging), and elevation, abbreviated "RICE." A **shin splint** is pain often caused by overuse of the muscles in the

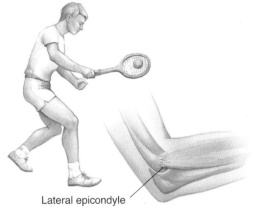

Lateral epicondyle

FIGURE 6-5   Tennis and golfer's elbow. Repetitive motions can cause an inflammation of the medial and lateral epicondyles, causing pain. *Asset provided by Anatomical Chart Co.*

lower leg. It may include a stress fracture (a small sliver or a crack in the bone) of the tibia or an inflammation of the periosteum. Shin splint is actually a collective term describing the pain rather than the condition. Its treatment may also include RICE.

Paralysis

Paralysis is the loss of sensation and voluntary muscle movement caused by injury or disease. The following terms name kinds of paralysis:

- **Hemiparesis**: slight paralysis of one side of the body
- **Myoparesis**: weakness or partial paralysis of a muscle
- **Paraplegia**: paralysis of both legs and the lower part of the body
- **Quadriplegia**: paralysis of all four extremities
- **Hemiplegia**: total paralysis of one side of the body

What is the difference between an abbreviation and an acronym? We speak each letter of an abbreviation, and we pronounce an acronym from the sound its letter combination makes. Because RICE spells a common word, it is often pronounced. Most acronyms do not start out as common English words, however, and although many of them eventually become common words, every acronym is unique. For example, if you ask 10 people on the street what radar stands for, 9 out of 10 of the "answers" will likely consist of blank stares. The word radar, which began life as an acronym meaning *radio detection and ranging*, is now a common English word. So, is RICE an acronym? Even though many health care workers treat it as an acronym, it remains an abbreviation and its pronunciation as a word includes the potential for confusing the general population.

Abbreviation Table   THE MUSCULAR SYSTEM

ABBREVIATION	MEANING
CTD	cumulative trauma disorder
DMD	Duchenne's muscular dystrophy
DTR	deep tendon reflexes
EMG	electromyography
IM	intramuscular
MG	myasthenia gravis
RICE	rest, ice, compression, elevation
ROM	range of motion

Study Table	THE MUSCULAR SYSTEM	
TERM AND PRONUNCIATION	**ANALYSIS**	**MEANING**
Structure and Function		
antagonist (an-TAG-oh-nihst)	a common English word	something (or in common use, someone) opposing or resisting the action of another
fascia (FASH-ee-ah)	the Latin word for band	fibrous sheath of connective tissue that covers a muscle
ligament (LIG-ah-ment)	from the Latin noun *ligamen* (string)	a type of muscle tissue connecting bones, cartilage, or other tissue structures
myocardial muscle (my-oh-CARD-ee-al)	*my/o* (muscle); *cardi/o* (heart); *-al* (adjective)	heart muscle
prime mover	two common English words	muscle that has the principal responsibility for a given movement
striated (STRY-ayted)	from the Latin verb *striare* (to groove)	adjective describing skeletal muscles
tendon (TEN-dun)	from the Latin verb *tendo* (stretch)	a type of muscle structure, such as the Achilles tendon, associated with appendicular muscles
tone, tonicity	from the Greek word *tonos*	tension present in resting muscles
Common Disorders		
amyotrophic lateral sclerosis (ay-my-oh-TROH-fik) or Lou Gehrig's disease	*a-* (deficient); *my/o* (muscle); lateral (side); *scler/o* (hard); *-osis* (abnormal condition)	a progressive degeneration of the nerve tracts of the spinal cord, causing muscular atrophy
asthenia (as-THEEN-ee-ah)	*a-* (deficient); *sthenos* (Greek word for strength)	weakness
atonia (AY-toh-nee-ah)	*a-* (deficient); *tonia* (tone)	flaccidity; lack of muscle tone; relaxation of muscle
atrophy (a-TROH-fee)	*a-* (deficient); *-trophy* (from the Greek word *trophé* meaning "nourishment")	wasting of the muscles
carpal tunnel syndrome	carpal (a wrist bone); tunnel (common English word); syndrome (a Greek word meaning "running together")	the tendons going through the carpal tunnel in the wrist become chronically swollen and inflamed
epicondylitis (EP-ih-KON-dih-LYE-tis)	*epi-* (around); *condyl* (rounded end surface of a bone); *-itis* (inflammation)	inflammation of the tissues around the elbow; golfer or tennis elbow

(continued)

TERM AND PRONUNCIATION	ANALYSIS	MEANING
fibromyalgia (FY-broh-MY-al-jee-ah)	*fibr/o* (fiber); *my/o* (muscle); *-algia* (pain)	a chronic disorder characterized by widespread aching and stiffness of muscles and soft tissues, accompanied by fatigue
hamstring injury	hamstring muscle	strain or tear of the hamstring muscle group (posterior femoral muscle group)
hemiparesis (hem-ee-PAH-ree-sis)	*hemi-* (half); *-paresis* (paralysis)	slight paralysis of one side of the body
hemiplegia (hem-ee-PLEE-jee-ah)	*hemi-* (half); *-plegia* (paralysis)	total paralysis of one side of the body
muscular dystrophy (DIS-tro-fee)	muscular (common English word); *dys-* (difficult); *-trophy* (from the Greek word *trophé* meaning "nourishment")	group of inherited muscle disorders that cause muscle weakness without affecting the nervous system
myasthenia gravis (MY-ahs-THEE-nee-ah GRA-viss)	*my/o* (muscle); asthenia (from the Greek word *astheneia* meaning "weakness")	MG; an immunologic disorder characterized by fluctuating weakness, especially of the facial and external eye muscle
myocele (MY-oh-seel)	*my/o* (muscle); *-cele* (hernia)	hernia of a muscle
myodynia (my-oh-DINN-ee-yuh); myalgia (my-AL-jee-a)	*my/o* (muscle); *-dynia* (pain); *-algia* (pain)	pain in a muscle
myoma (my-OH-muh)	*my/o* (muscle); *-oma* (tumor)	benign neoplasm of muscle tissue
myoparesis (MY-oh-pah-REE-sis)	*my/o* (muscle); *-paresis* (paralysis)	weakness or partial paralysis of a muscle
myositis (my-oh-SY-tihs)	*my/o* (s) (muscle); *-itis* (inflammation)	inflammation of muscle
myospasm (MY-oh-spaz-uhm)	*my/o* (muscle); *-spasm* (involuntary motion)	involuntary contraction of a muscle
paralysis (pah-RAL-ih-sis)	*para-* (not normal); *-lysis* (loosening)	loss of sensation and voluntary muscle movements caused by an injury or disease
paraplegia (PAR-ah-PLEE-jee-ah)	*para-* (not normal); *-plegia* (paralysis)	paralysis of both legs and the lower part of the body
periostitis (PEHR-ee-os-TY-tihs)	*peri-* (around); *oste/o* (bone); *-itis* (inflammation)	inflammation of the periosteum or the covering that surrounds the bone
plantar fasciitis (FASH-ee-eye-tis)	plantar (sole of the foot); fasci- (from *fascia*, Latin for band); *-itis* (inflammation)	inflammation of the plantar fascia causing heel pain
quadriplegia (kwah-drah-PLEE-jee-ah)	*quadri* (four); *-plegia* (paralysis)	paralysis of all four extremities

TERM AND PRONUNCIATION	ANALYSIS	MEANING
rotator cuff injury	rotator cuff (four muscles in the shoulder); injury (common English word)	inflammation of the rotator cuff in the shoulder caused by overuse
shin splint	two common English words used in an uncommon expression	term given to describe pain in the anterior portion of the lower leg during running, walking, and other similar activities
tenalgia (tehn-AL-jee-uh), tenodynia (ten-oh-DINN-ee-uh)	*ten/o* (tendon); *-algia* (pain); *-dynia* (pain)	pain in a tendon
tendonitis (ten-doe-NY-tiss); also sometimes spelled tendinitis (TEN-dih-NY-tiss)	*tendon/o* (tendon); *-itis* (inflammation)	inflammation of a tendon
Practice and Practitioners		
kinesiology (kih-nee-see-AWL-uh-jee)	*kinesi/o* (movement); *-logy* (study of)	study of muscle motion
kinesiologist (kih-nee-see-AWL-uh-jist)	*kinesi/o* (movement); *-logist* (one who studies)	a specialist in kinesiology
myology (my-AWL-uh-jee)	*my/o* (muscle); *-logy* (study of)	study of muscles
orthopedic (or-thoh-PEE-dik)	*orth/o* (straight); *pedics* (child); note: the word was coined in the 18th century, originating with the study of skeletal disorders in children	pertaining to orthopedics or the study of the musculoskeletal system
orthopedic surgeon (or-thoh-PEE-dik)	*orth/o* (straight); *pedics* (child); surgeon (common English word)	a physician in the field of orthopedics (can be MD or DO)
neurologist (new-ROL-oh-gist)	*neur/o* (nerve); *-logist* (one who studies)	a physician who diagnoses and treats disorders of the nervous system
Diagnosis and Treatment		
electromyography (ee-LEK-troh-my-OG-rafee)	*electr/o* (electricity); *my/o* (muscle); *-graphy* (process of writing)	abbreviation is EMG; records the strength of muscle contractions by means of electrical stimulation
myectomy (my-EKK-tuh-mee)	*my/o* (muscle); *-ectomy* (excision)	excision of part of a muscle
physical therapy (PT)	common English phrase	treatment to prevent disability and restore function through the use of heat, exercise, and massage to improve circulation, strength, flexibility, and muscle strength

(continued)

TERM AND PRONUNCIATION	ANALYSIS	MEANING
RICE (an abbreviation, not an acronym, which is nevertheless sometimes pronounced "rice")	abbreviation derived from rest, ice, compression, and elevation	treatment used for common muscular disorders (hamstring injuries, sprains, strains, etc.)
skeletal muscle relaxants	*skelet/o* (skeleton); *-al* (adjective suffix); relaxant: that which relaxes	medications used to reduce muscle spasm
tenontoplasty (teh-NON-toe-plass-tee); tendinoplasty (TEN-dih-no-plass-tee); tendoplasty (TEN-doe-plass-tee); tenoplasty (TEN-oh-plass-tee)	*tenont/o, tendin/o, tend/o, ten/o* (tendon); *-plasty* (surgical repair)	surgical repair of a tendon
tenorrhaphy (TEN-oh-raff-ee)	*ten/o* (tendon); *-rrhaphy* (suturing)	suturing of a tendon
tenotomy (ten-AW-tuh-mee); also sometimes tendotomy (ten-DAW-tuh-mee)	*ten/o* (tendon); *-tomy* (incision)	incision into a tendon

EXERCISES

EXERCISE 6-1 DEFINING TERMS THAT NAME MUSCLE MOVEMENTS

Thoroughly study Table 6-2 before attempting this exercise. Write a definition describing each of the movements listed. Check your answers with Table 6-2 or the answer key in Appendix A.

MOVEMENT	DEFINITION
1. inversion	_____
2. dorsiflexion	_____
3. abduction	_____
4. adduction	_____
5. plantar flexion	_____
6. supination	_____
7. rotation	_____
8. eversion	_____
9. extension	_____
10. flexion	_____
11. pronation	_____

EXERCISE 6-2 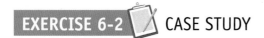 CASE STUDY

PHYSICAL THERAPY PROGRESS NOTE

CHIEF COMPLAINT: Cervical neck pain with limited movement and right shoulder pain with limited ROM.

PROGRESS: The patient states that he is the same as he was the last time he was in for therapy.

AGGRAVATING FACTORS: Working.

PAIN/DISCOMFORT LEVEL: The patient states that the pain is 5/10.

TREATMENT: Treatment today consisted of moist heat and ultrasound of the cervical spine; therapeutic exercise to the neck and shoulder for 45 minutes.

PATIENT'S PROGRESS: The patient is doing well with his cervical spine exercises. His neck flexion and neck extension and rotation are relatively improved. His radiating pain is reduced. His right shoulder is very painful. He has pain on flexion and abduction. He has pain on resisted abduction. He has rotator cuff tendonitis, probably caused by impingement.

The patient was put on a four-step treatment approach to decrease pain and increase neck and shoulder movement. He was advised to limit the use of his right arm as much as possible for 2 weeks, use ice and NSAIDs for pain, and keep his arm in a sling. He demonstrated improved ROM following his therapy. He was advised to use the exercise program on a regular basis.

QUESTIONS

1. What medical terms are associated with the patient's limited neck movements? Define each one.

   _____

   _____

   _____

2. What does "tendonitis" mean?

   _____

   _____

3. Explain what ROM is.

   _____

   _____

4. What does NSAID stand for?

   _____

   _____

EXERCISE 6-3 WRITE THE ABBREVIATION

Write the corresponding abbreviation in the blank space to the right.

1. electromyography   _____

2. cumulative trauma disorder   _____

3. Duchenne's muscular dystrophy   _____

4. range of motion   _____

5. deep tendon reflexes   _____

6. intramuscular   _____

7. myasthenia gravis   _____

8. rest, ice, compression, elevation   _____

EXERCISE 6-4 WORD BUILDING

Use the word elements listed to build the terms defined.

-algia	hemi-	-logy	para-	tendin/o
-cele	-itis	muscul/o	-paresis	ten/o
fasci/o	kinesi/o	my/o	-pathy	-tomy
fibr/o	-logist	neur/o	-plegia	-trophy

1. Incision into a tendon   _____

2. Physician who diagnoses and treats diseases of the nervous system   _____

3. Paralysis of both legs and the lower part of the body   _____

4. Hernia of a muscle   _____

5. Slight paralysis of one side of the body   _____

6. Inflammation of the fascia   _____

7. Pain resulting from movement   _____

8. A chronic disorder characterized by widespread aching   _____

9. Any disease of the muscle   _____

10. Inflammation of a muscle   _____

EXERCISE 6-5 FILL IN THE BLANK

Fill in the blank with the correct answer.

1. What are the three types of muscles?

   _____

2. Name two medical specialists who treat disorders of the muscular system.

   _____

3. What is the difference between a paraplegic and a hemiplegic?

   _____

4. Identify and define the word elements in the term "amyotrophic."

   _____

5. What is a prime mover when that phrase is used in connection with the muscular system?

   _____

   _____

6. What is the medical term for tennis elbow?

   _____

7. What does the abbreviation EMG stand for?

   _____

   _____

8. Define "muscular dystrophy."

   _____

   _____

9. What does each letter in RICE stand for?

   _____

   _____

10. What is the term, which is also the Latin word for string, that names what connects bones to bones to support muscles?

   _____

EXERCISE 6-6   TRUE OR FALSE

Circle the correct answer.

1. Plantar fasciitis can cause heel pain.
   True   False

2. Duchenne's disease is a type of arthritis.
   True   False

3. An antagonist is a muscle that opposes or resists the action of another muscle.
   True   False

4. Tennis elbow is another name for myositis.
   True   False

5. Shin splints may be caused by periostitis.
   True   False

6. Myoparesis is contraction of the muscle.
   True   False

7. Myocardium is the heart muscle.
   True   False

8. Tendons attach bone to bone.
   True   False

9. Kinesi/o is a root word for movement.
   True   False

EXERCISE 6-7 CROSSWORD PUZZLE: THE MUSCULAR SYSTEM

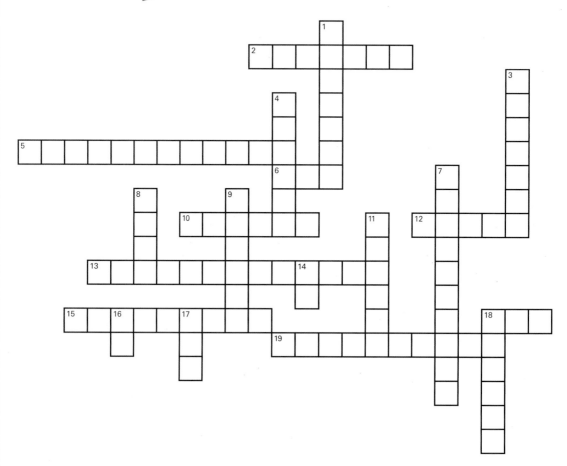

ACROSS

2. suffix for incomplete paralysis
5. widespread muscle aches, fatigue, unknown cause
6. abbreviation for Duchenne's muscular dystrophy
10. suffix for paralysis
12. lack of muscle tone
13. tennis elbow
15. muscle group in the back of the thigh
18. abbreviation for straight leg raises
19. heart muscle

DOWN

1. triangular shoulder muscle
3. wasting of tissue
4. prefix meaning "four"
7. opposes a prime mover
8. prefix meaning "half"
9. fibrous band that connects muscle to bone
11. band of connective tissue that covers the muscle
14. abbreviation for intramuscular
16. root word for muscle
17. abbreviation for range of motion
18. hollow internal organ muscle type

CHAPTER 6 QUIZ

Multiple Choice

1. The three types of muscle tissue are:
   a. smooth, cardiac, deltoid
   b. cardiac, epicardium, skeletal
   c. cardiac, skeletal, smooth
   d. skeletal, trapezius, deltoid

2. Physicians in which of the following medical specialty(ies) take care of muscular disorders?
   a. neurology
   b. orthopedic
   c. neurology and orthopedics
   d. chiropractic and orthopedics

3. Kinesiology is the study of:
   a. dance
   b. movement
   c. aerobics
   d. athletics

4. A quadriplegic is paralyzed in _____ limbs.
   a. one
   b. two
   c. three
   d. four

5. Carpal tunnel syndrome involves the _____.
   a. wrist
   b. knee
   c. elbow
   d. ankle

6. A muscle antagonist is a:
   a. muscle that resists the action of another
   b. muscle that has the principal responsibility for a given movement
   c. type of muscle that connects one muscle to another
   d. none of the above

7. A muscular disease, usually diagnosed by age 3 to 5 years, that requires wheelchair confinement by age 12; this disorder is characterized by progressive weakness.
   a. myasthenia gravis
   b. multiple sclerosis
   c. muscular dystrophy
   d. paraplegia

Fill in the Blank

8. Pointing the toes downward is called _____.

9. _____ is the term for weakness.

10. A hernia of a muscle is called _____.

11. _____ causes intense pain in the heel region upon walking.

12. A(n) _____ records the strength of muscle contractions.

13. The surgical repair of a tendon is called _____.

14. _____ is the study of muscles.

15. Muscle pain is called _____.

Define

16. antagonist _____

17. myoparesis _____

18. DTR _____

19. RICE _____

20. abduction _____

7   *The Nervous System*

LEARNING OBJECTIVES

Upon completion of this chapter, you should be able to:

- Name the major parts and functions of the nervous system.
- Define nervous system terms from your understanding of word elements.
- Name the parts of a nerve.
- Name the major divisions of the nervous system.
- Build, spell, and pronounce medical terms that relate to the nervous system.
- Define the terms that name disorders and treatment procedures related to the nervous system.
- Interpret selected abbreviations used in connection with the nervous system.
- Define the terms introduced in this chapter.

INTRODUCTION

The nervous system, one of the most complex systems in the body, coordinates the body's involuntary and voluntary actions. The nervous system works in conjunction with the endocrine system to maintain **homeostasis**, a term that means "a state of equilibrium."

The nervous system has two main divisions: the **central nervous system (CNS)** and the **peripheral nervous system (PNS)** (Fig. 7-1). The CNS consists of the brain and spinal cord. The PNS, which may be divided into **somatic** and **autonomic nervous subsystems**, controls skeletal muscles by means of the cranial and spinal nerves (Fig. 7-2).

WORD ELEMENTS FOUND IN NERVOUS SYSTEM TERMS

Table 7-1 lists most of the elements that make up nervous system terms. Some suffixes already learned may also be listed.

STRUCTURE AND FUNCTION

Nerve tissue, together with its associated connective tissue and blood vessels, make up both the CNS and the PNS. Nerve tissue is composed of fundamental units called **neurons**, which are separated, supported, and protected by **neuroglia**. Neurons carry electrical messages that coordinate the exchange of information between the body's internal and external environments, and the neuroglia offer protection and support to the nerve tissue.

The three principal parts of a neuron cell are its **cell body**, **dendrites**, and **axon** (Fig. 7-3). The cell body contains the nucleus and receives impulses from other cells through the dendrites. The dendrites, which project outward from the cell body, act as antennae that receive and transmit messages between the neuron and muscles, skin, or other neurons. The cell body passes these messages to the axon, which conducts electrical impulses away from the cell body. The connecting points for these message transfers are called **synapses**. **Synaptic** (adjective form of synapse) connections can occur between two nerve cells. The stimulus between the two cells is usually a chemical called a **neurotransmitter**. For example, hormones are typical neurotransmitters.

Groups of neuron cell bodies within the PNS are called **ganglia** (singular: **ganglion**). Groups of neuron cell bodies within the CNS are called **nuclei** (singular: **nucleus**). Groupings of axons are called **nerves** wherever they occur in the body.

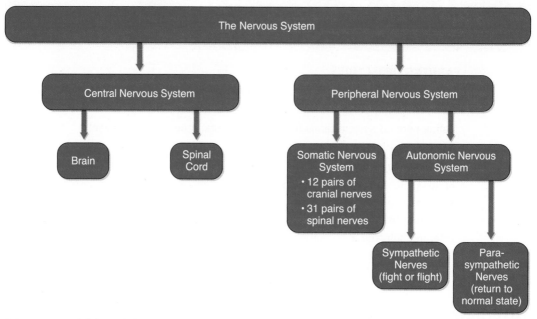

FIGURE 7-1   Divisions of the nervous system. The flow chart identifies the two main divisions of the nervous system: central and peripheral. Furthermore, it identifies how the peripheral nervous system is divided into the somatic and autonomic nervous systems and the main functions each performs.

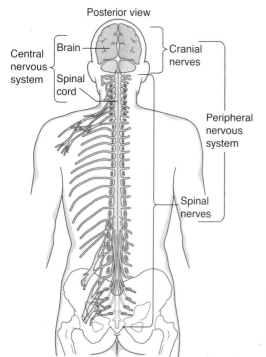

FIGURE 7-2   Posterior view. Divisions of the nervous system. The central nervous system is further divided into the brain and spinal cord. The cranial and spinal nerves are shown here as part of the peripheral nervous system. *From Cohen BJ. Medical Terminology: An Illustrated Guide. 5th ed. Philadelphia, PA: Lippincott Williams & Wilkins; 2007.*

Element	Function	Refers to
arachn/o	root	spider
cephal/o	root	head
cerebell/o	root	the cerebellum
cerebr/o	root	the cerebrum; also, the brain in general
cortic/o	root	outer layer or covering
encephal/o	root	brain
gangli/o, ganglion/o	root	ganglia (singular: ganglion)
gli/o	root	glue
hydr/o	root	water
iatr/o	root	physician; to treat
-mania	suffix	suffix meaning "morbid attraction to" or "impulse toward"
meningi/o	root	a membrane
ment/o	root	referring to the mind
-mnesia	suffix	memory
myel/o	root	in connection with the nervous system, refers to the spinal cord and medulla oblongata
neur/o	root	a nerve cell; nervous system
-oid	suffix	like
-paresis	suffix	weakness, loss of movement
-phasia	suffix	speech
-phobia	suffix	suffix meaning "morbid or unreasonable fear"
-plegia	suffix	paralyzed
psych/o	root	referring to the mind
schiz/o	root	to split
spin/o	root	referring to the spinal cord

TABLE 7-1 WORD ELEMENTS COMMON WITHIN NERVOUS SYSTEM TERMS

Word Elements Exercise FILL IN THE BLANKS

After studying Table 7-1, write the meaning of each of the elements listed in the corresponding blank space to the right.

1. -paresis _____

2. cortic/o _____

3. ment/o _____

4. -plegia _____

5. -mnesia _____

6. iatr/o _____

7. -phobia _____

8. encephal/o _____

(continued)

9. cerebr/o _____

10. hydr/o _____

11. meningi/o _____

12. gangli/o, ganglion/o _____

13. -mania _____

14. myel/o _____

15. neur/o _____

16. arachn/o _____

17. schiz/o _____

18. cephal/o _____

19. psych/o _____

20. -oid _____

21. cerebell/o _____

22. spin/o _____

23. -phasia _____

24. gli/o _____

Do you find some of the foregoing terms and definitions confusing? If so, you are not alone. For example, calling groups of neuron cell bodies nuclei or referring to groups of axons as nerves (a synonym for neurons) tends to defy visual conception. It is indeed hard to envision cell bodies and axons "disembodied" from their neurons and, apparently, acting independently. The reason for this terminology, however, is that axons may extend outward for a meter or more from their respective cell bodies, and dendrites likewise jut outward and may branch out multiple times, thus forming treelike clusters. Realization of these characteristics of neurons may help you visualize the complex nature of the nervous system and see the reasons for the terminology used.

Axons are covered by the **myelin sheath**, a white fatty material that provides protection and electrical insulation. Neurons are grouped together to carry out the highly complex sensing and processing actions required for everything we do.

Central Nervous System

The CNS is the body's control center. All messages originate and/or terminate either in the brain or in the spinal cord. The brain and spinal cord also interpret the messages and determine the body's responses.

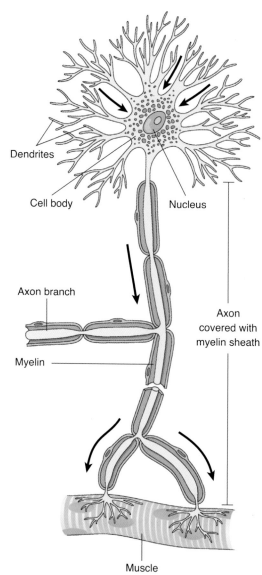

Dendrites

Cell body

Nucleus

Axon branch

Axon covered with myelin sheath

Myelin

Muscle

FIGURE 7-3 **Motor neuron.** The neuron is the basic functional unit of the nervous system. The arrows show the direction of the nerve impulse. Note the myelin sheath that covers the axon of the nerve. *From Cohen BJ. Medical Terminology: An Illustrated Guide. 5th ed. Philadelphia, PA: Lippincott Williams & Wilkins; 2007.*

☐ Frontal lobe ☐ Temporal lobe
☐ Parietal lobe ☐ Occipital lobe

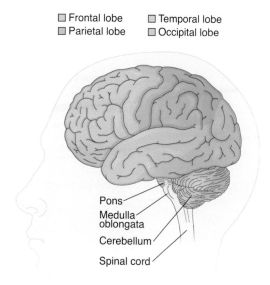

Pons
Medulla oblongata
Cerebellum
Spinal cord

FIGURE 7-4 **Lateral view of the brain, external surface.** The four main lobes (frontal, parietal, temporal, and occipital) are shown in this figure along with the major structures of the brain. *Modified from Cohen BJ. Medical Terminology: An Illustrated Guide. 5th ed. Philadelphia, PA: Lippincott Williams & Wilkins; 2007.*

The brain is one of the largest organs in the body and is responsible for most activities, both mental and physical. For example, sections of the brain control bodily functions, such as breathing and temperature regulation, while also controlling walking and all other deliberate activities.

The brain is separable into left and right hemispheres each with four lobes: **frontal, parietal, occipital**, and **temporal** (Fig. 7-4). The names of the lobes relate to their location relative to the skull (i.e., frontal relates to the front part of the head, parietal refers to the sides of the head, occipital identifies the back of the head, and temporal refers to the temples or area posterior to the eyes on the side of the head).

The major parts of the brain include the following (Fig. 7-5):

- **Cerebrum**: The cerebrum, the largest part of the brain, is where memories and conscious thoughts are stored. It also directs some willed bodily movements. An outer layer of gray matter called the **cerebral cortex** protects both hemispheres of the cerebrum. Please note, once again, that although groups of neuron cell bodies that exist within the PNS are called ganglia, groups of neuron cell bodies within the CNS are normally called nuclei (singular: nucleus).
- **Cerebellum**: The cerebellum, like the larger cerebrum situated above it, also inhabits both hemispheres. The cerebellum helps us perform learned body movements smoothly and helps us maintain our equilibrium.

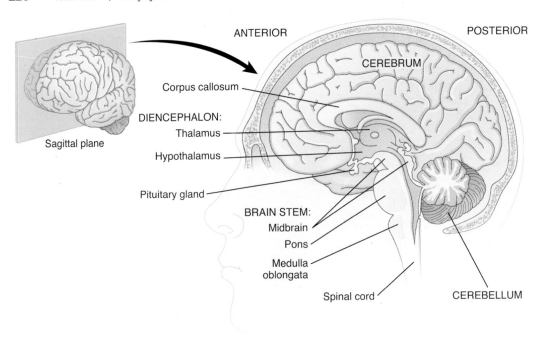

FIGURE 7-5   Sagittal section of the brain. The major parts of the interior brain structures are shown. *From Cohen BJ. Medical Terminology: An Illustrated Guide. 5th ed. Philadelphia, PA: Lippincott Williams & Wilkins; 2007.*

- **Diencephalon**: The diencephalon contains both the **thalamus** and the **hypothalamus**. The thalamus processes sensory information. The hypothalamus, which is the hormone and emotion center of the brain, controls autonomic functions such as heart rate, dilation of blood vessels, and hormone secretion.
- **Brain stem**: The brain stem contains the **mesencephalon** (or **midbrain**), the **pons** (which is a Latin word meaning "bridge"), and the **medulla oblongata**. The mesencephalon processes visual and audible sensory information. Visual tracking, such as moving the eyes to read or follow a moving object, is an example of a midbrain function. It also transmits hearing impulses to the brain. The pons passes information to the cerebellum and the thalamus to control subconscious somatic activities such as regulating respiration. The medulla oblongata sends sensory information to the thalamus to direct the autonomic functions of the heart, lungs, and other organs of the body. The cavities between the brain stem and the cerebrum are called **ventricles**.

The spinal cord and the brain communicate continuously with one another. The messages exchanged produce all the actions and functions that make life pleasurable, painful, and even possible. In the average-sized adult, the spinal cord is about a foot-and-a-half long and a half-inch wide. It is surrounded by membranes called **spinal meninges**, which absorb physical shocks that could otherwise damage neural tissue (Fig. 7-6). The outer layer of the brain and spinal cord consists of **dura mater**, a dense collection of collagen fibers. The middle layer is called the **arachnoid layer**, which is thin, delicate, and weblike. The inner layer, also called the **pia**, is in direct contact with brain tissue.

Peripheral Nervous System

The PNS includes 12 pairs of cranial nerves and 31 pairs of spinal nerves that run along the periphery of the body (see Fig. 7-2). The cranial and spinal nerves convey directions from the CNS to the PNS and carry information from the PNS back to the CNS.

The PNS is divided into two subsystems: the **somatic nervous system** and the **autonomic nervous system** (see Fig. 7-1). Conscious and habitual actions are called somatic, which comes from a Greek word meaning "body." Because some organs, such as the heart and lungs, work on

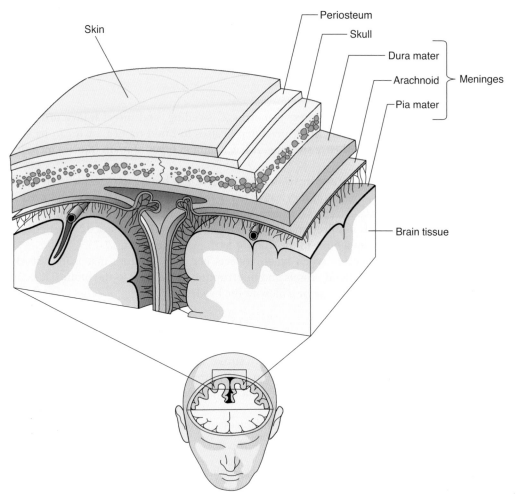

FIGURE 7-6 **Meninges.** The three protective layers of the meninges and adjacent tissues are shown. *Modified from Cohen BJ. Medical Terminology: An Illustrated Guide. 5th ed. Philadelphia, PA: Lippincott Williams & Wilkins; 2007.*

their own, their performance is said to be autonomic. The noun **autonomy** is a common English word that means "self-sufficient."

The autonomic nervous system may be further subdivided into the **sympathetic** and **parasympathetic nervous systems**. The sympathetic nerves stimulate "fight-or-flight" actions by increasing heart rate and dilating airways during periods of stress. The parasympathetic nerves counterbalance such changes and return the body to a homeostatic state when the danger has passed.

 Quick Check: Main Parts of the Nervous System

Fill in the blanks.

1. The CNS consists of the _____ and the _____.

2. The nervous system works in conjunction with the endocrine system to maintain _____, a term that means "a state of equilibrium."

3. The major parts of the brain include the cerebrum, cerebellum, diencephalon, and _____ _____.

DISORDERS OF THE NERVOUS SYSTEM

Disorders of the nervous system can result from trauma, vascular injury, tumors, systemic degenerative diseases, and seizures. Behavioral disorders are treated as a separate category.

Brain Trauma

Head injuries can produce skull fractures, hemorrhage, swelling, and direct injury to the brain itself. Brain injury may be relatively mild, involving bruises to brain tissues, or it can be severe, causing tissue destruction and massive swelling. A few common types of brain injuries include the following:

- **Concussion** (cerebral concussion: violent shaking of the brain) may result from a fall or blow to the head. A concussion may cause temporary loss of consciousness followed by a short period of amnesia. Dizziness, nausea, and headache are common with a concussion.
- **Subdural hematoma** is a collection of blood trapped in the subdural space beneath the dura mater. It may result from a blow to the front or back of the head (Fig. 7-7).
- **Epidural hematoma** occurs when blood collects between the dura mater and the skull, causing pressure on the blood vessels and interrupting blood flow to the brain. This condition is caused by a skull fracture or a blow to the head.

Vascular Insults

A vascular insult is an injury to the blood vessels.

- **Cerebrovascular accident**: Also known as a stroke, a cerebrovascular accident results from oxygen deprivation caused by a blockage in or rupture of a blood vessel.
- **Transient ischemic attack**: A transient ischemic attack is a temporary interruption in the blood supply to the brain.
- **Aneurysm**: An aneurysm is a localized dilation of an artery caused by weakness in the vessel wall or heart chamber (Fig. 7-8).

Doesn't the word "insult" refer to a verbal attack, such as when someone calls someone else a name that causes hurt feelings? Yes, it does, but in the phrase "vascular insult," it means something else. The Latin verb *insulto* literally means "to physically jump on." So a vascular insult is a physical event related to that Latin meaning.

Tumors

Tumors are lesions or neoplasms that may cause localized dysfunction, producing an increase in **intracranial pressure**. Tumors may be benign or malignant. Two examples of tumors occurring in the nervous system include **astrocytomas** and **meningiomas**.

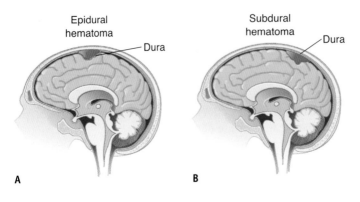

Epidural hematoma — Dura

Subdural hematoma — Dura

A   B

FIGURE 7-7 Epidural and subdural hematoma. A. Epidural hematoma occurs with a traumatic brain injury when blood accumulates between the dura and the skull. **B.** Subdural hematoma occurs within the dura layer. *From Cohen BJ. Medical Terminology: An Illustrated Guide. 5th ed. Philadelphia, PA: Lippincott Williams & Wilkins; 2007.*

Systemic Degenerative Diseases

Degenerative diseases develop slowly over time. A progressive deterioration may start out affecting individual body actions and end up involving other body systems. Examples of systemic degenerative diseases include **multiple sclerosis**, **Parkinson's disease**, and **Alzheimer's disease**.

- Multiple sclerosis is a progressive degenerative disease with symptoms caused by **demyelination**, a patchy loss of the myelin sheath.
- Parkinson's disease usually develops after age 60 years and occurs with the loss of the neurotransmitter **dopamine**, which inhibits transmission of nerve impulses.
- Alzheimer's disease is a degenerative, eventually fatal condition involving atrophy of the cerebral cortex, producing a progressive loss of intellectual function.

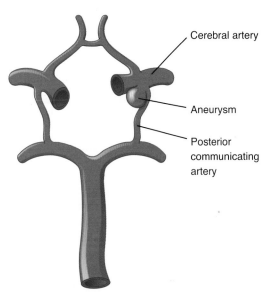

FIGURE 7-8 Cerebral aneurysm. The circle of arteries that supply blood to the brain is called the circle of Willis named after Thomas Willis, an English physician. (It is located near the center of the brain.) The aneurysm is a bulge or weakening of the artery. *Reprinted with permission from Porth CM. Pathophysiology. 6th ed. Philadelphia, PA: Lippincott Williams & Wilkins; 2002:443.*

Seizure Disorders

A seizure occurs when there is an abnormal uncontrolled burst of electrical activity in the brain. Seizures may result from trauma, tumors, fevers, medications, or other causes. Some seizures go unnoticed when the signs are vey subtle. Other seizures can cause loss of consciousness or involuntarily body movements.

Epilepsy is a chronic disorder characterized by recurrent seizures that result from the excessive discharge of neurons in the brain. Two basic types of epileptic seizures are **grand mal seizures** and **petit mal seizures**. A grand mal seizure is severe and characterized by alternating contraction and relaxation of muscles, which produces jerking movements of the face, trunk, and/or extremities. A petit mal seizure is a milder form of seizure that lasts only a few seconds and does not include convulsive movements.

Behavioral Disorders

Some behavioral disorders are related to the nervous system. They may be caused by physical changes, substance abuse, medications, or any combination thereof. The categories include anxiety, mood, and psychotic disorders.

- **Anxiety disorders** are characterized by feelings of apprehension or uneasiness, sometimes associated with the anticipation of danger. Common examples include **obsessive-compulsive disorder**, which may be signaled by repetitive behaviors; **posttraumatic stress disorder**; and the various **phobias**, which are persistent, irrational fears of specific situations or things.
- **Mood disorders** include **depression**, which is characterized by loss of interest or pleasure in activities; and **bipolar** (formerly called **manic-depressive**) **disorder**, which alternates between manic and depressive episodes.
- **Psychotic disorders** are more serious than anxiety or mood disorders because they feature a loss of contact with reality and a deterioration of normal social functioning. An example of a psychosis is **schizophrenia**, which may manifest itself as **paranoia**, withdrawal, hallucinations, and/or delusions.

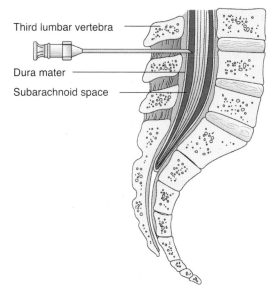

Procedures and Practitioners

When evaluating the health of a person's nervous system, medical professionals use various procedures. Sometimes, a patient's mental health is determined by a qualified professional observing and talking with the patient. Other times, diagnostic tests to evaluate the condition of the brain and its activity are employed. Some diagnostic procedures are listed in the following:

- **Computerized tomography** is a noninvasive radiologic test that uses a computer to produce cross-sectional images of the soft tissue structures of the brain and spinal cord. This procedure can reveal problems such as brain tumors, aneurysms, etc.
- **Magnetic resonance imaging** uses radio waves and a very strong magnetic field to produce images of the neural soft tissues. It is used to visualize disease-related changes in the brain or spinal cord that conventional X-ray procedures

FIGURE 7-9   Lumbar puncture. Insertion of a needle between the third and fourth or fourth and fifth lumbar vertebrae to withdraw cerebrospinal fluid. *From Cohen BJ. Medical Terminology: An Illustrated Guide. 5th ed. Philadelphia, PA: Lippincott Williams & Wilkins; 2007.*

would be unable to detect. For example, magnetic resonance imaging is able to isolate damaged areas of the brain caused by multiple sclerosis.

- **Electroencephalography**: The electroencephalogram is a written record of the brain's electrical activity. It is used to document increased electrical events of the brain caused by seizures.
- **Lumbar puncture** requires the insertion of a needle into the subarachnoid space between the third and fourth or fourth and fifth lumbar vertebrae to withdraw cerebrospinal fluid for analysis (Fig. 7-9).

The medical specialists who diagnose and treat the nervous system are **neurologists**, **neurosurgeons**, and **psychiatrists**. Neurologists and neurosurgeons work with patients who experience disorders of the neuromuscular system, whereas psychiatrists treat behavioral and mental health disorders. The health care professional with an advanced academic degree who treats mental and behavioral disorders is a **psychologist**.

Abbreviation Table THE NERVOUS SYSTEM	
ABBREVIATION	**MEANING**
ADHD	attention deficit hyperactivity disorder
CNS	central nervous system
CVA	cerebrovascular accident
ECT	electroconvulsive therapy
EEG	electroencephalography
ICP	intracranial pressure
IQ	intelligence quotient
LOC	level of consciousness

In the figure: Third lumbar vertebra, Dura mater, Subarachnoid space

ABBREVIATION	MEANING
LP	lumbar puncture
MS	multiple sclerosis
OBS	organic brain syndrome
OCD	obsessive-compulsive disorder
PERRLA	pupils equal, round, and reactive to light and accommodation
PNS	peripheral nervous system
PTSD	posttraumatic stress disorder
SAD	seasonal affective disorder
TENS	transcutaneous electrical nerve stimulation
TIA	transient ischemic attack

Study Table THE NERVOUS SYSTEM

TERM AND PRONUNCIATION	ANALYSIS	MEANING
Structure and Function		
autonomic nervous system (aw-to-NOM-ik) (ANS)	autonomy (self-sufficiency); -ic (adjective suffix)	the parts of the PNS that carry messages between the CNS and organs that function autonomously
arachnoid mater (ah-RAK-noyd MAY-turh)	from the Greek word *arachne* (spider, cobweb); -oid (resemblance)	delicate weblike layer of the meninges; middle layer
axon (AX-ohn)	*axo-* (axis); -n noun ending	the part of a neuron that conducts electrical impulses
brain stem	common English words	the part of the brain that controls functions, including heart rate, breathing, and body temperature; includes midbrain, pons, and medulla oblongata
cell body	common English words	one of the three parts of a neuron cell; the other two are the axon and dendrites
central nervous system (CNS)	common English words	the subdivision of the nervous system that includes the brain and spinal cord
cerebellum (SERR-uh-bell-uhm)	*cerebr/o* (brain)	the part of the brain that controls the skeletal muscles
cerebral cortex (seh-REE-bruhl KOR-tex)	*cerebr/o* (brain); -al (adjective suffix)	the gray matter surrounding the cerebrum
cerebrospinal fluid (seh-REE-bro-SPY-nuhl)	*cerebr/o* (brain); from Latin word *spina*; fluid (common English word)	the fluid in and around the brain and spinal cord

(continued)

TERM AND PRONUNCIATION	ANALYSIS	MEANING
cerebrum (seh-REE-bruhm)	*cerebr/o* (brain)	the largest part of the brain; controls conscious thought and stores memories
dendrite (DEN-dryte)	from the Greek word (relating to a tree)	one of two processes extending from a neuron cell body; the other is the axon
diencephalon (dy-en-SEFF-uh-lohn)	*di-* (two); *encephal/o* (of or relating to the brain); *-on* (noun suffix)	the part of the brain containing both the thalamus and the hypothalamus
dura mater (DOO-ruh MAY-tuhr)	Latin words meaning "hard mother"	the outer meninges, the fibrous membrane protecting the CNS
frontal lobe (FRUN-tahl)	common English words	the front part of the brain from which voluntary muscle movements and other sensory and motor tasks are directed
ganglion (GANG-lee-ohn); plural: ganglia	a Greek word meaning "swelling" or "knot"	a group of neuron cell bodies grouped together in the PNS
hypothalamus (HY-po-thal-uh-muhs)	*hypo-* (below, deficient); from the Greek word *thalamus* (a bed, a bedroom)	the hormone and emotion center of the brain that controls autonomic functions
leptomeninx (LEPP-toh-ME-ninks)	*lepto-* (light, slender, thin frail); meninx is plural form of *mening/o* (membrane)	collective term for the arachnoid mater and pia mater
medulla oblongata (meh-DUH-luh ohb-lohng-GAH-tuh)	a Latin word (marrow); from the Latin *oblongatus* (oblong)	the part of the brain stem that sends sensory information to the thalamus to direct the autonomic functions of the heart, lungs, and other viscera
meninges (meh-NIHN-jees)	*mening/o* (membrane)	Three-layer membrane surrounding brain and spinal cord
mesencephalon (mez-ehn-SEFF-ah-lon)	*mes/o* (middle); *encephal/o* (brain); *-on* (noun suffix)	the middle part of the brain between the diencephalon and the pons; also called the midbrain
myelin sheath (MY-eh-lin sheeth)	*myel/o-* (bone marrow; spinal cord)	a fatty white envelope of cells providing protection and electrical insulation to neurons
nerve	common English word	a whitish, cordlike structure composed of one or more bundles of nerve fibers outside the CNS, together with their connective tissues and nourishing blood vessels
neuroglia (nuhr-o-GLEE-uh)	*neur/o* (nerve); from the Greek *glia* (glue)	cells within both the CNS and PNS, which, although they are external to neurons, form an essential part of nerve tissue

TERM AND PRONUNCIATION	ANALYSIS	MEANING
neuron (NUHR-ohn)	*neur/o* (nerve); *-on* (noun suffix)	a nerve cell, including the cell body and its axon
neurotransmitter (NOO-roh-TRANS-mitt-ehr)	*neur/o* (nerve); from the Latin *trans* (across); *mittere* (to send)	chemical released by the presynaptic cell that is then picked up by the postsynaptic cell to effect an action
nucleus (NEW-klee-uhs); plural: nuclei (NEW-klee-eye)	a Latin word meaning "kernel"	a group of neuron cell bodies grouped together in the CNS
occipital lobe (AWK-sihp-ih-tuhl lobe)	from Latin word *occiput* (back of the head)	the part of the brain that processes information from the sense of sight and other sensory and motor tasks
parietal lobe (pah-RY-uh-tuhl lobe)	from the Latin adjective *parietalis* (walls); *-al* (adjective suffix)	the part of the brain that processes information from the sense of touch and other sensory and motor tasks
peripheral nervous system (puh-RIFF-uh-ruhl) (PNS)	*peri-* (surrounding); from the Greek word *pherein* (to carry); nervous system (common English words)	made up of neurons, neuroglia, and associated tissue, including the cranial and spinal nerves and the sensory and motor nerves that extend throughout the body
pia mater (PEE-ah MAY-turh)	Latin words meaning "tender mother"	inner layer of the meninges
pons (POHNS)	a Latin word meaning "bridge"	the part of the brain stem that passes information to the cerebellum and the thalamus to regulate subconscious somatic activities
psychomotor (SY-ko-mo-tuhr)	*psych/o* (of the mind); from the Latin word *motor* (mover)	an adjective used to indicate the relation between psychic activity and muscular movement
somatic nervous system (so-MAT-ik)	*somat/o* (body, bodily); *-ic* (adjective suffix)	the parts of the PNS that carry impulses for conscious rather than habitual activity
spinal nerves (SPY-nahl)	from the Latin word *spina* (spine)	the 31 pairs of nerves located along the spinal column
synapse (SIH-naps)	*syn-* (together); from the Greek word *hapto* (clasp)	the connecting point between nerve cells or between a nerve cell and a receptor or effector cell
temporal lobe (TEM-puh-ruhl lobe)	from the Latin word *temporalis* (time, temple)	the part of the brain that processes information from the senses of hearing, smell, and taste, and other sensory and motor tasks
thalamus (THAL-uh-muhs)	from the Greek word *thalamus* (bed, bedroom)	part of the brain that processes sensory information
ventricles (VEN-trik-uhls)	from the Latin word *ventriculus*, dim. of *venter* (belly)	cavities between the cerebrum and brain stem

(continued)

TERM AND PRONUNCIATION	ANALYSIS	MEANING
Common Disorders		
Alzheimer's disease (ALZ-hy-mur)	named after German physician Alois Alzheimer, who first described it in 1906	a disease that may begin in late middle life, characterized by progressive mental deterioration that includes loss of memory and visual and spatial orientation
amnesia (am-NEE-zah)	*a-* (without); *-mnesia* (memory)	loss of memory
aneurysm (AN-ur-izm)	from the Greek *ana* (up) and *eurys* (broad)	localized dilation of an artery due to vessel wall weakness
anxiety disorder	common English words	a feeling of apprehension or uneasiness that results from anticipation of danger
aphasia (uh-FAY-jhah)	*a-* (absence of); from the Greek word *phases* (speech)	loss of speech
astrocytoma (A-stroh-sy-TOH-mah)	from the Greek word *astron* (star); *cyt/o* (cell); *-oma* (tumor)	star-shaped tumor that usually develops in the cerebrum; frequently in people younger than 20 years old
ataxia (ah-TAK-see-ah)	*a-* (without); from the Greek word *taxis* (order)	lack of muscular coordination
bipolar disorder	*bi-* (twice, double); from the Latin word *polus* (the end of an axis)	disorder characterized by manic episodes alternating with depressive episodes
cerebral thrombosis (seh-REE-bruhl throm-BO-sihs)	*cerebr/o* (brain); *-al* (adjective suffix); *thromb/o* (of or relating to a blood clot); *-sis* (abnormal condition)	blood clot in the brain
cerebrovascular accident (seh-REE-bro-VAS-ku-lahr) (CVA)	*cerebr/o* (brain); *vascul/o* (blood vessel); *-ar* (adjective suffix)	a synonym for *cerebral stroke*, an acute clinical event, related to impairment of cerebral circulation, lasting more than 24 hours
cerebrovascular disease (seh-REE-bro-VAS-ku-lahr)	*cerebr/o* (brain); *vascul/o* (blood vessel); *-ar* (adjective suffix)	brain disorder involving a blood vessel
delirium (duh-LEER-ee-uhm)	from the Latin word *deliro* (to be crazy)	impaired consciousness
delusion (deh-LOO-shun)	from the Latin word *ludere* (to play)	false belief or wrong judgment despite evidence to the contrary
dementia (duh-MEN-shah)	from Latin *de* (apart, away); *mens* (mind)	impaired intellectual function
depression	from the Latin word *depressio*	prolonged period where there is a loss of interest or pleasure in almost all activities

TERM AND PRONUNCIATION	ANALYSIS	MEANING
dysphasia (DISS-fay-jhah)	*dys-* (bad, difficult); from the Greek word *phases* (speaking)	impaired speech
encephalitis (en-seff-uh-LY-tiss)	*encepal/o* (of or pertaining to the brain); *-itis* (inflammation)	inflammation of the brain
epidural hematoma (EH-pih-dur-ahl hee-mah-TOH-ma)	*epi-* (above); dural (relating to the dura mater); *hemat/o* (blood); *-oma* (tumor)	a collection of blood in the space between the skull and dura mater
epilepsy (EPP-ih-lepp-see)	from the Greek *epilepsia* (seizure)	CNS disorder often characterized by seizures
glioblastoma (GLY-oh-blass-TOH-mah)	*glio* (glue); from the Greek word *blastos* (germ); *-oma* (tumor)	a cerebral tumor occurring most frequently in adults
glioma (gly-OH-muh)	*glio-* (glue); *-oma* (tumor)	tumor of glial tissue
grand mal seizure (grahn-mahl SEEZ-yuhr)	French words meaning "big illness"	type of severe seizure with tonic-clonic convulsion
hallucination (hah-LOO-sih-nay-shun)	from the Latin word *alucinor* (to wander in mind)	subjective perception of an object or voice when no such stimulus exists
hemiparesis (heh-mee-puh-REE-suhs)	*hemi-* (one-half); *-paresis* (slight paralysis)	partial paralysis of one side of the body
hemiplegia (hehm-ee-PLEE-jee-ah)	*hemi-* (one-half); *-plegia* (paralysis)	paralysis of one side of the body
Huntington's disease (HUN-ting-tuhn)	named after American physician George Huntington who described the disorder in 1872	hereditary disorder of the CNS
hydrocephalus (hy-dro-SEFF-uh-lehs)	*hydro-* (water); *cephal/o* (of or pertaining to the head)	excessive cerebrospinal fluid in the brain
hyperesthesia (hy-per-ess-THEE-zyuh)	*hyper-* (extreme or beyond normal); *esthesi/o* (sensation)	abnormal sensitivity to touch
kleptomania (klep-toh-MAY-knee-yah)	from the Greek word *klepto-* (to steal); from the Latin *-mania* (insanity)	uncontrollable impulse to steal
meningioma (meh-nihn-jee-OH-muh)	*mening/o* (membrane); *-oma* (tumor)	benign tumor of the meninges
meningitis (meh-nihn-JY-tiss)	*mening/o* (membrane); *-itis* (inflammation)	inflamed meninges
multiple sclerosis (skleh-RO-sihs)	multiple (from the English word meaning "many"); *scler/o* (hardness); *-osis* (abnormal condition)	disease of the CNS characterized by the formation of plaques in the brain and spinal cord

(continued)

TERM AND PRONUNCIATION	ANALYSIS	MEANING
myasthenia gravis (MY-ahs-THEE-nee-ah GRA-viss)	*my/o* (muscle); *astheneia* (weakness)	muscle weakness, lack of strength
myelitis (my-eh-LY-tiss)	*myel/o* (bone marrow or spine); *-itis* (inflammation)	inflammation of the spinal cord
myelomeningocele (MY-loh-mih-NIHN-gee-oh-seel)	*myel/o* (bone marrow or spine); *meningi/o* (membrane); *-cele* (hernia)	protrusion of the membranes of the brain or spinal cord through a defect in the cranium or vertebral column
neuralgia (nuh-RALL-jah)	*neur/o* (nerve); *-algia* (pain)	pain in a nerve
neuropathy (nuh-ROP-ah-thee)	*neur/o* (nerve); *-pathy* (disease)	a disease involving the cranial, central, or autonomic nervous systems
obsessive-compulsive disorder (OCD)	common English words	type of anxiety disorder characterized by persistent thoughts and impulses with repetitive responses that interfere with daily activities
paralysis (pah-RALL-ih-sihs)	*para-* (abnormal, alongside); *-lysis* (destruction)	loss of one or more muscle functions
paranoia (pahr-ah-NOY-ya)	*para-* (abnormal, alongside); from Greek word *noeo* (to think)	a serious mental disorder characterized by unreasonable suspicion or jealousy, along with a tendency to interpret everything others do as hostile
paraplegia (pahr-ah-PLEE-jee-ah)	*para-* (abnormal, alongside); *-plegia* (paralysis)	paralysis of the lower extremities and, often, the lower trunk of the body
paresthesia (per-ess-THEE-zyuh)	*para-* (abnormal); *esthesi/o* (sensation)	numbness
Parkinson's disease (PAR-kin-suhn); also Parkinson's, parkinsonism	named for English physician James Parkinson, who described it in 1817	disease of the nerves in the brain due to an imbalance of dopamine
petit mal seizure (petty-mahl SEEZ-yuhr)	French words meaning "small illness"	milder form of seizure lasting only a few seconds and does not include convulsive movements; also known as *absence seizures*
phobia (FOH-bee-ah)	*phob/o* (exaggerated fear); *-ia* (noun suffix)	a fear of something that is not a hazard from a statistical point of view
plegia (PLEE-jee-uh)	*-plegia* (paralysis)	paralysis
poliomyelitis (pohl-ee-oh-MY-eh-LY-tiss)	*polio-* (denoting gray color); *myel/o* (bone marrow or spine); *-itis* (inflammation)	inflamed gray matter of the spinal cord

TERM AND PRONUNCIATION	ANALYSIS	MEANING
psychosis (sy-KO-sihs)	*psych/o* (of or pertaining to the mind); *-sis* (condition of)	a serious disorder involving a marked distortion of, or sharp break from, reality; general term covering severe mental or emotional disorders
quadriplegia (kwad-rih-PLEE-jee-ah)	*quadr/i* (four); *-plegia* (paralysis)	paralysis of all four limbs
schizophrenia (skits-oh-FREN-ee-ah)	*schiz/o* (denoting split or double sided); from the Greek word *phren* (mind)	a severe mental illness characterized by auditory hallucinations, paranoia, and an inability to distinguish reality from fiction
seizure (SEE-zhur)	common English word	sudden disturbance in brain function sometimes producing a convulsion
somnambulism (sahm-NAM-bu-lih-sm)	from Latin words *somnus* (sleep) and *ambulo* (walk); *-ism* (a medical condition)	sleep walking
subdural hematoma (SUB-dur-ahl hee-mah-TOH-ma)	*sub-* (beneath); *dura* (hard); *-al* (adjective suffix); *hemat/o* (blood); *-oma* (tumor)	a collection of blood trapped in the space beneath the dura mater, between the dura and arachnoid layers of the meninges
syncope (SIN-kuh-pee)	from the Greek word *syncope* (a cutting short, a swoon)	fainting
transient ischemic attack[a] (TRANS-ee-ent IH-skee-mik)	from Greek *isch*, a root (to restrict), and the suffix *-emia* (blood)	temporary interruption in the blood supply to the brain
vertigo (VER-tih-goh)	from the Latin word *verto* (turn)	dizziness
Practice and Practitioners		
neurologist (nuhr-AWL-ih-gihst)	*neur/o* (nerve); *-logist* (practitioner)	a medical specialist who treats nervous system disorders
neurology (nuhr-AWL-uh-jee)	*neur/o* (nerve); *-logy* (the study of)	medical specialty dealing with the nervous system
neurosurgeon (NOO-roh-sur-juhn)	*neur/o* (nerve); from the Greek word *kheirourgos* (working or done by hand)	surgeon who specializes in operations on the nervous system
psychiatrist (sy-KY-ah-trist)	*psych/o* (of or pertaining to the mind); *iatr/o* (of or pertaining to medicine or a physician); *-ist* (one who specializes in)	a medical doctor who specializes in the diagnosis and treatment of psychological disorders
psychologist (sy-KOL-oh-jist)	*psych/o* (of or pertaining to the mind); *-logist* (one who studies a certain field)	a (nonmedical) doctor of psychology who specializes in the diagnosis and treatment of psychological disorders

(continued)

TERM AND PRONUNCIATION	ANALYSIS	MEANING
Diagnosis and Treatments		
antianxiety agent	*anti-* (against); from the Greek word *angho* (to squeeze, embrace, throttle)	drug used to suppress anxiousness and relax muscles
anticonvulsant agent	*anti-* (against); from the Latin *con* (with) and *vulsus* (to tear up)	drugs used to decrease seizure activity
antipsychotic agent	*anti-* (against); *psych/o* (of or pertaining to the mind); *-tic* (adjective suffix)	drug given to patients to affect behavior and treat psychiatric disorders
craniectomy (KRAY-nee-ek-tuh-mee)	*crani/o* (cranium); *-ectomy* (excision)	excision of part of the skull
craniotomy (KRAY-nee-aw-tuh-mee)	*crani/o* (cranium); *-tomy* (cutting operation)	incision into the skull
electroconvulsive therapy (ECT) or electroshock therapy (EST)	*electr/o* (electric); from the Latin words *con* (with) and *vulsus* (to tear up)	a controlled convulsion produced by passing an electric current through the brain
electroencephalography (ee-LEK-tro-en-sef-ah-LAH-grah-fee) (EEG)	*electr/o* (electric); *encephal/o* (brain); *-graphy* (process of recording)	record of the electrical potential of the brain
lobotomy (lo-BAWT-uh-mee)	*lob/o* (lobe); *-tomy* (cutting operation)	incision into a lobe
lumbar puncture (LP)	from the Latin word *lumbus* (lion)	insertion of a needle into the subarachnoid space between the third and fourth or fourth and fifth lumbar vertebrae to withdraw fluid for diagnosis
magnetic resonance imaging (MRI)	common English words	uses radio waves and a very strong magnetic field to produce images of the soft tissue
myelography (my-eh-LOG-rah-fee)	*myel/o* (bone marrow or spine); *-graphy* (process of recording)	radiography of the spinal cord and nerve roots
neuroplasty (NURR-oh-plass-tee)	*neur/o* (nerve); *-plasty* (repair)	surgery to repair a nerve
sedatives or hypnotics	from the Latin *sedeo* (sit); from the Greek word *hypnotikos* (causing one to sleep)	drugs used to induce calming effect or sleep

[a]The transient ischemic attack, abbreviated TIA, is, from a terminology perspective, related more to the cardiovascular system, and you will note that it is repeated in that chapter for the sake of logic.

EXERCISES

EXERCISE 7-1 📋 FIGURE LABELING: NEURON

Label the parts of the motor neuron. Select from the terms listed in the table.

axon branch	cell body	muscle	nucleus
axon covered with myelin sheath	dendrites	myelin sheath	

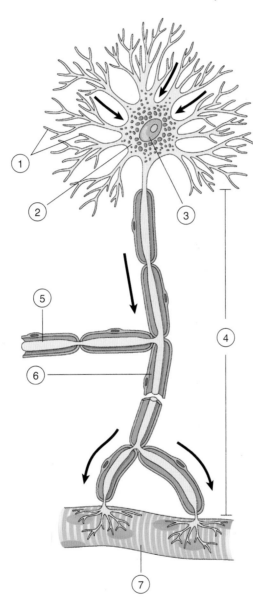

1. _____   4. _____   6. _____

2. _____   5. _____   7. _____

3. _____

EXERCISE 7-2 📋 CASE STUDY

Read the following excerpt from an emergency room record and answer the questions.

CHIEF COMPLAINT: Mental status changes and aphasia.

BRIEF HISTORY: J.D. is an 85-year-old female who presents to the emergency department with difficulty talking. Her daughter states that J.D. has had garbled speech for the past few days, repeatedly says, "How do you do?" and answers the same to any questions asked. This has happened in the past, but the daughter says her mother has always "gotten better." This morning J.D. woke up and has weakness on the right side of her body. There are no other modifying factors or associated signs or symptoms.

ASSESSMENT: Probable history of TIA; now CVA with resulting dysphasia and right hemiparesis.

1. What is a TIA? _____

2. What does the acronym CVA represent? _____

3. Break up the medical term *dysphasia* and define its word elements. _____

_____

4. What does the root word *paresis* mean? _____

5. What is the difference between *hemiparesis* and *hemiplegia*? _____

_____

6. Break up the term *hemiplegia* and define the word elements. _____

_____

EXERCISE 7-3 📋 WORD PARTS

Fill in the blanks with the proper roots.

1. The root for "nerve" is _____.

2. The root for "spinal cord" is _____.

3. The suffix for "to cut" is _____.

4. The root for "head" is _____.

5. The suffix for "speech" is _____.

6. The root for "to split" is _____.

7. Name a root and a suffix for "mind": _____ and _____.

EXERCISE 7-4 WORD ELEMENTS

Break each of the following terms into its word elements: root, prefix, and suffix. Then define each term.

Example   *cerebrospinal*

roots: cerebro and spino, suffix: al

adjective referring to the brain and spinal cord

1. *psychosis*

   _____

   _____

2. *electroencephalography*

   _____

   _____

3. *astrocytoma*

   _____

   _____

4. *cerebrovascular*

   _____

   _____

5. *hemiplegia*

   _____

   _____

6. *hydrocephalus*

   _____

   _____

7. *encephalitis*

_____

_____

8. *epidural*

_____

_____

9. *psychiatrist*

_____

_____

10. *meningioma*

_____

_____

EXERCISE 7-5   MATCHING

Match the term in the first column with its definition in the second column.

1. _____ cerebrum

2. _____ cerebral cortex

3. _____ brain stem

4. _____ somatic nerves

5. _____ pons

6. _____ autonomic nerves

7. _____ meningomyelocele

8. _____ neuralgia

9. _____ convulsion

10. _____ syncope

A. accumulation of fluid on the brain

B. nerve pain

C. contains the mesencephalon (midbrain), pons, and medulla oblongata

D. dizziness

E. hernia of the meninges and the spinal cord

F. outer layer of the cerebrum

G. fainting

H. smallest part of brain

I. contact point between two nerves

J. involuntary nerves

11. _____ vertigo

K. largest part of the brain

12. _____ hydrocephalus

L. inflammation of a nerve

13. _____ neuritis

M. seizure

14. _____ synapse

N. voluntary nerves

EXERCISE 7-6 SPELL CHECK

Circle the correct spelling of the medical term.

1. _____ is the loss, due to brain damage, of the ability to speak or write or to comprehend the written or spoken word.

   Aphasia   Afasia   Aphazia   Aphesia

2. _____ is a type of psychosis that may manifest itself as paranoia, withdrawal, or psychotic symptoms.

   Skitzophrenia   Schizofrenia   Schizophrenia   Skizophrenia

3. _____ are the potent chemicals in the synaptic space between neurons.

   Nuerotransmiters   Neurotransmiters   Neurotransmitters   Neuritransmitters

4. _____ _____ is a collection of blood in the subdural space.

   Subdaral hemitoma   Subdural hemitonia   Subdural henitoma   Subdural hematoma

EXERCISE 7-7 ✎ WRITE THE ABBREVIATION

Write the corresponding abbreviation in the blank space to the right.

1. intelligence quotient   _____

2. posttraumatic stress disorder   _____

3. peripheral nervous system   _____

4. transcutaneous electrical nerve stimulation   _____

5. central nervous system   _____

6. multiple sclerosis   _____

7. cerebrovascular accident   _____

8. pupils equal, round, and reactive to
    light and accommodation   _____

9. lumbar puncture   _____

10. seasonal affective disorder   _____

11. transient ischemic attack   _____

12. organic brain syndrome   _____

13. attention deficit hyperactivity disorder   _____

14. electroconvulsive therapy   _____

15. electroencephalography   _____

16. intracranial pressure   _____

17. level of consciousness   _____

18. obsessive-compulsive disorder   _____

EXERCISE 7-8 CROSSWORD PUZZLE: THE NERVOUS SYSTEM

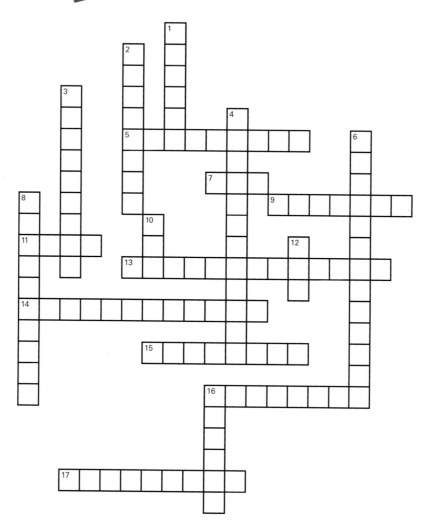

ACROSS

5. part of the nervous system containing the midbrain, pons, medulla oblongata
7. abbreviation for obsessive-compulsive disorder
9. manic-depressive
11. bridge
13. paranoia, withdrawal from reality, chronic psychosis
14. space between the arachnoid and pia mater
15. drug used to induce sleep
16. processes visual and audible sensory information in the brain
17. nerve glue

DOWN

1. extreme persistent and irrational fear
2. largest part of the brain
3. false beliefs
4. nonphysician who treats behavior disorders
6. perception in the absence of a stimulus; seeing and hearing things
8. prolonged period with a loss of interest
10. abbreviation for level of consciousness
12. abbreviation for magnetic resonance imaging
16. white fatty sheath covering nerves

◀ **CHAPTER 7 QUIZ**

Abbreviations

Write out the term for the following abbreviations.

1. TIA = _____

2. PERRLA = _____

3. LP = _____

4. EEG = _____

5. MS = _____

6. OBS = _____

Multiple Choice

7. Which term means paralysis on **one side** of the body?
   - a. diplegia
   - b. paraplegia
   - c. monoplegia
   - d. hemiplegia

8. Which of the following terms means a disease of the CNS characterized by the formation of plaques in the brain and spinal cord?
   - a. amyotrophic lateral sclerosis
   - b. Parkinson's disease
   - c. multiple sclerosis
   - d. poliomyelitis

9. To what does the term *cerebrocranial* refer?
   - a. brain and cranium
   - b. cerebellum and cranium
   - c. cerebrum and brain
   - d. cerebrum and cerebellum

10. The axon is one of two processes that extend from a neuron cell body. What is the other?
    - a. effector
    - b. dendrite
    - c. neurotransmitter
    - d. ganglia

11. Which of the following means accumulation of blood under the outermost meningeal layer?
    - a. epidural hematoma
    - b. intracerebral hematoma
    - c. subdural hematoma
    - d. cerebral concussion

12. Which of the following means hardening of the brain?
    - a. multiple sclerosis
    - b. encephalosclerosis
    - c. encephalomyelopathy
    - d. epilepsy

13. What is cerebral meningitis?
    - a. inflammation of the cerebellum
    - b. inflammation of the medulla
    - c. inflammation of the meninges of the brain
    - d. inflammation of the meninges of the spinal cord

14. Which part of the nervous system conducts impulses to skeletal muscle and is under *conscious* control?
    a. autonomic
    b. central

    c. somatic
    d. afferent

15. _____ is the loss, due to brain damage, of the ability to comprehend written or spoken speech.
    a. aphazia
    b. aphesia

    c. aphasia
    d. apazia

Fill in the Blank: Disorders of the Nervous System

Use the terms listed below to fill in the blanks.

agnosia	epilepsy	myasthenia gravis	paraplegia
ataxia	hyperesthesia	myelitis	poliomyelitis
cerebral thrombosis	laminectomy	myelomeningocele	somnambulism
convulsion	meningitis	neuralgia	syncope
dementia	multiple sclerosis	neurosis	vertigo

16. Abnormal sensitivity to touch is called _____.

17. The name for "inflamed" gray matter of the spinal cord is _____.

18. Impaired intellectual function is called _____.

19. The demyelinization of the spinal cord nerves is called _____.

20. The protrusion of the meninges and spinal cord tissue through a spina bifida is called a/an _____.

21. The term for a blood clot in the brain is _____.

22. _____ is characterized by a lack of muscular coordination.

23. CNS disorder often characterized by seizures is termed _____.

24. _____ is synonymous with fainting.

25. Pain in a nerve is _____.

8 *The Endocrine System*

INTRODUCTION

The **endocrine system** consists of glands that produce special chemicals called **hormones**. Working together with the nervous system, endocrine glands maintain **homeostasis** (chemical balance) within the body. The nervous system also contributes to this process by either stimulating or delaying hormone release according to an intricate feedback mechanism.

Endocrinology is the medical practice of treating **endocrine** and hormonal disorders. The practitioner, an **endocrinologist**, specializes in caring for patients with endocrine diseases and hormonal dysfunctions that may involve sexual development, body growth, or other bodily functions.

WORD ELEMENTS FOUND IN ENDOCRINE SYSTEM TERMS

Table 8-1 lists most of the elements that make up endocrine system terms. Suffixes already learned are also listed.

STRUCTURE AND FUNCTION

There are nine primary glands in the endocrine system (Fig. 8-1); this chapter covers seven of them: **pituitary**, **thyroid**, **parathyroid**, **adrenal**, **pancreas**, **ovaries**, and **testes**. The hormonal secretions and primary functions of each of these glands are noted in Table 8-2.

The other two primary endocrine glands are the **pineal** and **thymus** glands. The pineal gland is located in the brain, and its secretory activity is only partially understood. Because scientific explanations were lacking, some philosophers advanced theories to explain its perceived purpose. René Descartes, for example, thought it might be a connecting point between the intellect and the rest of the body. The thymus gland, located beneath the sternum and above the trachea, works in conjunction with the immune system (see Chapter 10).

What do the words endocrine and hormone actually mean? Endocrine glands are so-called because they secrete hormones directly into the bodily fluids that surround them and eventually find their way into the bloodstream. In other words, endocrine gland secretions do not travel through ducts. Glands that direct their secretions through ducts are called exocrine glands. The word *hormone* comes from Greek and means "to urge on or set in motion." So, a hormone is a chemical "messenger" transported through blood to other parts of the body. When the hormone reaches its target destination, the "message" has been delivered and can be acted upon.

TABLE 8-1 WORD ELEMENTS USED IN FORMING ENDOCRINE SYSTEM TERMS

Element	Function	Refers to
acr/o	root	extremities
aden/o	root	gland
adren/o, adrenal/o	root	adrenal glands
calc/i	root	calcium
crin/o	root	to separate or secrete
endocrin/o	root	endocrine
gluc/o, glyc/o	root	sugar, glucose, glycogen
hypophys/o	root	pituitary gland
-ine	suffix	suffix used in the formation of names of chemical substances
-megaly	suffix	enlargement
-oma	suffix	tumor
pancreat/o	root	pancreas
parathyr/o, parathyroid/o	root	parathyroid gland
thyr/o, thyroid/o	root	thyroid gland
-tropin (from the Greek word *trophe*)	suffix	suffix meaning "nourishment" or "stimulation"

Word Elements Exercise FILL IN THE BLANKS

Study Table 8-1, and then without referring to it again, write the definition of each of the following word elements in the space to the right.

1. endocrin/o _____

2. hypophys/o _____

3. adren/o, adrenal/o _____

4. -ine _____

5. -tropin (from the Greek word *trophe*) _____

6. -oma _____

7. pancreat/o _____

8. acr/o _____

9. aden/o _____

10. thyr/o, thyroid/o _____

11. -megaly _____

12. gluc/o, glyc/o _____

13. crin/o _____

14. parathyr/o, parathyroid/o _____

15. calc/i _____

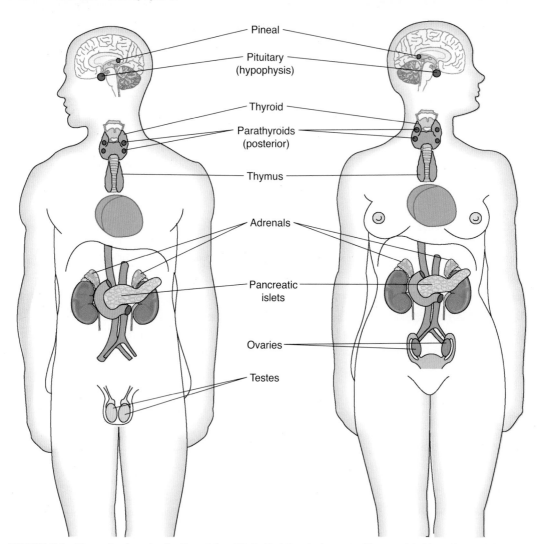

FIGURE 8-1   The endocrine glands. *From Cohen BJ.* Medical Terminology: An Illustrated Guide. *5th ed. Philadelphia, PA: Lippincott Williams & Wilkins; 2007.*

Pituitary Gland

The pituitary gland, also known as the **hypophysis**, is located at the base of the brain below the hypothalamus. It controls the activities of the other endocrine glands by releasing special hormones that regulate glandular functions. The pituitary gland is divided into an anterior lobe called the **adenohypophysis** and a posterior lobe called the **neurohypophysis**.

The adenohypophysis secretes several hormones essential for the development of sex glands, muscles, bones, thyroid gland, and other organs. The neurohypophysis secretes two hormones produced in the hypothalamus, the **antidiuretic hormone** and **oxytocin**. The antidiuretic hormone helps the body regulate fluid balance by reducing urination. Oxytocin stimulates labor during childbirth and promotes milk release during lactation. Studies of its effects on males have not, thus far, been conclusive.

Thyroid Gland

The thyroid is a butterfly-shaped gland that wraps around the larynx (Fig. 8-2). Its main jobs are to regulate the body's metabolism and calcium levels. The thyroid produces **triiodothyronine**, **thyroxine**, and **calcitonin**.

TABLE 8-2 SUMMARY OF THE ENDOCRINE GLANDS, HORMONES, AND HORMONE FUNCTIONS

Gland	Hormone	Hormone Function
pituitary		master gland; regulates activities of other glands
anterior lobe	growth hormone (GH)	growth and development of bones, muscles, other organs
	thyroid-stimulating hormone (TSH)	growth and development of thyroid gland
	adrenocorticotropin hormone (ACTH)	growth and development of adrenal cortex
	follicle-stimulating hormone (FSH)	stimulates production of sperm in the male and growth of ovarian follicles in the female
	luteinizing hormone (LH)	stimulates the production of testosterone in the male and secretion of estrogen and progesterone in the female
	prolactin hormone (PRL)	stimulates milk secretion in the mammary glands
	melanocyte-stimulating hormone (MSH)	regulates skin pigmentation
posterior lobe	antidiuretic hormone (ADH)	stimulates the reabsorption of water by the kidney tubules
	oxytocin	stimulates the uterus to contract during labor and delivery
thyroid	thyroxine (T_4)	influences growth and development, both physical and mental
	triiodothyronine (T_3)	maintenance and regulation of metabolism
	calcitonin	decreases the blood level of calcium
parathyroid	parathormone (PTH)	increases the blood level of calcium
adrenal		consists of outer portion (cortex) and inner portion (medulla)
cortex	cortisol (hydrocortisone)	regulates carbohydrates, proteins, fat metabolism; anti-inflammatory effect; helps the body cope during stress
	aldosterone	regulates water and electrolyte balance
	androgen (sex hormone)	development of secondary male sex characteristics
medulla	epinephrine (adrenaline)	acts as a vasoconstrictor, cardiac stimulant (increases heart rate and cardiac output), and antispasmodic; releases glucose into the blood (giving the body a spurt of energy)
	norepinephrine (noradrenaline)	acts as a vasoconstrictor; elevates blood pressure and heart rate
pancreas (islets of Langerhans)	insulin	transports glucose into the cells; decreases blood glucose levels
	glucagon	promotes release of glucose by liver; increases blood glucose levels
ovaries	estrogen	promotes growth, development, and maintenance of female sex organs
	progesterone	prepares uterus for pregnancy; promotes development of mammary glands
testes	testosterone	promotes growth, development, and maintenance of male sex organs

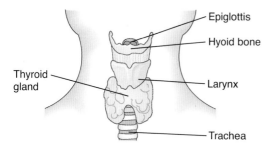

FIGURE 8-2   **The thyroid gland.** The thyroid gland is a two-lobed, butterfly-shaped gland that is located on the anterior surface of the upper trachea. It secretes a number of hormones that affect both metabolism and calcium levels in the blood. *Modified from Cohen BJ. Medical Terminology: An Illustrated Guide. 5th ed. Philadelphia, PA: Lippincott Williams & Wilkins; 2007.*

Parathyroid Gland

There are four **parathyroid glands** consisting of a superior and inferior pair, which are located on the posterior surface of the thyroid gland (Fig. 8-3). The hormone **parathormone**, also called **parathyrin** and abbreviated **PTH**, helps maintain correct calcium levels in the blood.

Adrenal Glands

The **adrenal glands** consist of two triangular-shaped glands, each one located on the top of a kidney. Their position on top of the kidneys has also earned them the name **suprarenal glands**. Each gland is divided into an outer part called the **adrenal cortex** and an inner part called the **adrenal medulla** (Fig. 8-4). The adrenal gland secretes the steroid hormones **cortisol** and **aldosterone**, which help the body cope with stress. It also produces **androgens**, which contribute to the development of male sex characteristics.

The adrenal medulla secretes **adrenaline**, also known as **epinephrine**, which stimulates the sympathetic nervous system.

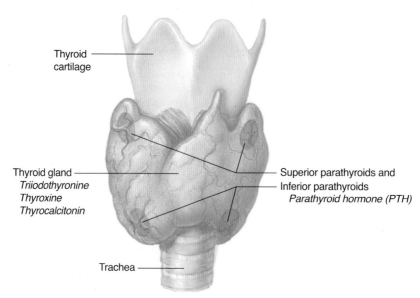

FIGURE 8-3   **The parathyroid glands.** The parathyroid (para- meaning "adjacent" or "near to") glands consist of four glands, a superior and inferior pair. These are located on the posterior surface of the thyroid gland. Their hormone secretion helps to regulate calcium balance.

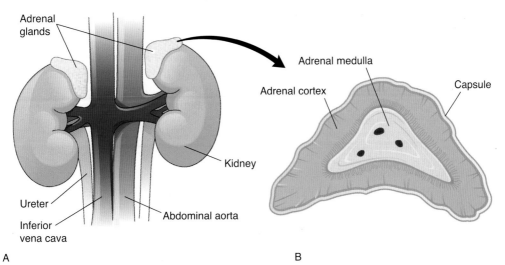

A   B

FIGURE 8-4 (**A, B**) **The adrenal glands.** The adrenal (ad- means "increase" or "move toward") or suprarenal (supra-means "above") glands are situated on top of the kidneys. They have two distinct regions, the cortex and medulla. Each secretes their own hormones. *From Cohen BJ. Medical Terminology: An Illustrated Guide. 5th ed. Philadelphia, PA: Lippincott Williams & Wilkins; 2007.*

Pancreas

The pancreas is a feather-shaped organ located behind the stomach. It contains clusters of special-ized cells called the **islets of Langerhans**, which produce **insulin** and **glucagon**. The function of the islet cells is to control blood sugar levels and glucose metabolism throughout the body.

Gonads

The ovaries and testes are the female and male gonads, respectively. This terminology is treated in Chapter 14.

DISORDERS AND TREATMENTS

Disorders of the endocrine system are almost always the result of an excess or deficit in hormone production. In other words, either too little or too much of a hormone causes a problem. If there is too little, replacement therapy is the normal treatment. If there is too much, surgery or radiation may be needed.

 Quick Check: A Few Facts about Glands

Fill in the blanks.

1. Another name for the pituitary gland is the _____.

2. Another name for the adrenal glands is the suprarenal glands because they are located _____.

3. Endocrine glands secrete hormones directly into _____.

Disorders of the Pituitary Gland

One cause of pituitary disorders can be a **benign adenoma** that causes too much of a hormone to be secreted. This condition may also destroy pituitary cells and cause too little hormone production.

Diabetes insipidus is caused by an insufficient amount of the antidiuretic hormone.

Gigantism is an abnormal overgrowth of the body or any of its parts, and **acromegaly** is enlargement of the extremities (mostly hands and feet). Both conditions are caused by excessive secretion of the growth hormone.

Disorders of the Thyroid Gland

As with other endocrine disorders, an excess or deficiency of thyroid hormone production creates an imbalance in the body, creating adverse effects on physical growth and function of tissues. **Hypothyroidism** is characterized by a decrease in thyroid function. **Hashimoto thyroiditis** is an autoimmune disorder. **Graves disease**, also known as a **toxic goiter**, is a type of **hyperthyroidism**.

What causes thyroid enlargement? Enlargement of the thyroid gland (goiter) is caused by a deficiency of iodine in the diet. This condition, no longer common in the United States, still affects populations in less developed parts of the world. The reason for its rarity in the United States is that in 1924, members of the Michigan State Medical Society championed the fight against goiter by convincing salt producers to include small amounts of iodine in their product. The discovery that goiter was a result of too little iodine in the diet had previously been noted by French physician J. B. Boussingault nearly a century earlier.

Disorders of the Adrenal Gland

Inflammatory conditions and viral infections involving the adrenal glands can cause a decrease in hormone production. Benign tumors are often the cause of increased hormone production from the adrenal glands.

Addison's disease is a progressive disorder caused by an insufficient amount of cortisol production in the adrenal gland or a failure of the pituitary gland to produce a stimulating hormone targeting the adrenal gland.

Cushing's syndrome is caused by an excessive amount of adrenal hormone secretion or by steroids administered as a treatment for other conditions.

The naming of disorders for persons who first identified them is a well-established practice. Recently, using the possessive form of the founder's name in the names of the disorders has been questioned, and one may, therefore, see and hear both Addison's disease and Addison disease. The problem is one of tradition versus logic. Those who eschew tradition in favor of logic say that Addison's disease is not something that 19th century British physician Thomas Addison contracted but rather a disorder he identified. Likewise, Harvey Cushing identified and did not contract Cushing's syndrome. Nevertheless, I chose to honor tradition over logic in this book, not because I value tradition over logic, but because looking up these disorders without the apostrophe on most, if not all, computer dictionaries will net a "not found" response.

There is an exception: Graves disease, although a traditional spelling, is not a true possessive. The rule for forming possessives specifies that this should be Graves disease. In this one case, therefore, tradition defies not only logic but also the rules of grammar and punctuation.

Disorders of the Pancreas

Diabetes mellitus is a major health problem that can produce lifelong effects. There are two main types: **Type 1 diabetes mellitus** is a metabolic disorder caused by insufficient production of insulin. Symptoms in the early stages include **glycosuria** (excess sugar in the urine) and **hyperglycemia** (excess sugar in the blood). **Type 2 diabetes mellitus** is an insulin-resistant disorder that occurs when the pancreas produces insulin but the body fails to use it effectively.

Treatment of Endocrine Disorders

Hormone replacement therapy is often used to correct endocrine disorders. Examples of disorders treatable by hormone replacement are hypothyroidism and diabetes mellitus. Corticosteroids may also be administered for their immunosuppressant and anti-inflammatory properties.

Abbreviation Table	THE ENDOCRINE SYSTEM
ABBREVIATION	**MEANING**
ACTH	adrenocorticotrophic hormone
ADH	antidiuretic hormone
BS	blood sugar
DM	diabetes mellitus
FBS	fasting blood sugar
FSH	follicle-stimulating hormone
GH	growth hormone
HbAlc	hemoglobin Alc (reflects average long-term glucose levels for 2 to 3 months before glucose blood level is drawn)
IDDM	insulin-dependent diabetes mellitus
LH	luteinizing hormone
MSH	melanocyte-stimulating hormone
NIDDM	non–insulin-dependent diabetes mellitus
PRL	prolactin
TSH	thyroid-stimulating hormone

Study Table — THE ENDOCRINE SYSTEM

TERM AND PRONUNCIATION	ANALYSIS	MEANING
Structure and Function		
adenogenous (ad-eh-NAW-jeh-nuhs)	*aden/o* (gland); *-genous* (originating)	originating in a gland
adenohypophysis (AD-eh-noh-hy-POFF-ih-sihs)	*aden/o* (gland); *hypophys/o* (pituitary gland)	the anterior pituitary gland
adrenal glands (ah-DREE-nahl); adrenal cortex, adrenal medulla	*adren/o* (adrenal glands); *cortex* (a Latin word meaning "bark"); *medulla* (a Latin word meaning "marrow, innermost part")	two glands, one located at the top of each kidney; adrenal cortex is the outer portion, adrenal medulla is the inner portion
adrenaline (ah-DREN-ah-lihn)	*adren/o* (adrenal glands); *-ine* (a suffix used to form names of chemical substances)	synonym for epinephrine, secreted from the adrenal medulla
adrenocorticotropic (ah-DREE-oh-KOR-tih-ko-TROH-pik) (ACTH)	*cortic/o* (from *cortex* [bark]); from the Greek word *trophe* (nourishment); *-in* (a suffix used to form names of biochemical substances)	pituitary secretion that stimulates the adrenal glands
androgen (AN-droh-jen)	*andro-* (masculine); *-gen* (suffix meaning "source of")	male hormone secreted by the adrenal cortex
aldosterone (al-DOSS-teh-rone)	ald (ehyd) + ster(ol) + *-one* (chemical suffix)	one of the corticosteroids, hormones produced by the adrenal glands
antidiuretic hormone (AN-tee-dy-uh-RET-ik) (ADH)	*anti-* (against); from the Greek *dia* (through); *-uresis* (urination)	hormone secreted by the posterior pituitary gland to prevent the kidneys from expelling too much water
calcitonin (kal-sih-TOH-nihn) (CT)	*calci-* (calcium); from the Greek *tonos* (to stretch); *-in* (suffix used to form names of biochemical substances)	hormone secreted by the thyroid to prevent too much calcium from absorbing into the bones
corticosteroids (KOR-tih-ko-STEHR-oyds)	*cortic/o* (from Latin word *cortex* [bark]); from steros (solid); *-oid* (resemblance to)	steroid produced by the cortices of the adrenal glands, cortisol
endocrine (EN-doh-krin)	*endo-* (within, inner); from the Greek word *krino* (to separate)	adjective describing a gland that delivers its secretions directly into bloodstream
epinephrine (EP-ih-NEFF-rihn)	*epi-* (upon); *nephr/o* (kidney); *-ine* (suffix used to form the names of chemical substances)	synonym for adrenaline, secreted from the adrenal medulla
estrogen (EHS-troh-jen)	from the Greek word *oistrus* (estrus); *-gen* (producing)	one of two hormones secreted by the ovaries

TERM AND PRONUNCIATION	ANALYSIS	MEANING
exocrine (EX-oh-krihn)	*exo-* (outside of); from the Greek word *krino* (to separate)	adjective describing a gland that delivers its secretions through a duct onto the skin or other epithelial surface
glucagon (GLOO-ka-guhn)	*gluc/o* (glucose); from the Greek word *ago* (to lead)	hormone secreted by the pancreas
gonadotropin (GO-nad-oh-TROH-pin) (FSH)	from the Greek word *gone* (seed); from the Greek word *trophe* (nourishment); *-in* (suffix used to form names of biochemical substances)	follicle-stimulating hormone; hormone promoting gonadal growth
gonadotropin (GO-nad-oh-TROH-pin) (ICSH)	from the Greek word *gone* (seed); from the Greek word *trophe* (nourishment); *-in* (suffix used to form names of biochemical substances)	interstitial cell-stimulating hormone; hormone promoting gonadal growth in the male
gonadotropin (GO-nad-oh-TROH-pin) (LH)	from the Greek word *gone* (seed); from the Greek word *trophe* (nourishment); *-in* (suffix used to form names of biochemical substances)	luteinizing hormone; stimulates ovulation
homeostasis	from two Greek words: *homos* (same) and *stasis* (existence)	tendency to equilibrium; remaining normal
hormone (HOHR-mohn)	from the Greek word *hormao* (to rouse or set in motion)	chemical messenger that is secreted by an endocrine gland directly into the bloodstream
hydrocortisone (hy-droh-KOR-tih-sone)	*hydro-* (water); *cortic/o* (from the Latin word *cortex* meaning "bark"); *-one* (chemical suffix)	an adrenal gland hormone secretion
hypophysis (hy-POFF-ih-sihs)	*hypophys/o* (pituitary gland)	synonym for pituitary gland
insulin (IN-soo-lihn)	from the Latin word *insula* (island)	one of two hormones produced in the pancreas
islets of Langerhans (EYE-lets LAN-gehr-hans)	after German pathologist Paul Langerhans, who described it in 1869; islets are the regions of the pancreas that contain its hormone-producing cells	clusters of specialized cells in the pancreas that secrete insulin
melanocyte-stimulating hormone (MEL-an-oh-syte) (MSH)	*melan/o* (black); *-cyte* (cell); from the Greek word *hormao* (to rouse or set in motion)	hormone secreted from the anterior pituitary gland

(continued)

TERM AND PRONUNCIATION	ANALYSIS	MEANING
melatonin (mel-ah-TONE-ihn)	melanophore + Greek *tonos* (to stretch); -*in* (suffix used to form names of biochemical substances)	hormone secreted by the pineal gland
neurohypophysis (NUHR-oh-hy-POFF-ih-sihs)	*neur/o* (nerve); *hypophys/o* (pituitary gland)	synonym for posterior pituitary gland
noradrenaline (nor-ah-DREN-ah-lihn)	*nor-* (chemical prefix); *adrenal/o* (adrenal glands); -*ine* (a suffix used to denote chemical substances)	synonym for norepinephrine; secreted from the adrenal medulla
norepinephrine (NOR-ehp-ih-NEFF-rihn)	*nor-* (chemical prefix); *epi-* (upon); from the Greek word *nephros* (kidney); -*ine* (a suffix used to denote chemical substances)	synonym for noradrenaline; secreted from the adrenal medulla
ovaries (OH-vayr-ees)	from the Latin word *ovum* (egg)	female gonads; two oval-shaped glands that are located in the pelvic cavity
oxytocin (ox-ih-TOH-sihn) (OXT)	from the Greek word *oxyto-kos* (swift birth); -*in* (suffix used to form names of bio-chemical substances)	hormone secreted by the posterior pituitary gland
pancreas (PAN-kree-uhs)	from the Greek word *pancreas* (sweet bread)	feather-shaped organ that lies posterior to the stomach
parathyroid gland (pahr-ah-THY-royd)	*para-* (prefix denoting in-volvement of two like parts; also denoting adjacent, along-side, near); *thyr/o* (thyroid gland)	secretes parathyroid hormone (PTH)
parathyroid hormone (pahr-ah-THY-royd), parathormone (PTH)	*para-* (prefix denoting involvement of two like parts; also denoting adjacent, along-side, near); *thyr/o* (thyroid gland); from the Greek word *hormao* (to set in motion)	a hormone secreted by the parathyroid gland
pineal gland (PIHN-ee-ahl)	from the Latin word *pinus* (pine); -*al* (adjective ending)	gland that secretes melatonin, an antioxidant that is other-wise not well understood
pituitary gland (pih-TOO-ih-tahr-ee)	from the Latin word *pituita*	synonym for hypophysis; master gland
progesterone (proh-JES-ter-ohn)	from the Latin *pro* (for); from the Latin *gestare* (to carry about)	one of two female hormones secreted by the ovary

TERM AND PRONUNCIATION	ANALYSIS	MEANING
prolactin (pro-LAK-tihn) (PRL)	from the Latin *pro* (for); from the Latin *lacteus* (milky)	a secretion of the anterior pituitary gland
suprarenal glands (SOO-prah-REEN-ahl)	*supra-* (above); *ren-* (kidney); *-al* (pertaining to)	another name for the adrenal glands
testes (TES-tees)	from the plural form of the Latin *testis* (testicle)	male gonads; two oval organs that lie in the scrotum
testosterone (teh-STAH-steh-rone)	from the Latin *testis* (testicle); ster(ol); *-one* (chemical suffix)	male hormone secreted by the testes
thyroid gland (THY-royd)	*thyr/o* (thyroid gland)	one of the four glands belonging solely to the endocrine system; located in the throat area
thyrotropin (thy-ROT-roh-pihn) (TSH)	*thyr/o* (thyroid gland); from the Greek *trophe* (nourishment); *-in* (suffix used to form names of biochemical substances)	thyroid-stimulating hormone
thyroxine (thy-ROK-sihn) (T_4)	*thyr/o* (thyroid gland); *-ine* (suffix used to form names of biochemical substances)	a secretion of the thyroid gland
triiodothyronine (try-EYE-oh-doh-THY-roh-neen) (T_3)	*tri-* (three); *iodo* (iodine); *thyr/o* (thyroid gland); *-ine* (a suffix used to form names of chemical substances)	another secretion of the thyroid gland that is often synthesized from thyroxine (T_4) by bodily organs
Common Disorders		
acromegaly (AK-roh-mehg-alee)	from the Greek *akron* (extremity); *-megaly* (enlargement)	enlargement of the extremities (mostly hands and feet) caused by excessive secretion of the growth hormone *after* puberty
Addison's disease	after the British physician, Thomas Addison, who first described the condition in 1855	a disorder characterized by a failure of the adrenal glands to produce hydrocortisone and, in some cases, aldosterone
adenitis (ad-eh-NY-tihs)	*aden/o* (gland); *-itis* (inflammation)	inflammation of a gland
adenohypophysitis (AD-eh-noh-hy-poff-ih-SY-tihs)	*aden/o* (gland); *hypophys/o* (pituitary gland); *-itis* (inflammation)	inflammation of the hypophysis
adrenalitis (ah-dree-nah-LY-tiss)	*adrenal/o* (adrenal glands); *-itis* (inflammation)	inflammation of an adrenal gland
adrenalopathy (ah-dree-nah-LOP-ah-thee); sometimes also adrenopathy (ah-dree-NOP-ah-thee)	*adrenal/o* (adrenal glands); *-pathy* (disease)	any disease of the adrenal glands

(continued)

TERM AND PRONUNCIATION	ANALYSIS	MEANING
adrenomegaly (ah-dree-noh-MEG-ah-lee)	*adren/o* (adrenal gland); *-megaly* (enlargement)	enlargement of the adrenal glands
Cushing's syndrome	named after Harvey Cushing, American physician, who described the disorder in 1932	a hormonal disorder caused by too much hydrocortisone
diabetes insipidus (DY-ah-BEET-ehs ihn-SIP-ih-duhs)	*diabetes*, a Greek word meaning "a compass," "a siphon"; *insipidus* (lacking flavor or zest)	condition brought about by the posterior pituitary's failure to produce enough antidiuretic hormone
diabetes mellitus, type 1 and type 2 (DY-ah-BEET-ehs meh-LY-tuhs)	*diabetes*, a Greek word meaning "a compass, a siphon"; *mellitus*, a Latin word meaning "sweetened with honey" or "honey-sweet"	condition brought about by insufficient production of insulin in the pancreas (type 1) or the failure of the body's cells to absorb glucose (type 2)
gigantism (JEYE-gan-tizm)	*giant* (common English word); *-ism* (condition)	abnormal overgrowth of the body due to excessive secretion of the growth hormone *before* puberty
glycosuria (GLY-koh-SYUR-ee-ah)	*glyc/o/s* (sugar); *-uria* (urine)	sugar in the urine
goiter (GOY-tuhr)	from the Latin word *gutter* (throat)	chronic enlargement of the thyroid gland
Graves disease	named after Robert James Graves (1796–1853), an Irish physician who first described exophthalmic goiter in 1835	a common form of hyperthyroidism resulting from overproduction of thyroxine caused by a false immune system response
Hashimoto's thyroiditis (Hah-shee-moh-toh)	Hashimoto (Japanese surgeon, 1881–1934); *thyr/o* (thyroid gland); *-itis* (inflammation)	an autoimmune disorder that attacks the thyroid gland causing hypothyroidism
hyperglycemia (hy-puhr-gly-SEEM-ee-ah)	*hyper-* (above normal); *glyc/o* (sugar); *-ia* (condition)	excessive sugar in the blood
hyperpituitarism (HY-puhr-pih-TOO-iht-ahr-izm)	*hyper-* (above normal); from the Latin word *pituita* (phlegm)	excessive hormone secretion by the pituitary gland
hyperthyroidism (HY-puhr-THY-royd-izm)	*hyper-* (above normal); *thyr/o* (thyroid); *-ism* (condition)	condition caused by an overactive thyroid; usually caused by an immune system disorder known as Graves disease
hypophysitis (hy-poh-fih-SY-tihs)	*hypophys/o* (pituitary gland); *-itis* (inflammation)	inflammation of the pituitary gland
hypopituitarism (hy-poh-pih-TOO-ih-tahr-izm)	*hypo-* (below normal); from the Latin word *pituita*; *-ism* (condition)	condition of diminished hormone secretion from the anterior pituitary gland

TERM AND PRONUNCIATION	ANALYSIS	MEANING
hypothyroidism	*hypo-* (below normal); thyroid refers to the thyroid gland; *-ism* (state of)	a decrease in thyroid function
pituitarism (pih-TOO-iht-ahr-izm)	from the Latin word *pituita*; *-ism* (condition)	any pituitary dysfunction
thyroaplasia (THY-roh-a-PLAY-zee-ah)	*thyr/o* (thyroid gland); aplasia from the Greek *a plassein* (not to form)	congenital condition characterized by low thyroid output
thyroiditis (thy-roy-DY-tihs)	*thyr/o* (thyroid gland); *-itis* (inflammation)	inflammation of the thyroid gland
thyromegaly (thy-roh-MEG-ah lee)	*thyr/o* (thyroid gland); *-megaly* (enlargement)	enlargement of the thyroid gland
Practice and Practitioners		
endocrinologist (en-do-krih-NOL-oh-jist)	*endocrin/o* (endocrine); *-logist* (one who specializes)	medical specialist in endocrinology
endocrinology (en-do-krih-NOL-oh-jee)	*endocrin/o* (endocrine); *-logy* (study of)	medical specialty of the endocrine system
Diagnosis and Treatments		
adenectomy (ad-eh-NEK-toh-mee)	*aden/o* (gland); *-ectomy* (excision)	excision of a gland
adenotomy (ad-eh-NOT-oh-mee)	*aden/o* (gland); *-tomy* (cutting operation)	incision of a gland
adrenalectomy (ah-dree-nah-LEK-toh-mee)	*adrenal/o* (adrenal glands); *-ectomy* (excision)	surgical removal of one or both adrenal glands
hypoglycemic (HY-poh-gly-SEE-mik)	*hypo-* (below normal); *glyc/o* (sugar); *-ic* (pertaining to)	drug used to lower blood sugar
hypophysectomy (HY-poh-fih-SEK-toh-mee)	*hypophys/o* (pituitary gland); *-ectomy* (excision)	surgical removal of the hypophysis (pituitary gland)
parathyroidectomy (PAHR-ahthy-royd-EK-toh-mee)	*parathyr/o* (parathyroid gland); *-ectomy* (excision)	surgical excision of the parathyroid gland
thyroidectomy (THY-royd-EK-toh-mee)	*thyr/o* (thyroid gland); *-ectomy* (excision)	excision of the thyroid gland
thyroparathyroidectomy (THY-roh-pehr-ah-THY-roy-DEK-toh-mee)	*thyr/o* (thyroid gland); *parathyr/o* (parathyroid gland); *-ectomy* (excision)	excision of the thyroid and parathyroid glands
thyrotomy (thy-ROT-oh-mee)	*thyr/o* (thyroid gland); *-tomy* (cutting operation)	surgery performed on the thyroid gland

EXERCISES

EXERCISE 8-1 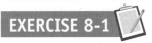 DEFINING ABBREVIATIONS

Study the Abbreviations Table and then write a definition for each of the following abbreviations without referring to the table again.

1. FSH   _____

2. FBS   _____

3. PRL   _____

4. ADH   _____

5. TSH   _____

6. DM   _____

7. MSH   _____

8. HbAlc   _____

9. LH   _____

10. NIDDM   _____

11. IDDM   _____

12. GH   _____

13. ACTH   _____

14. BS   _____

EXERCISE 8-2 FIGURE LABELING: THE ENDOCRINE SYSTEM

The endocrine glands

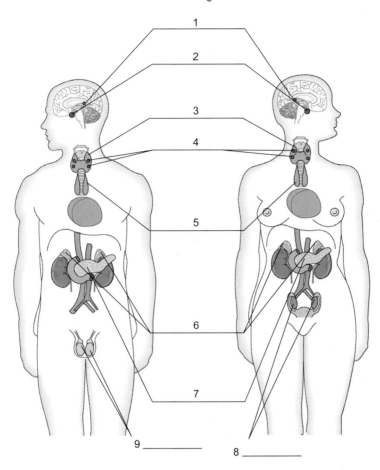

Select the endocrine gland from the list and place it by the corresponding number.

1. _____   adrenals

2. _____   ovaries

3. _____   pancreatic islets

4. _____   parathyroids

5. _____   pineal

6. _____   pituitary (hypophysis)

7. _____   testes

8. _____   thymus

9. _____   thyroid

EXERCISE 8-3 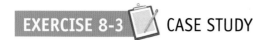 CASE STUDY

ENDOCRINOLOGY OFFICE CONSULTATION

After reading the case study, answer the following questions.

OFFICE NOTE: This 59-year-old woman has previously been in good health. On a routine physical examination, she was noted to have a thyroid nodule on the right lobe of the thyroid. She complained of hoarseness, dysphasia, local tenderness, and a slight enlargement on the right side of her neck. She also admits to an increase in activity and inability to sleep throughout the night.

On physical examination, the right side of the neck was visibly enlarged, and a nodule was felt; it was noted that the patient's eyes were bulging outward. A blood test to check her thyroid hormone blood levels indicated a high value of TSH. No other modifying factors or associated signs or symptoms were present.

1. In the last sentence of the opening paragraph, what does "admits to increase in activity" mean?

   _____

2. What does dysphasia mean? _____

3. What is a medical term for an "enlargement of the thyroid gland"? _____

4. What is TSH? _____

5. Rewrite the sentence: "On physical examination, the right side of the neck was visibly enlarged, and a nodule was felt; it was noted that the patient's eyes were bulging outward."

   _____

EXERCISE 8-4 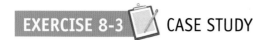 SPELL CHECK

Circle the correct spelling of the medical term.

1. An _____ is a physician who specializes in caring for patients with endocrine diseases and hormonal dysfunctions.

   enocreenologist   endokrineologist   endocrineologist   endocrinologist

2. A medication that can be taken orally to lower the blood sugar is called a _____.

   hypogysemic   hyperglycemic   hypoglycemic   hyperglysemik

3. _____ is one of the hormones produced in the pancreas that regulates blood sugar.

   insullin   insulin   insalin   insulen

4. One of the main disorders of the pancreas is called _____.

   diabetes mellitus   diabetis mellitus   diabetis melletes   diabetes melitus

EXERCISE 8-5 DISORDERS AND SYMPTOMS OF THE ENDOCRINE SYSTEM

Match the terms listed with the definitions below.

acromegaly   endogenous   polyuria
Cushing's syndrome   glycosuria   thyromegaly
diabetes mellitus (DM)   hyperglycemia

1. originating from within the body _____

2. enlargement of extremities caused by overproduction of the growth hormone in adults _____

3. lack of or insufficient insulin production from the pancreas _____

4. enlarged thyroid gland, also referred to as *goiter* _____

5. abnormally high levels of glucose in the blood _____

6. excessive and frequent urination _____

7. sugar in the urine _____

8. excessive amount of adrenal hormone present _____

EXERCISE 8-6 WORD BUILDING: THE ENDOCRINE SYSTEM

Use *adren/o* to build the medical words meaning:

1. enlargement of the adrenal gland _____

2. surgical removal of an adrenal gland _____

3. disease of the adrenal glands _____

Use *thyr/o or thyroid/o* to build the medical words meaning:

4. condition of minimal functioning of the thyroid gland _____

5. inflammation of the thyroid gland _____

6. incision of the thyroid gland _____

7. enlargement of the thyroid gland _____

Use *pancreat/o* to build the medical words meaning:

8. tumor of the pancreas _____

9. inflammation of the pancreas _____

10. originating in the pancreas _____

EXERCISE 8-7   CROSSWORD PUZZLE: THE ENDOCRINE SYSTEM

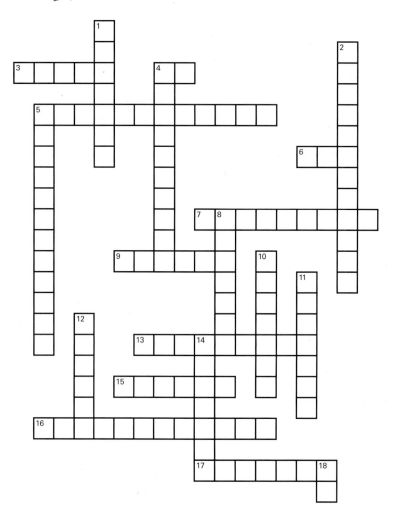

ACROSS

3. female gonad
4. abbreviation for growth hormone
5. oral medication used to treat type 2 diabetes
6. abbreviation for fasting blood sugar
7. master gland
9. autoimmune disorder resulting in hyperthyroidism; exophthalmos and goiter
13. condition caused by excess growth hormone in children
15. male gonads
16. located on the dorsal surface of the thyroid gland
17. gland located on the top of the kidney

DOWN

1. T_3 and T_4 are secreted from which gland?
2. hormone secreted by the male gonad
4. excess sugar in the urine
5. low blood sugar
8. hormone not produced in type 1 diabetes
10. a syndrome resulting from excess secretion of adrenal cortex; obesity, hirsutism, weakness
11. chemical secreted by an endocrine gland
12. enlarged thyroid
14. tumor of a gland
18. abbreviation for luteinizing hormone

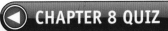 **CHAPTER 8 QUIZ**

Multiple Choice

1. The master gland is known as the:
   a. pituitary gland
   b. thymus gland
   c. thyroid gland
   d. pineal gland

2. The ovaries produce which two hormones?
   a. insulin and glucagon
   b. estrogen and progesterone
   c. testosterone and thymosin
   d. T_3 and T_4

3. Endocrine means:
   a. to cringe from within
   b. to secrete within
   c. to cry inside
   d. disease of the gland

4. Oversecretion of the pituitary growth hormone in an adult produces a condition called:
   a. hyperthyroidism
   b. Simmond's disease
   c. acromegaly
   d. tetany

5. _____ is an enlargement of the thyroid gland.
   a. hypothyroidism
   b. goiter
   c. thyroidectomy
   d. Addison's disease

6. A chemical secreted from an endocrine gland is called a/an:
   a. hormone
   b. lymph
   c. neurotransmitter
   d. insulin

7. Hypersecretion of the *growth hormone* may cause:
   a. insulin
   b. cretinism
   c. hypothyroidism
   d. gigantism

8. _____ is associated with excessive hormone secretion from the adrenal cortex.
   a. Cushing's syndrome
   b. Conn's syndrome
   c. goiter
   d. gigantism

9. The two-lobed gland in the neck is called the:
   a. Adam's apple
   b. thymus
   c. pituitary
   d. thyroid

Matching

Select the best definition from Column 2 to match the term in Column 1.

TERM	DEFINITION

10. _____ adrenalopathy

11. _____ hyperpituitarism

12. _____ adenogenous

13. _____ antidiuretic hormone

14. _____ adrenaline

15. _____ master gland, hypophysis

16. _____ calcitonin

17. _____ goiter

18. _____ parathyroid gland

19. _____ thyrotropin (TSH)

20. _____ thyromegaly

21. _____ adenohypophysitis

22. _____ thyroparathyroidectomy

A. synonym for epinephrine

B. thyroid-stimulating hormone, secreted by the anterior pituitary

C. enlargement of the thyroid gland

D. disease of the adrenal glands

E. synonym for pituitary gland

F. hormone secreted by the thyroid

G. originating in a gland

H. excision of the thyroid and parathyroid glands

I. hormone secreted by the posterior pituitary

J. secretes PTH (parathyroid hormone)

K. excessive pituitary secretion

L. inflammation of the anterior pituitary gland

M. chronic enlargement of the thyroid

9 *The Cardiovascular System*

LEARNING OBJECTIVES

Upon completion of this chapter, you should be able to:

- Identify and define the medical terms associated with the cardiovascular system and its functions.
- Define terms associated with disorders, procedures, and treatments related to the cardiovascular system.
- Recognize and define the word elements that make up cardiovascular system terms.
- Identify and interpret selected abbreviations related to the cardiovascular system.
- Spell and pronounce medical terms that relate to the cardiovascular system.

INTRODUCTION

The **cardiovascular system** comprises the heart, the blood, and all the blood vessels, which carry blood to all parts of the body (Fig. 9-1). The blood vessels include all the **arteries**, **veins**, and **capillaries**, which taken together form a transportation system that delivers oxygen and nutrients to the body's cells. The cardiovascular system also helps regulate body temperature and collects waste products from the cells.

This chapter covers medical terms naming anatomical components, major functions, disorders, treatments, and procedures associated with the cardiovascular system.

WORD ELEMENTS FOUND IN CARDIOVASCULAR SYSTEM TERMS

Table 9-1 lists most of the elements that make up cardiovascular system terms. Suffixes and prefixes that may already have been learned are also listed.

STRUCTURE AND FUNCTION

The Heart

The heart is a four-chambered hollow organ with three layers. The innermost layer is called the **endocardium**. The middle layer, which is the actual heart muscle and the thickest of the three layers, is called the **myocardium**. The outer layer of the heart is called the **epicardium**, which is surrounded by the **pericardium**, a sac that surrounds the heart (Fig. 9-2).

The heart acts as a double pump separated by a wall called a **septum**. The right side pumps deoxygenated blood to the **lungs** where it picks up oxygen, and the left side of the heart pumps the oxygenated blood to all other parts of the body through the entire body. This delivery system operates through the four chambers of the heart. The four chambers are as follows:

- **Right atrium**: upper right chamber that receives blood from all body parts except the lungs; the **interatrial septum** separates the right and left **atria** (plural of atrium).
- **Right ventricle**: lower right chamber that receives blood from the right atrium and pumps it to the lungs; the **interventricular septum** separates the right and left ventricles.
- **Left atrium**: upper left chamber that receives oxygen-rich blood as it returns from the lungs.
- **Left ventricle**: lower left chamber that pumps blood to all parts of the body.

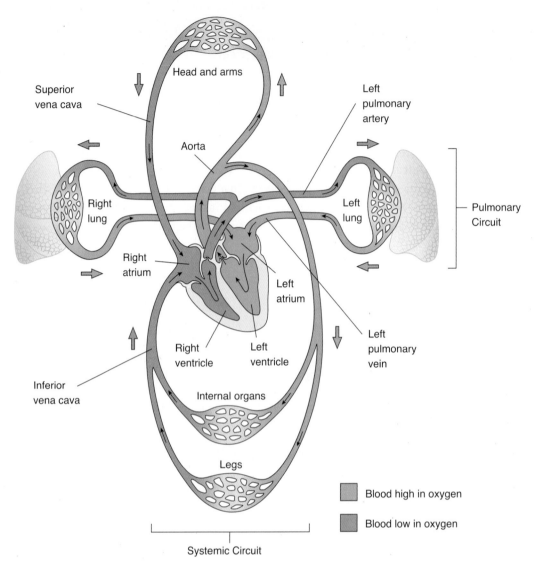

FIGURE 9-1 **The cardiovascular system.** The cardiovascular system consists of blood flow in a closed system of vessels. Oxygen content is exchanged in the pulmonary circuit, and blood rich in oxygen (red vessels) is returned to the left side of the heart. The pulmonary circuit carries blood to and from the lungs, and the systemic circuit carries blood to and from all other parts of the body. The vessels depicted in *red* signify blood that is high in oxygen; the vessels depicted in *blue* signify blood that is low in oxygen. *From Cohen BJ.* Medical Terminology: An Illustrated Guide. *5th ed. Philadelphia, PA: Lippincott Williams & Wilkins; 2007.*

Blood Flow through the Heart

Blood flow through the heart is directed by one-way valves located at the entrance and exit to each of the ventricles. The **atrioventricular** valves are found at the entrance to the ventricles and are so named because they come between the atria and ventricles. The right atrioventricular valve is also known as the **tricuspid valve** because it has three cusps or flaps that open and close. It controls the opening between the right atrium and right ventricle. The **left atrioventricular** valve is located between the left atrium and left ventricle and is called the **bicuspid** or **mitral valve**. It has two cusps or flaps that control blood flow.

Element	Function	Refers to
TABLE 9-1		**WORD ELEMENTS THAT FORM TERMS RELATING TO THE CARDIOVASCULAR SYSTEM**
angi/o	root	vessel
aort/o	root	aorta
arteri/o	root	artery
ather/o	root	fatty
atri/o	root	atrium
brady-	prefix	slow
cardi/o	root	heart
coron/o	root	crown; encircling, such as in the coronary blood vessels encircling the heart
-ectasis	suffix	dilation
electr/o	root	electrical
-emia	suffix	blood
endo-	root	inner, inside
-gram	suffix	written record
hem/o, hemat/o	root	blood
isch	root	restricted, narrowed
my/o	root	muscle
peri-	prefix	around, surrounding
phleb/o	root	vein
-stenosis	suffix	a narrowing
tachy-	prefix	fast
thromb/o	root	clot
valv/o, valvul/o	root	valve
varic/o	root	dilated; from the Latin word *varix* (a dilated vein)
vas/o	root	vessel
ven/o	root	vein
ventricul/o	root	ventricle

Word Elements Exercise — FILL IN THE BLANKS

After studying Table 9-1, write the word element that corresponds with each definition.

1. root meaning vein _____

2. root meaning heart _____

3. root meaning vessel _____

4. root meaning inner, inside _____

5. prefix meaning fast _____

6. root meaning clot _____

(continued)

  7. prefix meaning around, surrounding   _____

  8. root meaning fatty   _____

  9. root meaning atrium   _____

10. suffix meaning written record   _____

11. suffix meaning blood   _____

12. root meaning muscle   _____

13. suffix meaning a narrowing   _____

14. root meaning blood   _____

15. root meaning artery   _____

16. root meaning vein   _____

17. root meaning valve   _____

18. root meaning aorta   _____

19. prefix meaning slow   _____

20. root meaning dilated   _____

21. root meaning crown   _____

22. suffix meaning dilation   _____

23. root meaning vessel   _____

24. root meaning electrical   _____

25. root meaning ventricle   _____

26. root meaning restricted, narrowed   _____

> Why does the biscuspid valve have a second name? Mitral valve is an alternate name of the bicuspid valve. This name comes from the valve's similarity to a miter, which is a tall ceremonial hat worn by some clergymen as a symbol of their office. Miter (British: mitre) is an English word.

The exit valves are named **semilunar** because the flaps resemble half moons. The exit point at the right ventricle is called the **pulmonary semilunar valve**, and it is located between the right ventricle and the pulmonary artery. The **aortic semilunar valve** is located between the left ventricle and the aorta.

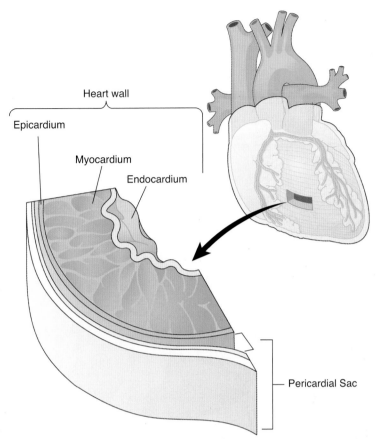

FIGURE 9-2 Layers of the heart and pericardium. The heart wall is composed of three layers: the epicardium (outer layer; epi- means "on top of"; cardi/o means "heart"), myocardium (heart muscle; my/o means "muscle"; cardi/o means "heart"), and endocardium (inner layer; endo- means "within"; cardi/o means "heart"). Note the thickness of the myocardial or "muscle" layer. The pericardial sac is actually composed of two layers and has fluid in the space between the layers. This fluid helps to reduce friction when the heart beats. *Modified from Cohen BJ. Memmler's The Human Body in Health and Disease. 10th ed. Philadelphia, PA: Lippincott Williams & Wilkins; 2005.*

Use the adjective "ventricular" only when you are absolutely sure of the meaning of the phrase you are uttering. The reason for caution is that the brain, as well as the heart, contains ventricles. Be careful, likewise, when combining the root "ventricul/o" with other word elements.

The pathway of blood through the heart is illustrated in Figure 9-3.

The Heartbeat

To pump blood effectively throughout the body, the heart must contract and relax in a rhythmic cycle. Electrical nerve impulses stimulate the myocardium and the chambers of the heart to contract and relax in sequence. The electrical conduction system of the heart includes the following (Fig. 9-4):

- **Sinoatrial node**: located in the upper posterior wall of the right atrium; sets the heartbeat; also called the pacemaker of the heart.
- **Atrioventricular node**: located on the bottom of the right atrium near the ventricle; transmits electrical impulses to the bundle of His.
- **Bundle of His**: located at the top of the interventricular septum and travels down along either side of the septum; transmits impulses to the Purkinje fibers.
- **Purkinje fibers**: peripheral fibers that end in the right and left ventricles; stimulation from the bundle of His causes excitation of the ventricular muscles, resulting in contraction.

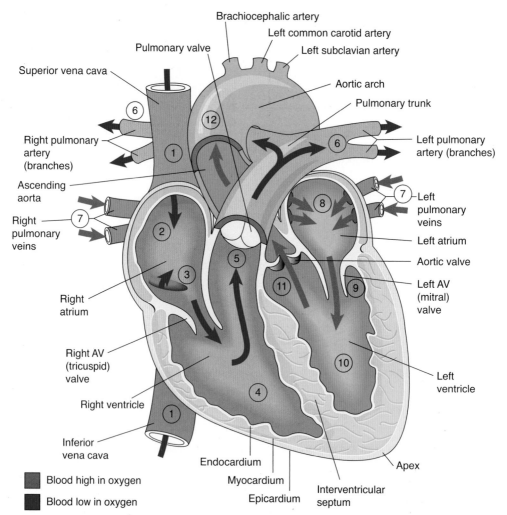

Superior vena cava

Pulmonary valve

Brachiocephalic artery

Left common carotid artery

Left subclavian artery

Aortic arch

Pulmonary trunk

Right pulmonary artery (branches)

Left pulmonary artery (branches)

Ascending aorta

Right pulmonary veins

Left pulmonary veins

Left atrium

Aortic valve

Right atrium

Left AV (mitral) valve

Right AV (tricuspid) valve

Left ventricle

Right ventricle

Inferior vena cava

Endocardium

Myocardium

Epicardium

Interventricular septum

Apex

Blood high in oxygen

Blood low in oxygen

FIGURE 9-3   The heart and pathway of blood flow. Deoxygenated blood returns from the body into the heart through the superior and inferior venae cavae. The pathway of the blood through the heart begins when blood is returned to the vena cava (#1) and exits the heart through the aorta (#12) to the rest of the body. Note: The right side of the heart is colored in *blue*, signifying deoxygenated blood. The left side of the heart is colored in *red* because it carries oxygenated blood. AV, atrioventricular. *From Cohen BJ. Medical Terminology: An Illustrated Guide. 5th ed. Philadelphia, PA: Lippincott Williams & Wilkins; 2007.*

Why bundle of His? Why not "bundle of His or Hers"? In 1893, German physician Wilhelm His figured out that a heartbeat starts in a particular group of atrioventricular fibers, which were, subsequently, named for him. A Czech anatomist/physiologist, Jan Evangelista Purkyně, likewise discovered the Purkinje (or Purkyne) fibers. Born in 1787, Purkyně contributed many other scientific discoveries to the world. For example, he was the first to show that fingerprints could be used to establish identity, and his studies of the human eye prefigured motion pictures.

Each heart contraction, called **systole**, is followed by a relaxation called **diastole**. These two phases make up the cardiac cycle and are illustrated in Figure 9-5.

Heart rate is determined by how many times the heart beats per minute. The blood that is forced through the vessels by contraction creates an increase in the artery pressure that can be felt by placing a finger at the radial artery located on the palm side of the wrist.

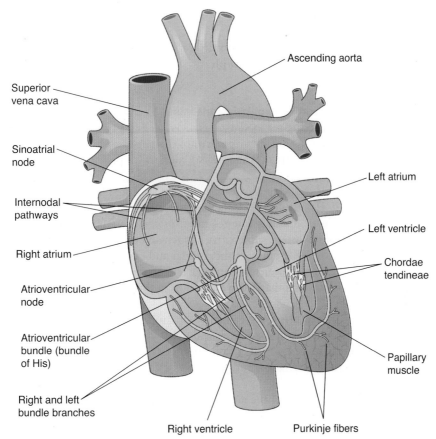

FIGURE 9-4 Electrical conduction system of the heart. The electrical stimulus begins in the sinoatrial node, also known as the pacemaker of the heart. The electrical stimulus moves from the sinoatrial node to the atrioventricular node, through the atrioventricular bundle of His, through the right and left bundle branches, and terminates in the Purkinje fibers where excitation of the ventricles occurs. *Modified from Cohen BJ*. Memmler's The Human Body in Health and Disease. *10th ed. Philadelphia, PA: Lippincott Williams & Wilkins; 2005.*

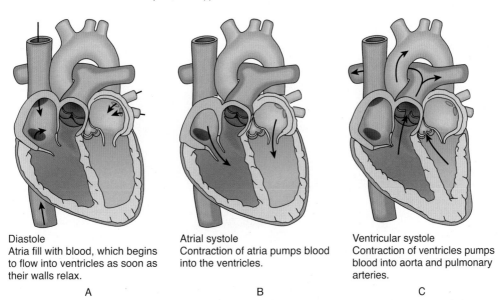

Diastole
Atria fill with blood, which begins to flow into ventricles as soon as their walls relax.

Atrial systole
Contraction of atria pumps blood into the ventricles.

Ventricular systole
Contraction of ventricles pumps blood into aorta and pulmonary arteries.

A   B   C

FIGURE 9-5 The cardiac cycle. A. Diastole: Ventricles relax as blood flows into the chambers. **B.** Atrial systole: Atria contract, pushing blood into the ventricles. **C.** Ventricular systole: Ventricles contract and pump blood into the pulmonary arteries and aorta. *From Cohen BJ*. Memmler's The Human Body in Health and Disease. *10th ed. Philadelphia, PA: Lippincott Williams & Wilkins; 2005.*

The electrical activity of the heart can be recorded on an **electrocardiogram**. The machine that does the recording is called an **electrocardiograph**.

The Blood and Blood Vessels

The blood vessels include the arteries, capillaries, and veins. Blood brings oxygen and nutrients to body cells and removes waste products. Blood itself is divisible into two main components: plasma, which is the liquid part, and the formed elements within the plasma. Blood plasma, which is clear and straw-colored, is composed mostly of water (91%), along with proteins and other nutrients in solution.

The names of blood vessels in the cardiovascular system are listed here:
- **Arteries**: thick-walled, elastic blood vessels that carry oxygenated blood away from the heart (note one exception: the pulmonary arteries carry unoxygenated blood).
- **Arterioles**: branches of the arteries that carry oxygenated blood to the capillaries.
- **Capillaries**: blood vessels that connect the arterial and venous systems; they are only one cell in thickness and exchange nutrients and waste material.
- **Venules**: branches of the veins that receive blood from the capillaries and transport it to the veins.
- **Veins**: blood vessels that return deoxygenated blood to the heart.

The **lumen** of a blood vessel is the opening through which blood flows. The nervous system can stimulate the lumen to be opened, a condition called **vasodilation**, or closed, a condition called **vasoconstriction**. Vasodilation and vasoconstriction each can have an effect on blood pressure.

Blood pressure is a measurement of the amount of pressure exerted against the walls of blood vessels. Blood pressure is recorded as a fractional number: **systolic** over **diastolic**. Systolic pressure occurs when the highest pressure is exerted against the vessel walls, and diastolic pressure occurs when the lowest pressure is exerted against the vessel walls. Blood pressure can be measured by several methods, but the most common is with an instrument called a **sphygmomanometer**, commonly called a blood pressure cuff (Fig. 9-6).

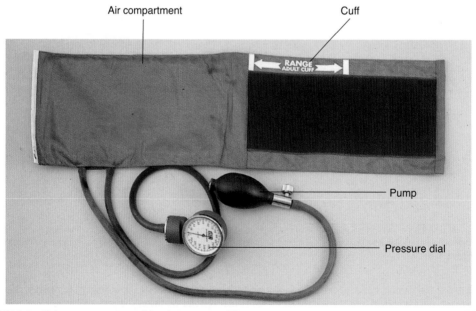

FIGURE 9-6 **Sphygmomanometer (blood pressure cuff).** *From Cohen BJ.* Medical Terminology: An Illustrated Guide. *5th ed. Philadelphia, PA: Lippincott Williams & Wilkins; 2007.*

TABLE 9-2 BLOOD TYPES AS DONORS AND RECIPIENTS		
Blood Type	**Can Donate to**	**Can Receive from**
A	A or AB only	A or O only
B	B or AB only	B or O only
AB (universal recipient)	AB only	A, B, AB, O
O (universal donor)	A, B, AB, O	O only

Elements of Blood

The formed elements in blood consist of **red blood cells** (**RBCs**), also called **erythrocytes**; **platelets**, also called **thrombocytes**; and **white blood cells** (**WBCs**), also called **leukocytes**. Each element has an important role, ranging from the transportation of oxygen to body cells to defense of the body against harmful organisms. The following list identifies the structure and function of each element:

- **Erythrocytes**: The main function of erythrocytes is to transport oxygen. The oxygen binds to **hemoglobin** (**Hb**), a protein.
- **Thrombocytes**: Also known as platelets, thrombocytes play an important role in the blood-clotting process. They are the smallest of the formed elements, roughly half the size of erythrocytes.
- **Leukocytes**: Leukocytes are the body's main defense against harmful organisms; there are five types of leukocytes: **neutrophils**, **eosinophils**, **basophils**, **lymphocytes**, and **monocytes**.

Blood Groups

The four major blood groups (types) are **A**, **AB**, **B**, and **O**. Blood type compatibility is an important consideration when blood is transferred from one person to another. Table 9-2 lists the blood type compatibilities for donors and recipients.

The presence or absence of a substance in a red blood cell is responsible for what is known as the **Rh factor**. The **Rh factor** is named for the first two letters in the word *rhesus*, a reference to the rhesus macaque, the blood of which was used in early experiments. A person whose blood contains the Rh factor is **Rh positive**. People with blood that does not contain the Rh factor are **Rh negative**.

PRACTICE AND PRACTITIONERS

The specialists who treat disorders of the cardiovascular system include **cardiologists**, **cardiovascular surgeons**, and **hematologists**. Cardiologists diagnose and treat heart disorders. Cardiovascular surgeons surgically correct disorders of the cardiovascular system. Hematologists treat disorders of the blood.

 Quick Check: Blood Vessels

Fill in the blanks.

1. The names of blood vessels in the cardiovascular system are **arteries**, **arterioles**, **capillaries**, **veins**, and **venules**, which receive blood from the capillaries and transfer it into the _____.

2. **Veins** are blood vessels that return deoxygenated blood to the _____.

3. Erythrocytes is another term for _____.

DISORDERS AND TREATMENTS

Disorders of the cardiovascular system, such as **coronary artery disease** and **thrombosis**, may involve the heart directly. Others include **anemia** and **leukemia**, which are blood disorders that affect the cardiovascular system. These disorders and others are listed in the following sections.

Coronary Artery Disease

One of the main causes of coronary artery disease is **atherosclerosis**, which is a progressive buildup of plaque that can cause the lumen of coronary arteries to narrow. When these plaques become thick and hard, they may also cause a loss of elasticity in the artery and impede blood flow to the heart muscle (Fig. 9-7). A deficiency of blood flow and oxygen to the myocardium is called **ischemia**.

One cause of plaque buildup in the coronary arteries is a condition called **hyperlipidemia**, which promotes blood clot formation.

Surgical procedures include the following:

- **Percutaneous transluminal coronary angioplasty** involves the insertion of a balloon-tipped catheter to open a blocked coronary artery (Fig. 9-8).
- **Arterial stent** includes the implantation of a stent, which is a mesh tube that is implanted into an artery to provide support (Fig. 9-9).
- **Coronary artery bypass graft**: open thoracic surgical procedure to graft another blood vessel to a blocked coronary artery (Fig. 9-10).
- **Endarterectomy** is the removal of the inner lining of a blocked artery.

Thrombosis

Thrombosis, also called a **thrombus**, in a blood vessel can impede blood flow to the myocardium and cause ischemia.

Myocardial Infarction

A **myocardial infarction** (**MI**), commonly called a heart attack, results from a lack of oxygen supply to the myocardium. Various diagnostic tests are used to identify abnormal cardiac function. Among these are an **electrocardiogram**, abbreviated ECG or EKG; **echocardiography** (ultrasonic examination of the heart); **cardiac catheterization** (insertion of a catheter and contrast dye into the coronary arteries to detect blockage); and a stress test.

A simple blood test to discover the presence of **troponin** may confirm a diagnosis of MI. Troponin is a protein released into the bloodstream when an MI occurs.

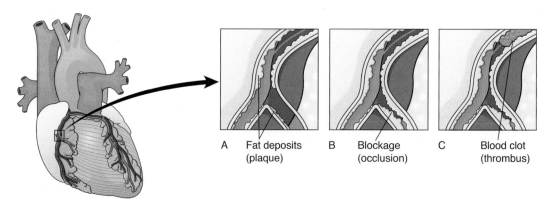

A   Fat deposits (plaque)   B   Blockage (occlusion)   C   Blood clot (thrombus)

FIGURE 9-7 Coronary atherosclerosis. Atherosclerosis (ather/o means "fatty"; scler/o means "hardening") is a progressive buildup of plaque that can cause the lumen of the coronary arteries, which nourish the myocardium to narrow. The formation of thrombi (plural for thrombus or clot) may occur as plaque accumulates in the lumen. *From Cohen BJ. Medical Terminology: An Illustrated Guide. 5th ed. Philadelphia, PA: Lippincott Williams & Wilkins; 2007.*

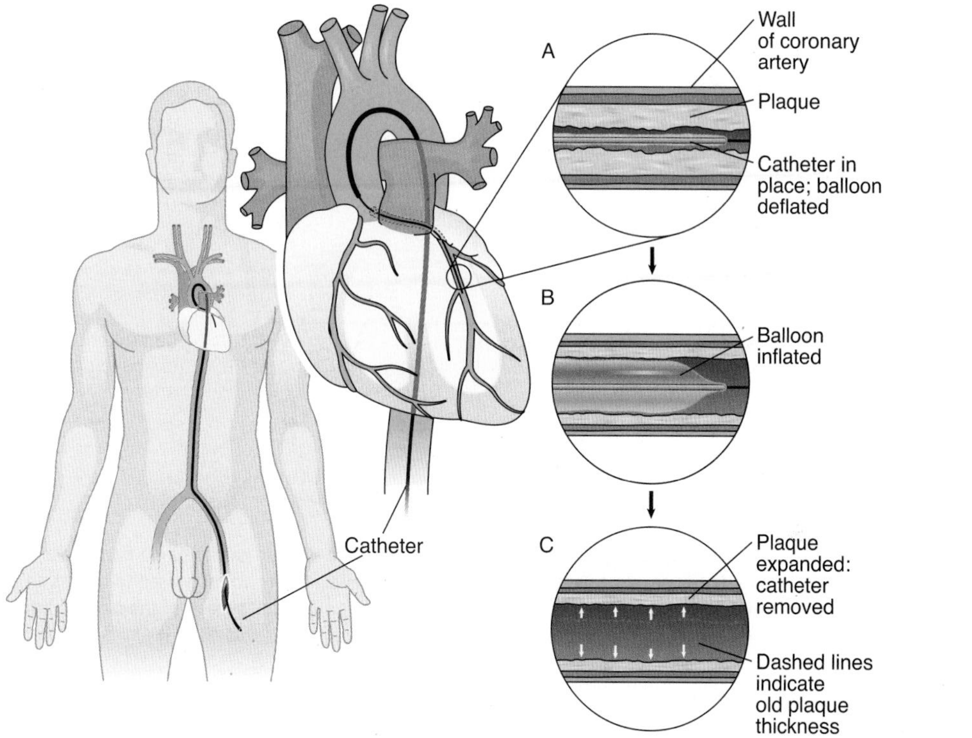

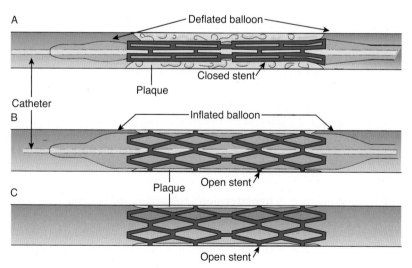

FIGURE 9-8 **Percutaneous transluminal coronary angioplasty. A.** Plaque deposits in the artery. **B.** Plaque buildup narrows the coronary vessel, impeding blood flow to the myocardium. **C.** The rough interior edges encourage clot formation in the artery. *From Cohen BJ. Medical Terminology: An Illustrated Guide. 5th ed. Philadelphia, PA: Lippincott Williams & Wilkins; 2007.*

FIGURE 9-9 **Arterial stent. A.** A balloon-tipped catheter is placed into the artery with the balloon deflated and the stent closed. **B.** When the stent is in the proper position of the narrowed artery, the balloon is inflated, causing the stent to open. **C.** The catheter is removed, and the stent remains in place. *From Cohen BJ. Medical Terminology: An Illustrated Guide. 5th ed. Philadelphia, PA: Lippincott Williams & Wilkins; 2007.*

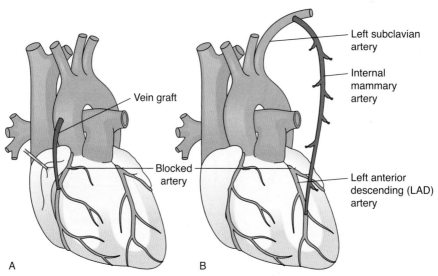

FIGURE 9-10   Coronary artery bypass graft. A. A segment of the saphenous vein carries blood from the aorta to a part of the right coronary artery that is distal to the occlusion. **B.** The internal mammary artery is used to bypass an obstruction in the left anterior descending coronary artery. The graft redirects the blood flow or "bypasses" the blocked artery. *Modified from Cohen BJ. Medical Terminology: An Illustrated Guide. 5th ed. Philadelphia, PA: Lippincott Williams & Wilkins; 2007.*

The acronym **MONA** is sometimes used to refer to standard emergency treatment for a suspected heart attack. M stands for morphine, O for oxygen, N for nitroglycerin, and A for aspirin.

Arrhythmias

An arrhythmia is any irregularity of the heart's rhythm, such as a slow or fast rate or extra beats. **Bradycardia** is a slower than normal heart rate, and **tachycardia** is a faster than normal rate. **Fibrillation** describes rapid, random, and ineffective contractions of the heart. Some arrhythmias are more serious than others. **Atrial fibrillation** occurs when the atria beat faster than the ventricles. This condition causes a quivering motion of the atria, which is usually not life threatening, although it can predispose the atria to thrombi formation. It affects many people and can often be controlled with drugs. Sustained **ventricular fibrillation**, which describes the condition in which the ventricles ineffectively pump blood, can be fatal.

    Cardioversion, a method of treatment for fibrillation, involves the application of an electric current to restore a normal heart rhythm. **Ablation therapy**, applying radiofrequency waves to the heart, is used to cure a variety of cardiac arrhythmias, such as some tachycardias and atrial fibrillation.

Hypertension

The term for high blood pressure is **hypertension** (abbreviated HTN). It occurs when the systolic reading exceeds 140 mmHg or the diastolic is greater than 90 mmHg. Over time, hypertension may lead to **arteriosclerosis** and/or **hypertrophy** of the left ventricle. When hypertension is related to another medical problem, such as a kidney disorder, it is called **secondary hypertension**.

Are atherosclerosis and arteriosclerosis the same ailment? Not exactly. A patient who has arteriosclerosis has hardening of the arteries caused by continuous high blood pressure. A patient with atherosclerosis has similar symptoms because his or her arteries have been narrowed by plaque buildup. So, a patient can have arteriosclerosis and not have atherosclerosis and vice versa. Both have the same symptoms, however, and some patients have both conditions.

Congestive Heart Failure

Congestive heart failure occurs when the heart cannot pump enough blood to meet the body's needs for oxygen and nutrients.

Blood Disorders

Any abnormality of the blood may be called a **dyscrasia**. There are three major types: **anemia**, **leukemia**, and **clotting disorders**:
- **Anemia** is caused by an abnormally low level of hemoglobin or low level of RBCs.
- **Leukemia** is characterized by an excessive increase in the number of WBCs.
- **Clotting disorders** include **hemophilia** (hereditary bleeding disorder), **thrombocytopenia** (an insufficient number of thrombocytes), and **disseminated intravascular coagulation** (extreme clotting caused by trauma or disease).

Abbreviation Table — THE CARDIOVASCULAR SYSTEM

ABBREVIATION	MEANING
A-fib	atrial fibrillation
AV	atrioventricular
BP	blood pressure
CABG	coronary artery bypass graft (open heart surgery)
CAD	coronary artery disease
CCU	cardiac care unit
CHF	congestive heart failure
CP	chest pain
DIC	disseminated intravascular coagulation
EKG or ECG	electrocardiogram, electrocardiograph, electrocardiography, cardiogram
Hb	hemoglobin (protein in the blood that carries oxygen)
HDL	high-density lipoprotein
HR	heart rate
HTN	hypertension
ICU	intensive care unit
LDL	low-density lipoprotein
MI	myocardial infarction
P	pulse
PTCA	percutaneous transluminal coronary angioplasty
RBC	red blood cell
SA	sinoatrial
SOB	shortness of breath
WBC	white blood cell
TIA	transient ischemic attack (This event affects the brain, which is part of the nervous system, and it is listed in Chapter 7. However, its effect on blood flow makes it relevant to the cardiovascular chapter as well. It is repeated here for that reason.)

Study Table / THE CARDIOVASCULAR SYSTEM

TERM AND PRONUNCIATION	ANALYSIS	MEANING
Structure and Function		
aorta (ay-OR-tah)	from the Greek word *aeirein* (to lift up or to be hung)	the main trunk of the systemic arterial system
aortic valve (ay-ORT-ik)	from the Greek word *aeirein* (to lift up or to be hung); from the Latin word *valva* (that which turns)	connects the left ventricle to the aorta
arteries (AR-tuh-rees)	from the Greek word *arteria* (windpipe)	the largest of the blood vessels that carry blood away from the heart
arterioles (ar-TEER-ee-oles)	from the Greek word *arteria* (windpipe)	the smallest arteries that connect with the capillaries
atria (singular: atrium) (AY-tree-ah; AY-tree-uhm)	a Latin word meaning "entry hall"	upper two of the four heart chambers, composed of the right atrium and left atrium
atrioventricular node (AY-tree-oh-ven-TRIK-u-lahr)	from the Latin word meaning "entry hall"; from the Latin *venter* (belly)	fibers located at the base of the right atrium near the ventricle that carry electrical stimulation to the bundle
basophil (BAY-soh-fil)	from the Greek *basis* and *philein* (to love)	a white blood cell with granules that stain with basic dyes
bicuspid or mitral valve (by-KUSS-pihd; MY-trahl)	*bi-* (two); from the Latin *cuspidem* (cusp or point); from the Latin *mitra* (turban); from the Latin word *valva* (that which turns)	connects the left atrium to the left ventricle
bundle of His	named for Swiss cardiologist Wilhelm His, Jr., who discovered the function of these cells in 1893	located at the top of the interventricular septum; carries electrical impulses from the atrioventricular node to Purkinje fibers
capillaries (KAP-ih-layr-ees)	from the Latin word *capillus* (hair)	the smallest of the blood vessels
cardiac cycle	*cardi/o* (heart); *-ac* (adjective ending)	a complete round of systole and diastole
diastole (dye-AS-toh-lee)	from the Greek word *diastole* (dilation)	relaxation phase of the heart
endocardium (en-doh-KAR-dee-uhm)	*endo-* (within); *cardi/o* (heart)	the inner surface of the heart
eosinophil (ee-oh-SIHN-oh-fil)	from the Greek words *eos* (dawn); *philein* (to love)	a white blood cell that stains with certain dyes
epicardium (ep-ih-KAR-dee-uhm)	*epi-* (on, upon); *cardi/o* (heart)	the outer covering of the heart

TERM AND PRONUNCIATION	ANALYSIS	MEANING
erythrocytes (er-RITH-ro-sites)	*erythr/o* (red); *-cyte* (cell)	red blood cells; abbreviated RBC
heart rate	common English words	the number of times per minute the heart contracts
hemoglobin (hee-mo-GLO-bihn)	*hem-* (blood); from the Latin *globus* (globe)	the protein that gives blood its red color; abbreviated Hb
inferior vena cava (VEE-nah KAV-ah)	*inferior*, a Latin word meaning "lower"; from the Latin words *vena* (vein); *cava* (hollow)	large vein that collects blood from the smaller veins of the lower body
left atrium (AY-tree-uhm)	a Latin word meaning "entry hall"	upper left heart chamber
left ventricle (VEN-trik-al)	from the Latin word *venter* (belly)	lower left heart chamber
leukocytes (LUKE-o-sytes)	*leuk/o* (white); *-cyte* (cell)	white blood cells; abbreviated WBC
mitral or bicuspid valve (MY-trahl; by-KUSS-pihd)	from the Latin word *mitra* (turban); from the Latin word *valva* (that which turns); *bi-* (two); from the Latin *cuspidem* (cusp or point)	connects the left atrium to the left ventricle
monocyte (MON-oh-site)	*mon/o* (single); *-cyte* (cell)	a relatively large white blood cell
myocardium (my-oh-KAR-dee-uhm)	*my/o* (muscle); *cardi/o* (heart)	the heart muscle, which includes nerves and blood vessels
neutrophil (NU-troh-fil)	from the Latin word *neuter* (neither); from the Greek word *philein* (to love)	a mature white blood cell normally constituting more than half of the total number of leukocytes
pericardial sac (pehr-ih-KAR-dee-ahl)	*peri-* (surrounding); *cardi/o* (heart); *-al* (adjective suffix)	another lining of the pericardium closest to the heart
pericardium (pehr-ih-KAR-dee-uhm)	*peri-* (surrounding); *cardi/o* (heart)	serous membrane lining the pericardial cavity
phagocyte (FAG-oh-site)	*phag/o* (eating, desiring); *-cyte* (cell)	a white blood cell capable of ingesting bacteria and other foreign matter
plasma (PLAZ-muh)	a Greek word meaning "something molded" or "created"	as differentiated from its non-medical context, the yellow fluid that makes up a bit more than half of whole blood by volume
platelets (PLATE-lets); also called thrombocytes (THROM-boh-sytes)	from the English word plate and the diminutive suffix *-let*	smallest of the formed elements; important in the coagulation process

(continued)

TERM AND PRONUNCIATION	ANALYSIS	MEANING
pulmonary artery (PULL-moh-nahr-ee)	*pulmon/o* (lung); from the Greek word *arteria* (windpipe)	vessel that carries deoxygenated blood from the right ventricle to the lungs
pulmonary valve (PULL-moh-nahr-ee)	*pulmon/o* (lung); from the Latin word *valva* (that which turns)	valve connecting the right ventricle and lungs
pulmonary veins (PULL-moh-nahr-ee vayns)	*pulmon/o* (lung); from the Latin word *vena* (blood vessel)	vessels that carry oxygenated blood from the lungs to the left atrium
pulse	from the Latin word *pulsum* (push, knock, drive)	rhythmic expansion and contraction of an artery produced by pressure of the blood moving through the artery
Purkinje fibers	named after Jan Evangelista Purkinje, who discovered them in 1839	fibers that carry stimulation throughout the ventricles
red blood cells	common English words	see erythrocyte
Rh factor	from rh(esus), so-called because the blood group was discovered in rhesus monkeys	an antigen, first discovered in the rhesus monkey; a person is either Rh positive or Rh negative
right atrium	a Latin word meaning "entry hall"	upper right heart chamber
right ventricle	from the Latin word *venter* (belly)	lower right heart chamber
septa (singular: septum) (SEPP-tah; SEPP-tuhm)	from the Latin word *saeptum* (a fence)	thin wall that separates cavities or masses; in the heart, septa separate the right atrium from the left atrium and the right ventricle from the left ventricle
sinoatrial node (SYE-noh-AY-tree-ahl)	from the Latin words *sinus* (bend, fold, curve) and *atrium* (entry hall)	known as the pacemaker of the heart; electrical impulse originates here
sinus rhythm (SYE-nus)	*sinus*, a Latin word meaning "bend," "fold," "curve"; from the Greek word *rhythmos* (measured flow or movement)	normal rhythm of the heartbeat
superior vena cava (VEE-nah KAV-ah)	*superior,* a Latin word meaning "higher"; from the Latin words *vena* (vein) and *cava* (hollow)	large vein that collects blood from the smaller veins of the upper body
systole (SIS-toh-lee)	a Greek word meaning "contraction"	contraction phase of the heart

TERM AND PRONUNCIATION	ANALYSIS	MEANING
tricuspid valve (try-KUSS-pihd)	*tri-* (three); from the Latin *cuspidem* (cusp or point)	valve connecting the right atrium to the right ventricle (right atrioventricular valve)
troponin (TROH-poh-nihn)	from the Greek word *trepein* (to turn)	a protein that is released into the bloodstream when a heart attack occurs
vascular (VASS-cue-lahr)	*vascul/o* (blood vessel); *-ar* (adjective suffix)	adjectival form of *vessel*
vasoconstriction (vaz-oh-CON-strik-shun)	*vas/o* (duct, blood vessel); from the Latin word *constringere* (to draw tight)	narrowing of the blood vessels
vasodilation (vaz-oh-DYE-lay-shun)	*vas/o* (duct, blood vessel); from the Latin word *dilatare* (to make wider, enlarge)	widening of the blood vessels
veins (VAYNS)	from the Latin word *vena* (vein)	the blood vessels that return blood from the tissues to the heart
venous (VEE-nuhs)	from the Latin word *vena* (vein)	adjectival form of *vein*
venules (VEE-nuhls)	from the Latin *venula* (diminutive form of *vena* [vein])	small veins
ventricle (VEN-trik-uhl)	from the Latin word *venter* (belly)	lower two of the four heart chambers, composed of the right ventricle and left ventricle
white blood cells	common English words	formed element in the blood that protects the body against harmful bacteria

Common Disorders

anemia (ah-NEE-mee-a)	from the Greek word *anaimia* (without blood)	abnormally low red blood cell count
aneurysm (AN-yur-iz-um)	from the Greek word *aneurysmos* (to dilate)	a localized dilation of an artery, cardiac chamber, or other vessel
angina pectoris (an JY-nah-pek-TOR-ihs)	from the Greek word *agkhone* (a strangling); also *angere* (anguish); *pectoris*, a Latin word meaning "chest"	pain in the chest due to ischemia
angiospasm (AN-jee-o-spaz-uhm)	*angi/o* (blood vessel); from the Greek word *spasmos* (spasm)	spasm in blood vessels
angiostenosis (AN-jee-o-steh-NO-siss)	*angi/o* (blood vessel); *-stenosis* (a narrowing)	narrowing of a blood vessel
arrhythmia (ah-RITH-mee-ah)	*a-* (without); from the Greek word *rhythmos* (measured flow or movement); *-ia* (condition)	abnormal rhythm; irregular heartbeat

(continued)

TERM AND PRONUNCIATION	ANALYSIS	MEANING
arteriosclerosis (ar-TEER-ee-o-sklu-RO-sis)	from the Greek word *arteria* (windpipe); *scler/o* (hardness); *-osis* (abnormal condition of)	hardening of the arteries
arteriospasm (ar-TEER-ee-o-spaz-uhm)	from the Greek word *arteria* (windpipe); from the Greek word *spasmos* (a spasm or convulsion)	spasm of an artery
arteriostenosis (ar-TEER-ee-oh-steh-NO-sihs)	from the Greek word *arteria* (windpipe); *-steno* (narrow); *-osis* (abnormal condition)	narrowing of an artery
arteritis (ar-tur-EYE-tihs)	from the Greek word *arteria* (windpipe); *-itis* (inflammation)	inflammation of an artery or arteries
atheroma (ath-er-OH-mah)	from the Greek word *ather* (groats, porridge); *-oma* (tumor)	fatty deposit or plaque within the arterial wall
atherosclerosis (ath-er-oh-skleh-ROH-sis)	from the Greek word *ather* (groats, porridge); *scler/o* (hardening); *-osis* (abnormal condition of)	hardening and narrowing of the arteries
atrial fibrillation (fih-brih-LAY-shun)	from the Latin word *atrium* (entry hall) *-al* (adjective suffix); from the Latin word *fibra* (fiber, string, thread)	rapid, random, ineffective contractions of the atrium
atriomegaly (AY-tree-oh-MEG-ah-lee)	from the Latin word *atrium* (hall); *-megaly* (enlargement)	enlargement of an atrium
bradycardia (bray-dee-KAR-dee-ah)	*brady-* (slow); *cardi/o* (heart); *-ia* (condition)	abnormally slow heartbeat
cardiac arrest (KAR-dee-ak)	*cardi/o* (heart); from the Latin words *ad* and *restare* (to stop, remain behind)	cessation of heart activity
cardiodynia (kar-dee-oh-DIN-ee-ah)	*cardi/o* (heart); *-dynia* (pain)	heart pain
cardiomalacia (kar-dee-oh-mah-LASH-ee-ah	*cardi/o* (heart); *-malacia* (softening)	softening of the heart
cardiomegaly (kar-dee-oh-MEG-ah-lee)	*cardi/o* (heart); *-megaly* (enlargement)	enlargement of the heart
cardiomyopathy (kar-dee-oh-my-AWP-uh-thee)	*cardi/o* (heart); *my/o* (muscle); *-pathy* (disease)	disease of the heart muscle (myocardium)
cardiopathy (kar-dee-AWP-uh-thee)	*cardi/o* (heart); *-pathy* (disease)	any heart disease
cardiorrhexis (kar-dee-oh-REX-ihs)	*cardi/o* (heart); *-rrhexis* (rupture)	rupture in the wall of the heart
carditis (kar-DY-tiss)	*cardi/o* (heart); *-itis* (inflammation)	inflammation of the heart

TERM AND PRONUNCIATION	ANALYSIS	MEANING
congestive heart failure	from the Latin word *congerere* (to bring together, pile up)	syndrome where the heart is unable to pump enough blood to meet the body's needs for oxygen and nutrients; as a result, fluid is retained and accumulates in the ankles and legs
disseminated intravascular coagulation (dih-SEMM-ihn-ayted ihn-tra-VASS-kyu-lahr koh-AG-yu-LAY-shun)	from the Latin *dis-* (in every direction); *seminare* (to plant, propagate); *intra-* (within); *vascul/o* (vessel); *-ar* (adjective suffix); coagulation (from the Latin verb *coagulo* [curdle])	widespread clotting and obstruction of blood flow to the tissues
dyscrasia (dys-KRAY-sha)	*dys-* (bad, difficult); from the Greek word *krasis* (mingling)	general term for a blood disorder
endocarditis (en-doh-kar-DY-tiss)	*endo-* (within); *cardi/o* (heart); *-itis* (inflammation)	inflammation of the endocardium
hemolysis (hee-MAWL-ih-sihs)	*hem/o* (blood); *-lysis* (destruction)	change or destruction of red blood cells
hemophilia (hee-mo-FEEL-ee-ya)	*hem/o* (blood); *-phil(ia)* (attraction)	congenital disorder impeding the coagulation process
hemorrhage (HEM-o-rij)	*hem/o* (blood); *-rrhage* (burst forth)	discharge of blood
hyperlipidemia (high-per-LIP-ih-DEE-mee-ah)	*hyper-* (above normal); *lip/o* (fat); *-demia* (from hema [blood])	elevated cholesterol, triglycerides, and lipoproteins in the blood
hypertension	*hyper-* (above normal); from the Latin word *tendere* (to stretch)	elevated blood pressure (>140/90 mmHg)
ischemia (is-KEE-mee-ah)	from the Greek word *iskhaimos* (a stopping of the blood); *-ia* (condition)	deficiency in blood supply to the tissues
myocardial infarction (my-oh-KAR-dee-ahl in-FARK-shun) (MI) (Note: MI is an abbreviation, not an acronym.)	*my/o* (muscle); *cardi/o* (heart); *-al* (adjective suffix); from the Latin word *infractionem* (a breaking)	heart attack
myocarditis (my-oh-kar-DY-tiss)	*my/o* (muscle); *cardi/o* (heart); *-itis* (inflammation)	inflammation of the heart muscle
pericarditis (pehr-ih-kar-DY-tiss)	*peri-* (surrounding); *cardi/o* (heart); *-itis* (inflammation)	inflammation of the pericardium
tachycardia (tak-ih-KAR-dee-ah)	*tachy-* (fast); *cardi/o* (heart); *-ia* (condition)	abnormally rapid heartbeat

(continued)

TERM AND PRONUNCIATION	ANALYSIS	MEANING
thrombocytopenia (THROM-boh-sigh-toh-PEE-nee-ah)	*thromb/o* (blood clot); *cyt/o* (cell); *-penia* (deficiency)	abnormal decrease in the number of thrombocytes or platelets
transient ischemic attack	isch: root from the Greek word for restricting or thinning; *-emia*, suffix referring to blood	transient ischemic attack
thrombus (THROM-bus)	*thromb/o* (blood clot)	blood clot attached to an interior wall of a vein or artery
valvulitis (valv-yu-LY-tiss)	from the Latin word *valva* (that which turns); *-itis* (inflammation)	inflammation of a heart valve
vasculitis (also angiitis)	*vascul/o* (blood vessel); *-itis* (inflammation)	inflammation of a vessel
vasoconstriction (VAZE-o-kon-STRIK-shun)	*vas/o* (duct, blood vessel); from the Latin word *constingere* (to draw tight)	narrowing of the arteries
vasodilation (VAZE-o-dy-LAY-shun) (also sometimes vasodilatation)	*vas/o* (vessel); from the Latin word *dilitare* (to make wider)	the widening of the arteries
Diagnosis and Treatment		
ablation (ah-BLAY-shun)	from the Latin words *ab-* (away); and *latus* (brought)	partial destruction of the pathway of the electrical conduction system of the heart to treat irregular heart rhythms
angiogram (AN-jee-o-gram)	*angi/o* (blood vessel); *-gram* (record or picture)	printed record obtained through angiography
angiography (an-jee-AWG-ruff-ee)	*angi/o* (blood vessel); *-graphy* (process of recording)	radiography of a blood vessel after injection of a contrast medium
antianginals	*anti-* (against); *angi/o* (blood vessel); *-al* (adjective suffix)	drugs used to treat chest pain
antiarrhythmics	*anti-* (against); *a-* (without); from the Greek word *rhythmos* (measured flow or movement)	drug used to treat rhythm abnormalities
cardiac catheterization (KATH-eh-ter-eye-zay-shun)	*cardi/o* (heart); *-ac* (pertaining to); from the Greek word *kathienai* (to let down, thrust in)	procedure where a catheter is inserted into an artery and guided into the heart; may be used for diagnosis of blockages or treatment

TERM AND PRONUNCIATION	ANALYSIS	MEANING
cardiac glycosides	*cardi/o* (heart); *-ac* (pertaining to); *glyc/o* (sugar) + *-ide*	drugs used to improve heart output by increasing the muscular contraction
cardiogram (KAR-dee-oh-gram) (Note: Associated terms are electrocardiogram [ee-LEK-troh-KAR-dee-oh-gram] and electrocardiograph [ee-LEK-troh-KAR-dee-oh-graf]; the abbreviation for any of them can be either EKG or ECG.)	*cardi/o* (heart); *-gram* (record or picture)	a graphic trace of electrical activity in the heart
cardioversion (KAR-dee-oh-VER-zhun)	*cardi/o* (heart); from the Latin word *vertere* (to turn)	use of electrical shock to restore the heart's normal rhythm
diuretic (DYE-ur-eh-tik)	from the Greek word *diouretikos* (prompting urine)	a drug used to increase urine production or urination
echocardiography (EK-oh-KAR-dee-AH-grah-fee)	from the Greek word *ekhe* (sound); *cardi/o* (heart); *-graphy* (process of recording)	ultrasonic procedure used to evaluate the structure and motion of the heart
nuclear stress test	common English words	assessment of blood flow through the heart through the use of a nuclear element injection while the patient exercises
sphygmomanometer (SFIG-moh-mah-NOM-eh-ter)	from the Greek words *sphygmos* (pulse), *manos* (thin), *metros* (measure)	instrument used to measure blood pressure
statins	from lovastatin, from *lo* + *vastatin* (stuff)	a type of cholesterol-lowering drug
stent	English word *stenting* refers to the process of stiffening	a device implanted into an artery to open and provide support to the arterial wall
ventricular fibrillation (ven-TRIK-yu-lahr fih-brih-LAY-shun)	from the Latin *ventriculus* (little belly); *-ar* (adjective suffix); from the Latin word *fibra* (fiber, string, thread)	irregular contractions of the ventricles; may be fatal unless reversed
Practice and Practitioners		
cardiologist (kar-dee-AWL-oh-jist)	*cardi/o* (heart); *-logist* (one who specializes)	heart specialist
cardiology (kar-dee-AWL-oh-jee)	*cardi/o* (heart); *-logy* (study of)	medical specialty dealing with the heart
hematologist (HEE-mah-tah-lo-gist)	*hemat/o* (blood); *-logist* (one who specializes)	blood specialist
hematology (HEE-mah-TAH-lo-jee)	*hemat/o* (blood); *-logy* (study of)	medical specialty dealing with blood

(continued)

TERM AND PRONUNCIATION	ANALYSIS	MEANING
Surgical Procedures		
angioplasty (AN-jee-o-plass-tee)	*angi/o* (blood vessel); *-plasty* (surgical repair)	surgical repair of a blood vessel
atrioseptoplasty (AY-tree-o-SEP-toh-plass-tee)	from the Latin words *atrium* (entry hall) and *saeptum* (fence); *-plasty* (surgical repair)	surgical repair of an atrial septum
cardiotomy (kar-dee-AW-tuh-mee)	*cardi/o* (heart); *-tomy* (cutting operation)	incision into the heart or incision into the cardia of the stomach
coronary artery bypass graft	from the Latin *cor* (heart); common English words	through an open chest, a graft (piece of vein or other heart artery) is implanted on the heart to bypass a blockage
endarterectomy (end-art-er-ECK-toh-mee)	*endo-* (within); *arteri/o* (artery); *-ectomy* (excision)	surgical removal of the lining of an artery
pericardiotomy (PEHR-ih-car-dee-AW-toh-mee)	*peri-* (surrounding); *cardi/o* (heart); *-tomy* (cutting operation)	incision into the pericardium
valvoplasty (VALV-oh-plass-tee); also valvuloplasty (VALV-yu-loh-plass-tee)	from the Latin word *valva* (that which turns); *-plasty* (surgical repair)	surgical repair of a heart valve
valvotomy (valv-AW-toh-mee); also valvulotomy (valv-yu-LAWT-oh-mee)	from the Latin word *valva* (that which turns); *-tomy* (cutting operation)	surgical removal of a blocked heart valve (stenosis of a heart valve) by cutting into it

EXERCISES

 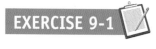 FIGURE LABELING: THE BLOOD FLOW THROUGH THE HEART

Label the parts of the heart using the terms listed.

aorta	left ventricle	pulmonary valve	right ventricle
aortic valve	mitral or bicuspid valve	pulmonary veins	superior and inferior venae cavae
left atrium	pulmonary arteries	right atrium	tricuspid valve

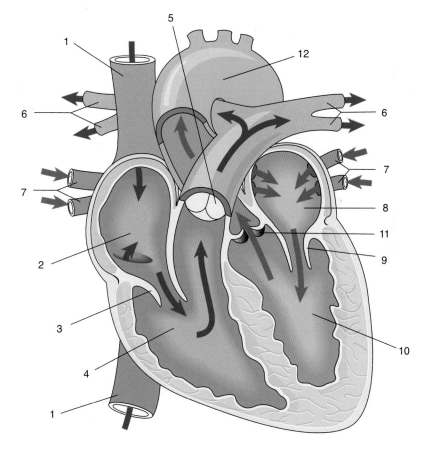

1. _____   7. _____

2. _____   8. _____

3. _____   9. _____

4. _____   10. _____

5. _____   11. _____

6. _____   12. _____

EXERCISE 9-2   CASE STUDY

BRIEF HISTORY: The patient is a 56-year-old male who had been complaining of recurrent chest pain when performing mild activities at home. The chest pain subsides when he lies down. He also has experienced shortness of breath (SOB) when carrying in the groceries and climbing up one set of stairs. He has a history of high blood pressure.

EMERGENCY ROOM VISIT: The patient arrives at the emergency room with angina pectoris that is relieved by rest, a blood pressure of 180/110 mmHg, and SOB. An EKG is performed that indicates the patient is having atrial arrhythmias and an MI. He is given aspirin and started on antiarrhythmics, diuretics, vasodilators, and oxygen. He is admitted to the CCU for observation and treatment.

DIAGNOSIS: Hypertension, an MI, and atrial fibrillation.

Answer the following questions using information learned in this chapter and found in the chapter tables.

1. Define angina pectoris. _____

2. What does the acronym SOB stand for? _____

3. What is hypertension? _____

4. What is an EKG? _____

5. What type of pharmacologic intervention is used with this patient? Define each drug classification. _____

   _____

6. What is an MI? What are the two roots in myocardial, and what do they mean?

   _____

   _____

7. Define atrial fibrillation. _____

EXERCISE 9-3 WORD BUILDING: THE CARDIOVASCULAR SYSTEM

Using this chapter and the knowledge you've gained from the previous chapters, complete this exercise. The word elements are provided in the table for you.

a-, an-	-ectomy	-lysis	-spasm
angio/o	-emia	-megaly	-stenosis
arteri/o	erythr/o	my/o	thromb/o
ather/o	-genic	-oma	-tomy
atri/o	hem/o; hemat/o	-penia	valv/o
cardi/o	-ic, -ia, -ac, -al, -ar, -ary -ous, -um	peri-	vas/o
-cyte	inter-	-philia	ven/o
-dilation	leuk/o	-rhythm	ventricul/o

1. originating in the heart _____

2. an incision into the atrium _____

3. a red blood cell _____

4. hereditary bleeding disorder caused by a deficiency of a clotting factor _____

5. spasm of a vein _____

6. removal of a blood clot _____

7. dilation of a vessel _____

8. enlargement of the heart _____

9. narrowing of an artery _____

10. fatty plaque _____

11. a white blood cell _____

12. the surgical removal of a valve _____

13. pertaining to the heart _____

14. destruction of red blood cells _____

15. between the ventricles _____

16. an abnormally low level of hemoglobin _____

17. heart muscle _____

18. removal of a fatty plaque _____

19. abnormal heart rhythm _____

EXERCISE 9-4   SPELLING

In the space provided, write the correct spelling of the misspelled terms.

1. throbcytpenia   _____

2. oyxgen   _____

3. mycardial   _____

4. iscemia   _____

5. artrectomy   _____

6. atriventrcular   _____

7. lukemia   _____

8. athrosclersis   _____

9. semiluner   _____

10. distolic   _____

EXERCISE 9-5   MATCHING

Match the term in Column B with the correct definition in Column A.

COLUMN A	COLUMN B
1. _____ pacemaker of the heart	A. ischemia
2. _____ electric current used to restore normal sinus rhythm	B. anemia
3. _____ surgical removal of the inner lining of an artery	C. cardioversion
4. _____ abnormality of the blood	D. SA node
5. _____ thrombocytes	E. hemoglobin
6. _____ a protein in the RBC	F. vasoconstriction
7. _____ deficiency of blood flow to an organ	G. tricuspid valve
8. _____ vessels are narrowed	H. endarterectomy
9. _____ low level of hemoglobin in the blood	I. platelets
10. _____ between the right atrium and right ventricle	J. dyscrasia

EXERCISE 9-6 📋 WRITE THE ABBREVIATION

1. coronary artery disease   _____

2. high-density lipoprotein   _____

3. intensive care unit   _____

4. congestive heart failure   _____

5. myocardial infarction   _____

6. electrocardiogram, electrocardiograph,   _____
   electrocardiography, cardiogram

7. percutaneous transluminal   _____
   coronary angioplasty

8. red blood cell   _____

9. atrioventricular   _____

10. shortness of breath   _____

11. pulse   _____

12. cardiac care unit   _____

13. hypertension   _____

14. atrial fibrillation   _____

15. coronary artery bypass graft   _____
    (open heart surgery)

16. sinoatrial   _____

17. transient ischemic attack   _____

18. disseminated intravascular coagulation   _____

19. chest pain   _____

20. low-density lipoprotein   _____

21. hemoglobin   _____

22. heart rate   _____

23. blood pressure   _____

24. white blood cell   _____

EXERCISE 9-7   CROSSWORD PUZZLE: THE CARDIOVASCULAR SYSTEM

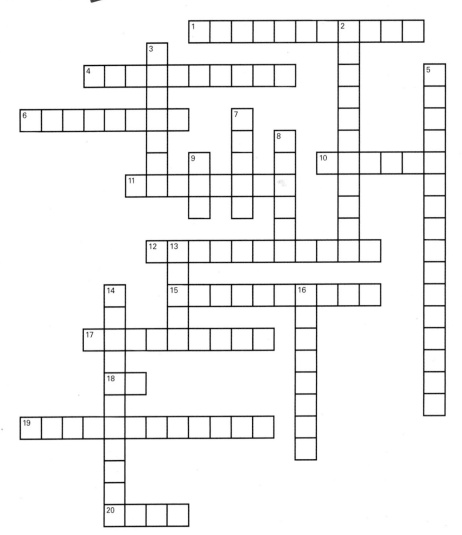

ACROSS

1. process of blood clotting
4. small arteries
6. blood clot
10. valve between the left ventricle and aorta
11. deficiency of oxygen to the tissues
12. smallest blood vessels
15. study of blood
17. any abnormality of the blood
18. abbreviation for hemoglobin
19. white cells ingest bacteria
20. suffix for blood

DOWN

2. another term for platelet
3. small veins
5. narrowing of blood vessels
7. swelling due to excessive fluid
8. fluid portion of the blood
9. abbreviation for congestive heart failure
13. root for "fatty"
14. red blood cell
16. malignant overgrowth of immature white blood cells

CHAPTER 9 QUIZ

Multiple Choice

1. A reduction in white blood cells is called:
   - a. eosinophil
   - b. polycythemia
   - c. leukopenia
   - d. anemia

2. An increase in red blood cells is called:
   - a. eosinophil
   - b. sickle cell
   - c. polycythemia
   - d. erythrocytopenia

3. Which of the following is a type of white blood cell?
   - a. thrombocyte
   - b. eosinophil
   - c. erythrocyte
   - d. platelet

4. What is the term that describes the destruction of bacteria by special white blood cells?
   - a. phagocytosis
   - b. leukocytosis
   - c. erythrocytosis
   - d. neutrophilosis

5. Platelets are also referred to as:
   - a. erythrocytes
   - b. thrombocytes
   - c. basophils
   - d. neutrophils

6. Oxygen-carrying pigment of red blood cells is called:
   - a. hematocrit
   - b. hemoglobin
   - c. leukemia
   - d. gamma globulin

7. The "universal recipient" is what blood type?
   - a. O
   - b. A
   - c. B
   - d. AB

8. Which of the following is a malignant disease of the hematopoietic organs (blood)?
   - a. leukemia
   - b. leukopenia
   - c. erythropenia
   - d. thrombosis

9. Which of the following terms describes hardened tissue?
   - a. sclerotic
   - b. thrombotic
   - c. occluded
   - d. fibrillated

10. What is the name of the artery that carries blood out of the heart to the lung?
    - a. jugular
    - b. venous
    - c. pulmonary
    - d. aorta

11. The study of the heart and heart conditions is called:
    - a. cardiology
    - b. cardiopathology
    - c. cardiopathy
    - d. myocardiology

12. An incision into a vein is called:
    - a. phlebitis
    - b. phlebotomy
    - c. phlebostomy
    - d. venitis

13. The heart muscle is supplied with blood vessels called:
    a. capillaries
    b. coronaries
    c. corpuscles
    d. carpals

14. The term for low blood pressure is:
    a. tachycardia
    b. bradycardia
    c. hypertension
    d. hypotension

15. The term for a rapid pulse rate is:
    a. hypertension
    b. tachycardia
    c. hypotension
    d. brachypnea

16. What is the function of a leukocyte?
    a. transports O_2
    b. manufactures Hgb
    c. initiates coagulation
    d. defends against disease

17. Which of the following means "one who studies cells"?
    a. hematology
    b. hematologist
    c. cytology
    d. cytologist

18. Which is the smallest blood vessel?
    a. artery
    b. arteriole
    c. vein
    d. capillary

19. Which of the following is characteristic of the artery in arteriostenosis?
    a. hardened
    b. soft
    c. dilated
    d. narrowed

20. What is the term for the area between the ventricles?
    a. intraventricular
    b. interdermal
    c. intracranial
    d. interventricular

10 *The Lymphatic System and Immunity*

LEARNING OBJECTIVES

Upon completion of this chapter, you should be able to:

- Define the terms that name the structures and functions of the lymphatic system.
- Define immunity.
- Define the terms that name the disorders and treatments of the lymphatic system.
- Build, spell, and pronounce medical terms that relate to the lymphatic system and immunity.

INTRODUCTION

The lymphatic system is a network of organs, tissues, and vessels spread throughout the body. Medically speaking, *immunity* refers to the body's capacity to resist disease, and some organizers of the body into systems prefer to call this capacity a system. Within such an organization, the immune system encompasses the lymphatic organs, tissues, and vessels. However, because the lymphatic system and the cardiovascular system share a capillary network, it makes at least some sense to use the name lymphatic system instead.

The lymphatic system distributes a fluid, called **lymph**, on a one-way path, whereas the cardiovascular system circulates blood within a closed system. Nevertheless, lymph is similar to blood in that it contains special cells called **lymphocytes**, which are a type of white blood cell that fights disease and infection.

A major function of the lymphatic system is to protect the body from infection. Its other two major functions are to maintain a balance of fluid and to absorb fats that are broken down in the digestive tract.

> What is lymph? Like blood plasma, lymph is a fluid that consists mostly of water. It also contains a low concentration of proteins in solution and, of course, lymphocytes. The word lymph is also used as an adjective in naming lymph vessels, lymph nodes, and so on. A second adjective, lymphatic, is most often used when referring either to the whole system or to some specific part of the system, such as the right lymphatic duct. Either adjective, however, is acceptable in any context.

WORD ELEMENTS FOUND IN LYMPHATIC SYSTEM TERMS

Table 10-1 lists most of the elements that make up lymphatic system terms. Suffixes and prefixes that may already have been learned are also listed.

STRUCTURE AND FUNCTION

The lymphatic system consists of lymph vessels, lymph, special lymphoid tissues called lymph nodes, and lymph organs. All of these structures play an important role in the body's immune responses. As mentioned previously, one of the other major functions of the lymphatic system is to

TABLE 10-1	WORD ELEMENTS USED TO FORM LYMPHATIC SYSTEM TERMS
Word Element	**Refers to**
an-	without
immun/o	immune system
lymphaden/o	lymph nodes
lymphangi/o	lymph vessels
lymph/o, lymphat/o	lymph or lymphatic system
-megaly	enlargement
phag/o	ingest or engulf
-phylaxis	protection
splen/o	spleen
thym/o	thymus
-oid	resembling
tonsill/o	lymph node, usually palatine tonsil

Word Elements Exercise   FILL IN THE BLANKS

Study Table 10-1 before attempting to complete this exercise. Then write a brief meaning for each of the word elements listed below.

1. immun/o   _____

2. phag/o   _____

3. -phylaxis   _____

4. -megaly   _____

5. tonsill/o   _____

6. splen/o   _____

7. an-   _____

8. lymphaden/o   _____

9. lymphangi/o   _____

10. lymph/o, lymphat/o   _____

11. thym/o   _____

12. -oid   _____

maintain fluid balance in the body. This function is accomplished through a complex network of structures composed of vessels and tissues. These structures are discussed first.

Lymphatic Structures

The lymph capillaries are similar to blood capillaries in that they are thin-walled tubes that carry fluid to larger vessels (Fig. 10-1). The fluid they carry is, of course, lymph, a clear yellowish liquid that is collected from tissues after it seeps out of capillaries of the cardiovascular system. Lymph contains lymphocytes, which attack and destroy foreign organisms. Lymph is picked up by the lymph vessels, filtered by the lymph nodes, propelled back into the venules, and then into the veins (Fig. 10-2).

Lymph nodes are small, bean-shaped structures that filter out harmful substances such as bacteria and viruses. When disease or infection is present, lymph nodes swell with lymph fluid, indicating that the lymphatic system is at work defending against an invading organism.

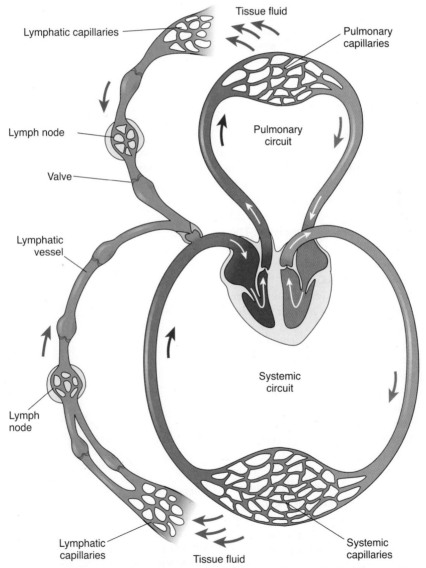

FIGURE 10-1 The lymphatic system in relation to the cardiovascular system. The lymphatic capillaries pick up the fluid in the tissues that exits from the blood capillaries. The fluid circulates in the lymph system and is returned to the blood vessels near the heart. *Modified from Cohen BJ, Taylor J. Memmler's Structure and Function of the Human Body. 8th ed. Baltimore, MD: Lippincott Williams & Wilkins; 2005.*

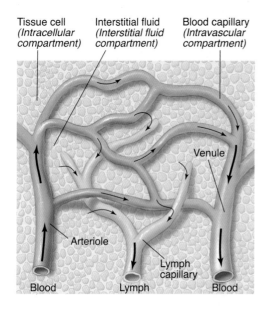

Tissue cell
(Intracellular
compartment)

Interstitial fluid
(Interstitial fluid
compartment)

Blood capillary
(Intravascular
compartment)

Venule

Arteriole

Lymph
capillary

Blood   Lymph   Blood

FIGURE 10-2 **Lymph flow.** Fluid travels from the arterioles to the venules. Some of the fluid that leaks out of the blood capillaries is left in the tissues (interstitial fluid). This fluid is picked up by the open-ended lymph capillaries and circulates in the lymph system as lymph. It travels in the lymphatic system until it is returned to the bloodstream. *From Premkumar K.* The Massage Connection Anatomy and Physiology. *Baltimore, MD: Lippincott Williams & Wilkins; 2004.*

Lymphatic Organs

There are four protective organs composed of lymphoid tissues that play a role in immunity. They are the **tonsils**, **spleen**, **thymus gland**, and the **appendix** (Fig. 10-3).

- The tonsils are located in the pharynx to filter out bacteria.
- The spleen is located in the upper left quadrant of the abdomen, where it filters bacteria from the blood and removes old blood cells by means of **hemolysis**. The process by which the lymphocytes engulf the bacteria and debris in the spleen is called **phagocytosis**.
- The thymus gland is located above the heart. Its job is to process lymphocytes and stimulate immunity.
- The appendix, which is attached to the large intestine, contributes to the development of immunity. The digestive system also includes **Peyer's patches**, which are small bundles of lymphoid tissue on the walls of the small intestine. Peyer's patches also protect against invading organisms (see Fig. 10-3).

The lymphatic organs are of paramount importance in immunity, which includes different types, such as **natural immunity**, **acquired immunity**, and **artificial immunity**. Natural immunity is passed on from mother to child before birth. Acquired immunity is obtained as a result of having had a disease of which a special "memory" remains. Artificial immunity, also called immunization, is acquired through vaccinations.

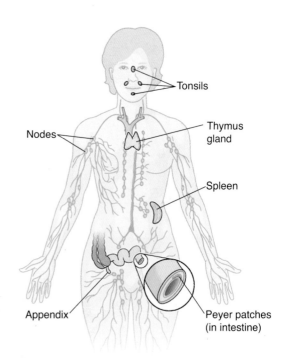

Tonsils

Thymus
gland

Nodes

Spleen

Appendix

Peyer patches
(in intestine)

FIGURE 10-3 **Location of lymphoid tissues and protective organs.** Lymph tissues and organs. Peyer's patches are found in the lining of the intestine and help to protect against invading organisms. *Modified from Cohen BJ.* Medical Terminology: An Illustrated Guide. *5th ed. Philadelphia, PA: Lippincott Williams & Wilkins; 2007.*

Quick Check: A Few Key Terms

Fill in the blanks.

1. Besides fighting infection, the lymphatic system maintains _____ _____ within the body.

2. The four protective lymphatic organs are the _____, _____, _____, and the _____.

3. Artificial immunity is also called _____.

PRACTICE AND PRACTITIONERS

Allergists specialize in diagnosing and treating altered immunologic and allergic conditions, and **hematologists** provide diagnosis and treatment of blood and blood-forming tissue disorders. An **immunologist** is a specialist who studies, diagnoses, and treats problems with immunity. **Oncologists** may become involved in the care of patients with tumors.

DISORDERS AND TREATMENTS

A primary function of the lymphatic system is to filter out harmful organisms. When bacteria spreads into the lymphatic system or when an injury to the body is not treated effectively, however, an infection can result in **lymphadenitis**. Lymph tissue swelling, called **lymphedema**, can result from infection or obstruction of the lymph vessels. **Lymphadenopathy** that produces enlarged lymph nodes is an indicator of possible infection. Lymph and immune disorders include the following:

- **Acquired immunodeficiency syndrome** is caused by the human immunodeficiency virus, an infectious process characterized by swollen lymph glands or lymphadenopathy.
- **Infectious mononucleosis** is an acute infection also caused by a virus.
- **Splenomegaly** may occur with other infectious diseases.
- **Anaphylaxis** is a life-threatening reaction to a foreign substance.
- **Hodgkin's lymphoma** is a malignant disease of the lymph nodes.
- **Rheumatoid arthritis** is an autoimmune disorder.
- **Systemic lupus** is a chronic inflammatory disorder that affects multiple body systems.

A range of treatments exists for treating lymphatic disorders. They include corticosteroids for relief of inflammation, immunosuppressants, and antiviral agents to reduce the body's reactions to foreign substances, and vaccination to offer artificial immunity.

Abbreviation Table THE LYMPHATIC SYSTEM AND IMMUNITY

ABBREVIATION	MEANING
AIDS	acquired immunodeficiency syndrome
CBC	complete blood count
HIV	human immunodeficiency virus
HLA	human leukocyte antigen
RA	rheumatoid arthritis
RIA	radioimmunoassay
SLE	systemic lupus erythematosus (usually shortened to lupus), an autoimmune disorder

Study Table | THE LYMPHATIC SYSTEM AND IMMUNITY

TERM AND PRONUNCIATION	ANALYSIS	MEANING
Structure and Function		
acquired immunity	common English words	resistance resulting from previous exposure to an infectious agent
allergen (AL-ur-jehn)	from the Greek word *allos* (other); *-gen* (producing)	an allergy-producing substance
antibody	*anti-* (against) + body	a molecule generated in specific opposition to an antigen
antigen (AN-tih-jehn)	*anti-* (against); *-gen* (producing)	substance that induces sensitivity or an immune response in the form of antibodies
appendix (ah-PEN-dicks)	from the Latin verb *appendum* (attach)	wormlike dead-end projection that is attached to the intestine
artificial immunity	common English words	immunization; immunity acquired from a vaccination
autoimmunity (aw-toh-ih-MYUN-iht-ee)	*auto-* (self) + immunity	literally, immune to oneself
inflammation (in-flah-MAAY-shun)	common English word	redness and irritation caused by injury or abnormal stimulation by a physical, chemical, or biologic agent
leukocyte (LUKE-oh-site)	*leuk/o* (white); *-cyte* (cell)	white blood cell
lymph (limf)	from the Latin word *lympha* (water, clear water, goddess of water)	fluid that flows through the lymphatic system; adjective synonymous with *lymphatic*
lymphatic system (lihm-FAT-tik)	*lymph/o* (lymph); *-atic* (adjective suffix)	collectively, the vessels, nodes, and capillaries that carry the lymph and its disease-fighting cells to the areas in which they are needed
lymphocyte (LIHM-foh-syte)	*lymph/o* (lymph); *-cyte* (cell)	white blood cell in the lymphatic system
macrophage (MAK-roh-fayj)	*macro-* (large); *phag/o* (ingest or engulf)	large phagocyte
microphage (MIKE-roh-fayj)	*micro-* (small); *phag/o* (ingest or engulf)	small phagocyte
monocyte (MON-oh-site)	*mono-* (single); *-cyte* (cell)	a type of white blood cell
natural immunity	common English words	resistance manifested by an individual who has not been immunized; immunity passed on from mother to fetus
neutrophil (NU-troh-fil)	*neutr/o* (neutral); *-phil* (love)	a granulocyte that is the chief phagocytic white blood cell

TERM AND PRONUNCIATION	ANALYSIS	MEANING
pathogen (PATH-oh-jehn)	*path/o* (disease); *-gen* (produce)	substance that produces disease
phagocyte (FAG-oh-syte)	*phag/o* (ingest or engulf); *-cyte* (cell)	white blood cell that clears away pathogens and debris
phagocytosis (FAG-oh-sy-toh-sis)	*phag/o* (ingest or engulf); *cyt/o* (cell); *-osis* (condition of)	process carried out by white blood cells
reaction (ree-AK-shun)	common English word	an action of an antibody on a specific antigen; also, in reference to immune responses, an abnormal or unwanted reaction
spleen (SPLEEN)	*splen/o* (spleen)	immune system organ that gets rid of damaged red blood cells and reclaims and stores iron
T cell	T (stands for thymus) + cell	cells that make up about 80% of lymphocytes; the T denotes their work with the thymus
thymus (THY-muhs)	*thym/o* (thymus)	immune system gland located behind the sternum
tonsil (TON-sihl)	*tonsill/o* (tonsil)	collection of lymph tissue; in common understanding, the lingual, pharyngeal, and (especially) palatine tonsils
Common Disorders		
anaphylaxis (an-ah-FIL-ax-ihs)	*ana-* (without); from the Greek word *phylaxis* (protection)	life-threatening reaction to a foreign substance; symptoms include blockage of air passages, decreased blood pressure, generalized edema
hemolysis (hee-MAWL-ih-sihs)	*hem/o* (blood); *-lysis* (destruction)	change or destruction of red blood cells
Hodgkin's lymphoma (HODJ-kin lim-FOH-mah)	named after English physician Thomas Hodgkin (1798–1866) who first described it; *lymph/o* (lymph or lymphatic system); *-oma* (tumor)	chronic malignant disease of the lymph nodes
immunodeficiency (IM-yu-noh-dee-FISH-ehn-see)	*immun/o* (immune system) + deficiency	impairment of the immune system
lymphadenitis (LIM-FAD-eh-NY-tiss)	*lymph/o* (lymph or lymphatic system); *aden/o* (gland); *-itis* (inflammation)	inflammation of a lymph node (or nodes)
lymphadenopathy (lim-fah-deh-NOP-ah-thee)	*lymph/o* (lymph or lymphatic system); *aden/o* (gland); *-pathy* (disease)	chronic or excessively swollen lymph nodes; any disease of the lymph nodes

(continued)

TERM AND PRONUNCIATION	ANALYSIS	MEANING
lymphangitis (lim-fan-JY-tihs); also sometimes lymphangiitis (lim-FAN-jee-EYE-tihs); see also lymphatitis	*lymphangi/o* (lymph vessel); *-itis* (inflammation)	inflammation of lymph vessels
lymphatitis (lim-fah-TY-tihs)	*lymph/o* (lymph or lymphatic system); *-itis* (inflammation)	inflammation of the lymph vessels or nodes
lymphedema (lim-feh-DEE-mah)	*lymph/o* (lymph or lymphatic system); from the Greek word *oidema* (a swelling tumor)	swelling of the subcutaneous tissues due to obstruction of lymph vessels or nodes
lymphoma (lim-FOH-mah)	*lymph/o* (lymph or lymphatic system); *-oma* (tumor)	tumor of lymph tissue
lymphopathy (lim-FOP-ah-thee)	*lymph/o* (lymph or lymph gland); *-pathy* (disease)	disease of the lymph vessels or nodes
splenitis (splee-NY-tihs)	*splen/o* (spleen); *-itis* (inflammation)	inflammation of the spleen
splenomegaly (splee-noh-MEG-ah-lee)	*splen/o* (spleen); *-megaly* (enlargement)	enlargement of the spleen
splenopathy (splee-NOP-ah-thee)	*splen/o* (spleen); *-pathy* (disease)	any disease of the spleen
systemic lupus erythematosus (sis-TEM-ik LOO-pahs er-RITH-ee-mah-TOH-suhs)	adjective form of the English word *system; lupus* (a Latin word meaning "wolf"); *erythematosus* (from the Greek word *erythema* meaning "flush")	an inflammatory connective tissue disorder with variable features; diffuse erythematous (red) butterfly rash on face
thymitis (thy-MY-tihs)	*thym/o* (thymus); *-itis* (inflammation)	inflammation of the thymus
tonsillitis (TAWN-sih-LY-tihs)	*tonsill/o* (tonsils); *-itis* (inflammation)	inflammation of a tonsil (commonly, the palatine tonsil)
Diagnosis and Treatment		
antiviral (an-ty-VIR-al)	*anti-* (against); from the Latin word *virus* (poison, sap of plants, slimy liquid)	drugs used to treat various viral infections or conditions
chemotherapy (KEE-moh-ther-ah-pee)	*chem/o* (chemical) + therapy, a common English word	treatment of malignancies using chemical agents and drugs (usually reserved for treatment of cancer)
corticosteroids (kor-tih-ko-STER-oyds)	from the Latin word *cortex* (bark); from the Greek *steros* (solid, stable)	hormonelike preparations used as anti-inflammatory agents; topical agents used for their immunosuppressive and anti-inflammatory properties

TERM AND PRONUNCIATION	ANALYSIS	MEANING
immunization (IM-u-ny-zay-shun)	*immun/o* (immune system); *-ization* (noun suffix)	process by which resistance to an infectious disease is induced
immunosuppressant (IM-yu-no-suh-PRESS-ant)	*immun/o* (immune system) + suppressant	something that interferes with the immune system
lymphangiography (lim-FAN-jee-OG-rah-fee)	*lymphangi/o* (lymph vessel); *-graphy* (process of recording)	radiography of the lymph vessels

Practice and Practitioners

allergist	from the Greek words *allos* (other, different, strange) and *ergon* (activity); *-ist* (one who specializes)	a medical practitioner who specializes in the diagnosis and treatment of allergies
hematologist (hee-mah-TAHL-oh-jist)	*hemat/o* (blood); *-logist* (one who specializes)	a medical practitioner who specializes in the diagnosis and treatment of blood disorders
immunologist (im-yu-NOL-oh-jist)	*immun/o* (immune system); *-logist* (one who specializes)	a medical practitioner specializing in the immune system
immunology (IM-yu-NOL-oh-jee)	*immun/o* (immune system); *-logy* (study of)	the medical specialty dealing with the immune system
oncologist (on-KOL-oh-jist)	from the Greek word *onkos* (mass, bulk); *-logist* (one who specializes)	a medical practitioner who specializes in the diagnosis and treatment of malignant tumors

Surgical Procedures

lymphadenectomy (lim-fah- deh-NEK-toh-mee)	*lymphaden/o* (lymph gland); *-ectomy* (excision)	excision of lymph nodes
lymphangiectomy (lim-FAN-jee-EK-tah-mee)	*lymphangi/o* (lymph vessel); *-ectomy* (excision)	excision of a lymph vessel
lymphangiotomy (lim-FAN-jee-OT-oh-mee)	*lymphangi/o* (lymph vessel); *-tomy* (cutting operation)	incision of a lymph vessel
splenectomy (splee-NEK-toh-mee)	*splen/o* (spleen); *-ectomy* (excision)	excision of the spleen
splenorrhaphy (splee-NOR-ah-fee)	*splen/o* (spleen); *-rrhaphy* (rupture)	suture of a ruptured spleen
splenotomy (splee-NOT-oh-mee)	*splen/o* (spleen); *-tomy* (cutting operation)	incision of the spleen
thymectomy (thy-MEK-toh-me)	*thym/o* (thymus); *-ectomy* (excision)	excision of the thymus
tonsillectomy (TAWN-sih-LEK-toh-mee)	*tonsill/o* (tonsil); *-ectomy* (excision)	excision of a tonsil

EXERCISES

| EXERCISE 10-1 | CASE STUDY

BRIEF HISTORY: A 16-year-old male complained to his parents of being extremely fatigued. He wasn't able to keep up with his school schedule or after school sport activities. His throat was sore and he noticed "lumps" in his neck and groin. He had a fever and loss of appetite. He recently began to complain of pain in his upper left belly.

OFFICE VISIT: A physician examined the patient and ordered blood tests. He noted lymphadenopathy in the cervical, axillary, and inguinal areas. He also observed an erythematous throat and determined that the spleen was enlarged.

DIAGNOSIS AND TREATMENT PLAN: The diagnosis was mononucleosis, an infectious disease caused by a virus. The prescribed treatment consisted of over-the-counter analgesics to reduce the abdominal pain, along with fluids and rest. Throat lozenges were prescribed to ease sore throat discomfort.

Answer the following questions and then try rewriting the report to make it more straightforward (that does not mean eliminating medical terms but rather using them concisely and as necessary). Compare your rewritten report with the version shown in Appendix A.

1. What does "lymphadenopathy" mean? _____

2. What is the medical term for an "enlarged spleen"? _____

3. What is mononucleosis? _____

4. Rewrite the report to reduce the amount of energy needed to gain a full understanding of the case.[a] _____

---

[a]The phrase "a 16-year-old male" could refer to a male dog, cat, horse, etc. In this sentence, we discover that the "male" complained to his parents, and at that point we can guess that the writer meant to say "a 16-year-old boy." However, the reader must process the entire sentence in order to know that. Read the entire report with the following fact in mind: writing and reading takes thought, and thought uses energy. A lazy, thoughtless writer demands more of the reader's time and energy than a careful, thoughtful writer does. One might contend that the increased demand is insignificant in a short report. However, even that slight increase illustrates something about this writer, and that "something" is that the adjectives *thoughtless* and *lazy* should not apply to a health care professional.

EXERCISE 10-2 | MATCHING

Match the term in Column B with the correct definition in Column A.

COLUMN A	COLUMN B
1. _____ enlarged spleen	A. lymphadenopathy
2. _____ specialty that deals with immune disorders	B. lymphedema
3. _____ artificially acquired immunity	C. phagocytosis
4. _____ life-threatening allergic reaction to a foreign substance	D. autoimmune
5. _____ disease of the lymph glands	E. splenomegaly
6. _____ accumulation of fluid in the intercellular tissues	F. lymphocyte
7. _____ the process of engulfing foreign materials	G. immunology
8. _____ protective lymph organ that is attached to the proximal end of the large intestine	H. anaphylaxis
9. _____ the body reacts to its own tissues	I. appendix
10. _____ specialized WBC of the immune system	J. immunization

EXERCISE 10-3 | WORD BUILDING: THE LYMPHATIC SYSTEM AND IMMUNITY

Use the following word elements to build the terms defined in the following.

aden/o	-graphy	-logist	-oma	thym/o
angi/o	immun/o	lymph/o	-pathy	
-cytosis	-itis	-megaly	phag/o	

1. inflammation of a lymph gland _____

2. tumor of a lymph gland _____

3. enlargement of the thymus _____

4. inflammation of a lymph vessel _____

5. disease of a lymph gland _____

6. specialist who studies and treats the immune system _____

7. radiographic procedure of the lymphatic system _____

8. process of a WBC engulfing a harmful organism _____

EXERCISE 10-4   WRITING THE ABBREVIATION

In the right hand column, write the abbreviation for each of the following phrases.

1. rheumatoid arthritis   _____

2. radioimmunoassay   _____

3. human leukocyte antigen   _____

4. systemic lupus erythematosus   _____
   (usually shortened to lupus),
   an autoimmune disorder

5. acquired immunodeficiency   _____
   syndrome

6. complete blood count   _____

7. human immunodeficiency virus   _____

EXERCISE 10-5 CROSSWORD PUZZLE: THE LYMPHATIC SYSTEM AND IMMUNITY

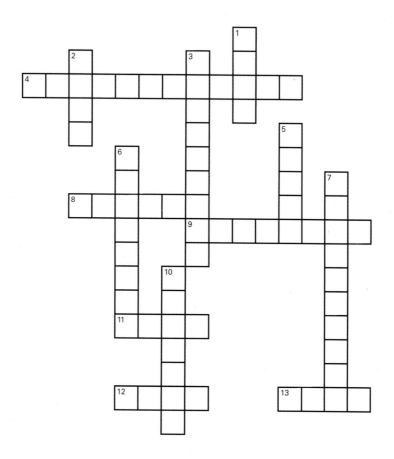

ACROSS

4. use of drug agents to treat malignancies
8. gland located in the chest that produces lymphocytes
9. protection against disease
11. acronym for acquired immunodeficiency syndrome
12. suffix meaning "blood"
13. root word for "gland"

DOWN

1. root word meaning "to ingest" or "engulf"
2. root word for "white"
3. destruction of red blood cells
5. root word for "spleen"
6. redness
7. disorder that results from an immune response to one's own tissues
10. disease of the lymphatic system that may spread

CHAPTER 10 QUIZ

True or False

Circle the best answer.

1. True   False   Hodgkin's lymphoma is a progressive disorder that is characterized by an enlarged spleen and lymph nodes.

2. True   False   The tonsils have no role in the immune system.

3. True   False   A reaction to poison ivy is an example of anaphylaxis.

4. True   False   SLE is an example of an autoimmune disease.

5. True   False   Hemolysis is a form of lymphatic cancer.

6. True   False   Splenomegaly is enlargement of the spleen.

7. True   False   An accumulation of lymph in the soft tissue is called lymphedema.

8. True   False   Drugs are or may be used to prevent or reduce the body's normal reactions to invasions of harmful organisms.

9. True   False   Peyer's patches are located in the back of the throat.

10. True   False   The axilla is one area where there is a concentration of lymph nodes.

11 *The Respiratory System*

LEARNING OBJECTIVES

Upon completion of this chapter, you should be able to:

- Identify and define the word elements of the respiratory system.
- Build, spell, and pronounce medical terms that relate to the respiratory system.
- Interpret abbreviations relating to the respiratory system.
- Define the terms naming the major parts of the respiratory system.
- Define terms naming disorders, treatments, and procedures related to the respiratory system.

INTRODUCTION

The respiratory system consists of the **nose** (**nasal cavity**), **pharynx, larynx, bronchi, bronchioles, alveoli**, and **lungs** (Fig. 11-1). The purpose of the respiratory system is to furnish oxygen to the body's cells and to remove carbon dioxide. Figure 11-2 is a diagram that shows the process of gas exchange, which is accomplished through external and internal respiration. **External respiration** is the process whereby air is brought into the lungs and oxygen and carbon dioxide (a waste product) are exchanged in the blood within the capillaries surrounding the alveoli. **Internal respiration** is the process whereby oxygen and carbon dioxide move between the blood and the body's cells.

WORD ELEMENTS USED IN RESPIRATORY SYSTEM TERMS

Please see Table 11-1.

STRUCTURE AND FUNCTION

The structures that make up the respiratory system are discussed in the following paragraphs.

The Nose

Air enters the body through the nose, which is lined with small hairs called **cilia**, and passes into the **nasal cavity** where it is warmed and moistened. **Mucus** coats the lining of the nasal cavity to filter out particles too small to be blocked by the cilia.

The Pharynx

The **pharynx**, also known as the throat, has three divisions: the **nasopharynx, oropharnyx**, and **laryngopharynx** (see Fig. 11-1). The nasopharynx is posterior to the nasal cavity, the oropharynx is the middle portion located behind the mouth, and the laryngopharynx is the lower portion behind the larynx. Associated with the pharynx are three pairs of lymphoid tissue called tonsils. The **adenoids**, also known as **pharyngeal tonsils**, are located in the nasopharynx; the **palatine tonsils** are in the oropharynx; and the **lingual tonsils** are at the base of the posterior portion of the tongue (Fig. 11-3). The tonsils are accessory organs that aid in filtering bacteria.

The Larynx

The **larynx** (voice box) is a cartilaginous structure located between the pharynx and trachea (Fig. 11-4). The larynx is held open by a number of cartilages, the largest being the thyroid cartilage

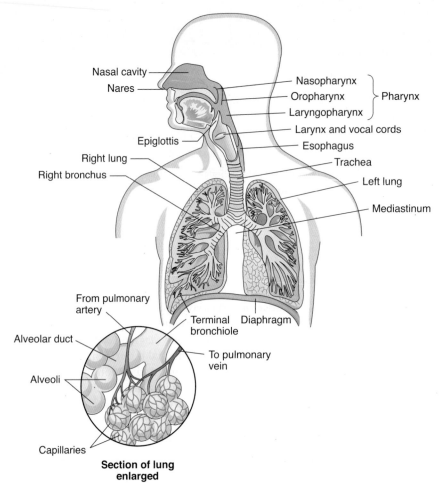

FIGURE 11-1 **The respiratory system.** An overview of the respiratory anatomical terms. The main structures include the nasal cavity, pharynx (three divisions), larynx, trachea, bronchi, bronchioles, and alveoli. Enlarged section of the terminal bronchiole shows the relationship between the alveoli and blood capillaries. External respiration occurs as oxygen moves from the alveoli into the blood and carbon dioxide moves from the blood out into the alveoli where it will be exhaled. *Modified from Cohen BJ*. Medical Terminology: An Illustrated Guide. *5th ed. Philadelphia, PA: Lippincott Williams & Wilkins; 2007.*

(Adam's apple). Also contained in the larynx are the **vocal cords** (Fig. 11-5). These folds of mucous membrane vibrate as air from the lungs flows over them to produce sound.

The space between the vocal cords is the **glottis**, which closes during swallowing to keep food out of the respiratory tract (see Fig. 11-5A). Note in Figure 11-5B that the glottis is open to allow breathed air to pass through. The little leaf-shaped cartilage located above the glottis is called the **epiglottis**, a flaplike structure that covers the larynx to prevent swallowed food from entering the trachea and lungs.

The Trachea

The **trachea** (windpipe) is a cartilaginous tube that extends from the pharynx to the main bronchi.

The Bronchi, Bronchioles, and Alveoli

The inferior portion of the trachea branches off into two major airways called the **right** and **left bronchi**. Air passes through the bronchi, which subdivide into increasingly smaller branches called

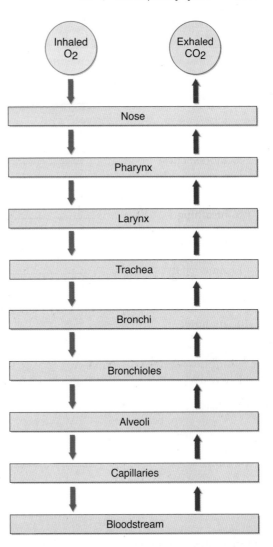

FIGURE 11-2 Pathway of inhaled/exhaled air.
(*Red arrows* indicate oxygenated air; *blue arrows* represent deoxygenated air.) Oxygen (O_2) enters the respiratory system through the nose and travels down through the larynx and pharynx and into the lungs where a gas exchange takes place. Oxygen moves into the bloodstream where it is carried to the cells and is exchanged with carbon dioxide (CO_2). The carbon dioxide passes back up through the respiratory structures and is exhaled.

TABLE 11-1	WORD ELEMENTS THAT MAKE UP TERMS RELATED TO THE RESPIRATORY SYSTEM	
Element	**Type**	**Meaning**
bronch/o, bronchi/o	root	bronchus
laryng/o	root	larynx
nas/o, rhin/o	root	nose
-oxia	suffix	oxygen
or/o	root	mouth, opening
pharyng/o	root	pharynx
-phonia	suffix	voice
phren/o	root	diaphragm
pleur/o	root	pleura
-pnea	suffix	breathing
pneum/o, pneumon/o	root	air, lung
pulmon/o	root	lung
sinus/o	root	sinus cavity
thorac/o, thorac/i, thoracic/o	root	thorax, chest
trache/o	root	trachea

Word Elements Exercise — CHOOSING AN ELEMENT

Study Table 11-1 carefully. Then write a word element in the blank on the right that matches the word on the left.

1. voice _____

2. trachea _____

3. thorax, chest _____

4. bronchus _____

5. breathing _____

6. larynx _____

7. sinus cavity _____

8. pleura _____

9. air, lung _____

10. nose _____

11. oxygen _____

12. pharynx _____

13. diaphragm _____

14. lung _____

15. mouth _____

bronchioles. The air terminates in the bronchial tree in tiny air sacs called **alveoli**.

The Lungs

The two lungs, one each located on either flank of the heart, are enclosed in the **pleura**, which is a membrane composed of two layers called the **parietal** and the **visceral** layers (Fig. 11-6). The parietal (outer) layer lines the thoracic cavity and forms the sac containing each lung. The visceral (inner) layer closely surrounds each lung. The right lung is slightly larger than the left and has three sub-units called the **superior lobe**, **middle lobe**, and **lower lobe**. The left lung has only two lobes: the **superior** and **inferior lobes**. The very top of each lung is called the **apex**. The lungs and airways bring in fresh, oxygen-enriched air and get rid of waste carbon dioxide made by the cells in the body.

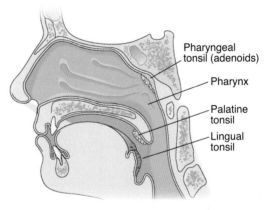

FIGURE 11-3 **The pharynx and tonsils.** The pharyngeal tonsil or adenoids are located in the nasopharyngeal region or upper portion of the throat. The palatine tonsils are located in the oropharynx or back of the mouth. The lingual tonsils are located at the base of the tongue. *From Cohen BJ. Medical Terminology: An Illustrated Guide. 5th ed. Philadelphia, PA: Lippincott Williams & Wilkins; 2007.*

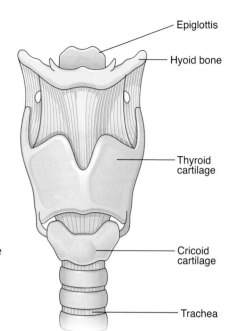

Epiglottis

Hyoid bone

Thyroid cartilage

Cricoid cartilage

Trachea

FIGURE 11-4 The larynx. The larynx (voice box) is a cartilaginous structure located between the pharynx and trachea. It is held open by a number of cartilages, the largest being the thyroid cartilage (Adam's apple). A little leaf-shaped cartilage located above the glottis is called the epiglottis (epi- means "upon"; glottis means "opening in the vocal cords"). This flaplike structure swings downward during swallowing to cover the larynx so food does not enter the trachea and the lungs. *From Cohen BJ. Medical Terminology: An Illustrated Guide. 5th ed. Philadelphia, PA: Lippincott Williams & Wilkins; 2007.*

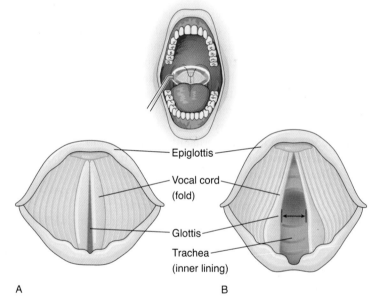

Epiglottis

Vocal cord (fold)

Glottis

Trachea (inner lining)

FIGURE 11-5 The vocal cords, a superior view. A. The glottis in a closed position. **B.** The glottis in an open position. *From Cohen BJ. Medical Terminology: An Illustrated Guide. 5th ed. Philadelphia, PA: Lippincott Williams & Wilkins; 2007.*   A

B

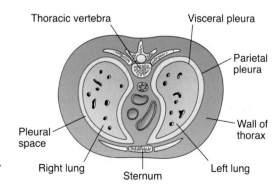

Thoracic vertebra

Visceral pleura

Parietal pleura

Pleural space

Wall of thorax

Right lung

Sternum

Left lung

FIGURE 11-6 Pleura. A horizontal cross-sectional view of the lungs illustrating the pleural linings and pleural space. The parietal pleura is the outer lining, whereas the visceral pleura is the inner lining. The space in between the two linings is called the pleural space. *Modified from Cohen BJ. Medical Terminology: An Illustrated Guide. 5th ed. Philadelphia, PA: Lippincott Williams & Wilkins; 2007.*

217

Quick Check: Defining Complex Terms by Deciphering Word Elements

In the caption for Figure 11-3, locate the word nasopharyngeal, then write and define each of its word elements.

PRACTICE AND PRACTITIONERS

Several different health care professionals diagnose and treat respiratory system disorders. A **pulmonologist** is a physician who specializes in **pulmonology**, which encompasses the lungs and their related organs and structures. Both **otolaryngologists** and **otorhinolaryngologists** diagnose and treat disorders of the ears, nose, and throat. **Respiratory therapists** are allied health care professionals who specialize in airway management, mechanical ventilation, and blood acid–base balance.

DISORDERS AND TREATMENTS

The pathway through which air moves in and out of the lungs needs to remain **patent** (a common English word that when used as a medical term means "physically open") in order for proper oxygen and carbon dioxide exchange to take place. When this pathway becomes partially blocked, the body's normal response is a sneeze or cough, which may produce **sputum**; **hemoptysis**, which is bloody sputum; or other secretions that need to be removed for optimal airway **patency**.

Abnormal breath sounds are another indication of respiratory disease. **Rales**, also known as crackles, are high-pitched popping sounds usually originating in the smaller airways. **Rhonchi** (singular: rhonchus) are low-pitched sounds that come from the larger airways. **Wheezing** or whistling sounds may indicate excessive secretions or partially obstructed airways, and **stridor** is a high-pitched squeaking sound that occurs when one breathes in. Breathing patterns and rates may also be altered by respiratory diseases. Normal breathing, **eupnea**, should be regular and effortless. The following is a list of abnormalities in respiration:

- **Tachypnea**: rapid rate of respiration (may be normal during exercise)
- **Bradypnea**: abnormal slowness of respiration
- **Apnea**: cessation of respiration; short periods of apnea normally occur during sleep
- **Dyspnea**: difficult or painful respiration
- **Orthopnea**: discomfort or difficulty in breathing while lying flat; difficulty is relieved by sitting up
- **Cheyne-Stokes**: a rhythmic respiratory pattern in which a variation in depth of respirations alternates with periods of apnea
- **Kussmaul breathing**: rapid deep respiration

A number of disorders affect the respiratory system. Some of them are briefly discussed under the following broad categories: infectious disorders, obstructive lung diseases, and expansion disorders.

Infectious Disorders

Following are a few of the infections (some common, some less so) that occur in the respiratory system:

infectious rhinitis (the common cold)
sinusitis
croup (Croup is also called **laryngotracheobronchitis**.)
epiglottitis (In very severe cases, treatment may include a **tracheostomy**.)
influenza (flu)
pneumonia
laryngitis

dysphonia (sometimes accompanies laryngitis)
pertussis (whooping cough)
tuberculosis

Obstructive Lung Diseases

Obstructive disease impairs airflow through the respiratory tree. The obstruction may be caused by an increased production of secretions or actual destruction of the lung tissues. **Cystic fibrosis**, **emphysema**, and **asthma** are well-known disorders that fall into this category.

Expansion Disorders

Adequate lung expansion is necessary for proper ventilation and gas exchange to take place. Some disease conditions place restrictions on the lung's capacity, thereby causing nonaeration of the lung tissues. **Atelectasis** and **pneumothorax** are two such disorders.

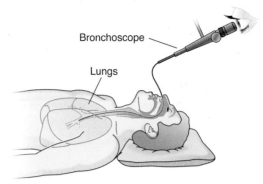

FIGURE 11-7   Bronchoscopy. Introduction of a bronchoscope through the nose that is then guided down into the bronchi. Visual examination (suffix -scopy means "visual examination") can be made of the bronchial tree, biopsies may be taken from the bronchi, and secretions may be removed for analysis or to reduce respiratory distress. *From Cohen BJ.* Medical Terminology. *4th ed. Philadelphia, PA: Lippincott Williams & Wilkins; 2003.*

Procedures and Treatments

Both invasive and noninvasive procedures are used to diagnose respiratory disorders. The noninvasive procedures include chest X-rays, lung scans, **pulse oximetry**, **arterial blood gases**, and computed tomography scans. Invasive procedures may include **thoracentesis** and **bronchoscopy** (Fig. 11-7). Respiratory therapists perform **pulmonary function tests** on patients to assess breathing and ventilation. Lung volumes are measured with a **spirometer**.

Abbreviation Table	THE RESPIRATORY SYSTEM
ABBREVIATION	**MEANING**
ABG	arterial blood gas
CF	cystic fibrosis
CO_2	carbon dioxide
COPD	chronic obstructive pulmonary disease
CXR	chest X-ray
ERV	expiratory reserve volume (as measured with test equipment)
IRV	inspiratory reserve volume (as measured with test equipment)
O_2	oxygen
PFT	pulmonary function test
R	respiratory rate
RV	residual volume (as measured with test equipment)
SOB	shortness of breath
T&A	tonsils and adenoids (also tonsillectomy and adenoidectomy)
TB	tuberculosis
TLC	total lung capacity (as measured with test equipment)
TV	tidal volume (as measured with test equipment)

Study Table | THE RESPIRATORY SYSTEM

TERM AND PRONUNCIATION	ANALYSIS	MEANING
Structure and Function		
alveoli (al-VEE-oh-lee); singular: alveolus	diminutive of the Latin word *alveus* (cavity, hollow)	small cavities in which oxygen is removed from the air delivered by the bronchioles (note: alveoli are also found in other body systems)
apex (AY-pex)	a Latin word meaning "summit," "peak," "tip"	word used to describe the upper tip of each lung
base	common English word	word used to describe the bottom of each lung
bronchi (BRON-kee); singular: bronchus (BRON-kuss)	*bronch/o-, bronch/i-* (bronchus)	tubes (right and left) branching off from the trachea and into the lungs
bronchiole (BRON-kee-ole)	*bronch/o-, bronch/i-* (bronchus)	very small branches of bronchi that extend into the lungs
cilia (SIHL-ee-ah)	plural of the Latin word *cilium* (eyelash, eyelid)	small hairs in the upper respiratory tract that sweep foreign matter and mucus out of the respiratory tract
diaphragm (DY-uh-fram)	from the Greek word *diaphragma* (partition, barrier)	the major muscle of respiration located at the base of the thoracic cavity
epiglottis (ep-ih-GLOT-ihs)	*epi-* (upon) + the Greek *glottis* (tongue, mouth of the windpipe)	a mucous membrane-covered, leaf-shaped piece of cartilage at the root of the tongue
external respiration	common English words	process whereby air is brought into the lungs, and oxygen and carbon dioxide (waste product) are exchanged in the blood within the capillaries of the alveoli
glottis (GLOT-is)	a Greek word meaning "tongue," "mouth of the windpipe"	vocal folds and apparatus of the larynx
internal respiration	common English words	process whereby the oxygen and carbon dioxide are exchanged at the cellular level
laryngopharynx (LAYN-in-go-FAYR-inx)	*laryng/o* (larynx); *-al* (adjective suffix); *pharyng/o* (pharynx)	lower portion of the pharynx
larynx (LAYR-inx)	*laryng/o* (larynx)	voice box, vocal cords
mediastinum (MEE-dee-ahs-TYN-um)	from the Latin word *mediastinus* (midway)	area between the lungs that houses the heart, aorta, trachea, esophagus, and bronchi
mucus (MYU-kus)	a Latin word meaning "slime," "mold"	clear secretion produced in the respiratory tract

TERM AND PRONUNCIATION	ANALYSIS	MEANING
nasal (NAY-zuhl)	*nas/o* (nose); *-al* (adjective suffix)	adjective referring to the nose
nasopharynx (NAY-zoh-FAYR-inx)	*nas/o* (nose); *pharyng/o* (pharynx)	upper portion of the pharynx
oropharynx (O-roh-FAYR-inx)	from the Latin word *oris* (mouth); *pharyng/o* (pharynx)	middle portion of the pharynx
patency (PAY-tehn-see)	from the Latin word *patere* (lie open, be open)	the state of being open
patent (PA-tehnt or PAY-tehnt)	from the Latin word *patere* (lie open, be open)	open; adjective form of patency
pharynx (FAYR-inx)	a Greek word meaning "throat"	passageway just below the nasal cavity and mouth
phrenic (FREN-ik)	from the Greek word *phren* (midriff, heart, mind)	adjective referring to the diaphragm; synonymous with diaphragmatic
pleura (PLU-rah)	a Greek word meaning "side of the body," "rib"	serous membrane that surrounds the lung; *parietal pleura* is the outer layer; *visceral pleura* is the inner layer
pulmonary (PULL-muhn-ayr-ee)	*pulmon/o* (lung); *-ary* (adjective suffix)	adjective frequently used to modify another term in or associated with the lungs
sputum (SPYOU-tum)	from the Latin word *spuere* (to spit)	thick mucus ejected through the mouth
trachea (TRAY-kee-uh)	from the Greek word *trakheia* (windpipe)	windpipe
vocal cords	common English words	folds of mucus membranes that are used in speech production
Common Disorders		
apnea (APP-nee-uh)	*a-* (without); *-pnea* (breathing)	absence of breathing
asthma (AZ-mah)	A Greek word meaning "a panting"	a lung disease characterized by reversible inflammation and constriction
atelectasis (at-eh-LEK-tah-sihs)	from the Greek word *ateles* (incomplete); *-ectasis* (expansion)	collapse of a lung or part of a lung, leading to decreased gas exchange
bradypnea (BRAH-dip-NEE-ah)	*brady-* (slow); *-pnea* (breathing)	abnormal slowness of respiration
bronchial pneumonia (BRAWN-kee-uhl nu-MO- nee-ah); also called *bronchopneumonia*	*bronchi/o* (bronchus); *-al* (adjective suffix); *pneumon/o* (air, lung)	inflammation of the smaller bronchial tubes
bronchiectasis (BRON-kee-EK-tay-sis)	*bronchi/o* (bronchus); *-ectasis* (expansion)	chronic dilation of the bronchi

(continued)

TERM AND PRONUNCIATION	ANALYSIS	MEANING
bronchiolitis (bron-kee-oh-LY-tihs)	*bronchi/o* (bronchus); *-itis* (inflammation)	inflammation of the bronchioles
bronchiostenosis (BRON-kee-oh-steh-NOH-sis)	*bronchi/o* (bronchus); *sten/o* (narrowing); *-osis* (abnormal condition of)	narrowing of the bronchial tubes
bronchitis (bron-KY-tihs)	*bronchi/o* (bronchus); *-itis* (inflammation)	inflammation of the mucous membrane of the bronchial tubes
bronchoconstriction (BRON-koh-kon-STRIK-shun)	*bronch/o* (bronchus) + constriction	the bronchi become narrowed or constricted
bronchodilation (BRON-ko-DYE-lay-shun)	*bronch/o* (bronchus) + dilation	the bronchi become more open or dilated
bronchopneumonia (BRON- koh-nu-MO-nee-uh); also called *bronchial pneumonia*	*bronch/o* (bronchus); *pneumon/o* (air, lung); *-ia* (condition)	inflammation of the smaller bronchial tubes
bronchospasm (BRON-ko-spaz-uhm)	*bronch/o* (bronchus) + spasm	abnormal contraction of bronchi
Cheyne-Stokes (SHAYN STOHKS)	named after John Cheyne, British physician, and William Stokes, Irish physician, who first described the disorder in the 19th century	a rhythmic respiratory pattern where there is a variation in depth of respirations alternating with periods of apnea
croup (krupe); laryngotracheobronchitis	obsolete English verb (to croak); *laryng/o* (larynx); *trache/o* (trachea); *bronchi/o* (bronchus)	a viral infection that causes swelling of the larynx and epiglottis; a barking noise is characteristic
cystic fibrosis (SIS-tik FYE-broh-sis)	from the Greek word *kystis* (bladder, pouch); from the Latin word *fibra* (fiber); *-osis* (abnormal condition)	genetic disorder in which the lungs become clogged with excessive amounts of abnormally thick mucus
dysphonia (DIS-fohn-ya)	*dys-* (difficult); *phon/o* (sound); *-ia* (condition)	difficult or painful speech
dyspnea (DISP-nee-uh)	*dys-* (difficult); *-pnea* (breathing)	difficult breathing
emphysema (ehm-fih-SEE-mah)	a Greek word meaning "swelling"	condition in which the alveoli are inefficient because of distension
hemoptysis (HEE-mop-ti-sis)	*hem/o* (blood); *-ptysis* (spitting)	blood-tinged frothy sputum
influenza (IN-flew-EN-zah); flu	an Italian word meaning "influence" (of planets or stars)	highly contagious viral infection of the upper respiratory tract that is spread by droplets
Kussmaul (KUHS-mowl)	named after 19th century German physician who first noted it among patients with advanced diabetes mellitus	rapid deep respirations that are characteristic of an acid–base imbalance (frequently seen in uncontrolled diabetes)

TERM AND PRONUNCIATION	ANALYSIS	MEANING
laryngitis (LAYR-ihn-jy-this)	*laryng/o* (larynx); *-itis* (inflammation)	inflammation of the larynx
laryngospasm (lah-RIHN-go-spaz-uhm)	*laryng/o* (larynx) + spasm	involuntary contraction of the larynx
laryngostenosis (lah-RIHN-go-steh-NO-sihs)	*laryng/o* (larynx); *sten/o* (narrowing); *-osis* (abnormal condition)	a narrowing of the larynx
orthopnea (or-THOP-NEE-ah)	*ortho-* (straight, correct); *-pnea* (breathing)	discomfort or difficulty in breathing while lying flat; difficulty is relieved by sitting up
pertussis (per-TUSS-ihs)	from the Latin *per-* (through) + *tussis* (cough)	an acute infectious inflammation of the larynx, trachea, and bronchi caused by *Bordetella pertussis*
pharyngitis (fair-in-JY-tihs)	*pharyng/o* (pharynx); *-itis* (inflammation)	inflammation of the pharynx
pharyngospasm (fah-RIN-goh-spas-uhm)	*pharyng/o* (pharynx) + spasm	involuntary contraction of the pharynx
phrenoplegia (freh-no-PLEE-jee-ah)	*phren/o* (diaphragm); *-plegia* (paralysis)	paralysis of the diaphragm
pneumolith (NOO-mo-lith)	*pneum/o* (air, lung); from the Greek word *lithos* (stone)	calculus in a lung
pneumonia (noo-MONE-yah) (synonym for *pneumonitis*)	*pneumon/o* (air, lung); *-ia* (condition)	inflammation of a lung caused by infection, chemical inhalation, or trauma
pneumonitis (noo-mo-NY-tihs) (synonym for *pneumonia*)	*pneumon/o* (air, lung); *-itis* (inflammation)	inflammation of a lung caused by infection, chemical inhalation, or trauma
pneumothorax (NOO-moh- thoh-rax)	*pneumon/o* (air, lung); from the Greek word *thorakos* (breastplate, chest)	accumulation of air in the pleural space
rales (RAYLS)	from the French word *raler* (to make a rattling sound in the throat)	abnormal breath sound; crackles
rhinitis (ry-NY-tihs)	*rhin/o* (nose); *-itis* (inflammation)	inflammation of the inner lining of the nasal cavity
rhinopathy (ry-NAW-pah-thee)	*rhin/o* (nose); *-pathy* (disease)	any disease of the nose
rhinorrhea (ry-no-REE-ah)	*rhin/o* (nose); *-rrhea* (discharge)	discharge from the rhinal mucous membrane
rhonchi (RON-kye)	from the Greek *rhonchos* (snore)	abnormal breath sound; low-pitched sonorous sounds
sinusitis (sy-nuh-SY-tihs)	*sinus/o* (sinus); *-itis* (inflammation)	inflammation of the respiratory sinuses

(continued)

TERM AND PRONUNCIATION	ANALYSIS	MEANING
stridor (STRY-dohr)	a Latin word meaning "harsh, high pitched"	high-pitched squeaking sound frequently associated with croup
tachypnea (TAK-ip-NE-ah)	*tachy-* (rapid); *-pnea* (breathing)	abnormal rapid respiration
tracheitis (tray-kee-EYE-tihs)	*trache/o* (trachea); *-itis* (inflammation)	inflammation of the trachea
tracheostenosis (TRAY-kee-oh-steh-NO-sihs)	*trache/o* (trachea); *sten/o* (narrowing); *-sis* (condition)	abnormal narrowing of the trachea
tuberculosis (tu-BURK-yu-loh-sihs)	from the Latin word- *tuberculum* (small swelling, pimple); *-osis* (abnormal condition)	disease caused by presence of *Mycobacterium tuberculosis*, most commonly affecting the lungs
wheezing (WEE-zing)	common English word	abnormal breath sounds; whistling sounds heard with upper airway obstruction

Diagnosis and Treatment

antihistaminic (anti-HISS-tah-MIN-ik)	*anti-* (against); from the Greek word *histos* (tissue); from the Latin *amine* (ammonia, compound); *-ic* (adjective suffix)	drug used to treat acute allergic reactions
antipyretic (anti-PYE-reh-tik)	*anti-* (against); from the Greek *pyretos* (fever); *-ic* (adjective suffix)	drug used to reduce fever
arterial blood gas	*arteri/o* (artery) + blood + gas, common English words	measures the partial pressures of oxygen and carbon dioxide in the arterial blood
bronchodilator (bron-ko-DYE-lay-tor)	*bronch/o* (bronchus); from the Latin word *dilatare* (to spread wide)	drug used to expand the bronchi
bronchoscope (BRON-ko-skope)	*bronch/o* (bronchus); *-scope* (instrument for viewing)	a device for visually inspecting the interior of a bronchus
bronchoscopy (bron-KOSS-ko-pee)	*bronch/o* (bronchus); *-scopy* (use of instrument for viewing)	inspection using a bronchoscope
decongestant (DEE-kon-jes-tant)	*de-* (away from, cessation); from the Latin word *congerere* (to bring together)	drug used to reduce edema and congestion
laryngoscope (lah-RIHN-go-skope)	*laryng/o* (larynx); *-scope* (instrument for viewing)	instrument with a light at the tip to aid in visual inspection of the larynx
laryngoscopy (LAYR-ihn-GOSS-koh-pee)	*laryng/o* (larynx); *-scopy* (use of instrument for viewing)	visual inspection of the larynx with the aid of a laryngoscope
pharyngoscope (fah-RIN-goh-skope)	*pharyng/o* (pharynx); *-scope* (instrument for viewing)	instrument with a light at the tip to aid in the visual inspection of the pharynx

TERM AND PRONUNCIATION	ANALYSIS	MEANING
pharyngoscopy (FAH-rihn-GAW-skoh-pee)	*pharyng/o* (pharynx); *-scopy* (use of instrument for viewing)	visual inspection of the pharynx with aid of a pharyngoscope
postural drainage (PAHS-chu-ral)	common English words	a physical therapy technique where the patient lies on his or her side on a decline to help drain the lungs
pulmonary function tests	*pulmon/o* (lung); *-ary* (adjective suffix) + function + tests, common English words	measurement of lung volumes to assess breathing and ventilation; instrument used is a spirometer
pulse oximeter (ahk-SIM-eh-tuhr)	from the Latin word *pellere* (to push, drive); from the Greek words *oxys* (sharp) and *metron* (measure)	a device that measures the oxygen saturation of arterial blood by reference to light wave lengths
pulse oximetry (ahk-SIM-eh-tree)	from the Latin word *pellere* (to push, drive); from the Greek words *oxys* (sharp) and *metron* (measure)	a small instrument is placed on a finger or thin body part that measures the oxygen saturation of arterial blood
rhinoscope (RY-noh-skope)	*rhin/o* (nose); *-scope* (instrument for viewing)	a small mirror with a thin handle; used in rhinoscopy
rhinoscopy (ry-NAW-skoh-pee)	*rhin/o* (nose); *-scopy* (use of instrument for viewing)	visual inspection of the nasal areas
Surgical Procedures		
bronchoplasty (BRAWN-koh-plass-tee)	*bronch/o* (bronchus); *-plasty* (surgical repair)	surgical repair of a bronchus
laryngectomy (LAYR-ehn-JEK-toh-mee)	*laryng/o* (larynx); *-ectomy* (excision)	excision of the larynx
laryngoplasty (lah-RIHN-go-plass-tee)	*laryng/o* (larynx); *-plasty* (surgical repair)	surgical repair of the larynx
laryngotomy (layr-ihn-GOT-oh-mee)	*laryng/o* (larynx); *-tomy* (cutting operation)	incision into the larynx
pharyngoplasty (fah-RIHN-go-plass-tee)	*pharyng/o* (pharynx); *-plasty* (surgical repair)	surgical repair of the pharynx
pharyngotomy (FAYR-ihn-GOT-oh-mee)	*pharyng/o* (pharynx); *-tomy* (cutting operation)	surgical incision into the pharynx
pneumonectomy (NOO-mo-NEK-toh-mee)	*pneumon/o* (air, lung); *-ectomy* (excision)	removal of pulmonary lobes from a lung
pneumonorrhaphy (noo-mo-NOR-ah-fee)	*pneumon/o* (air, lung); *-rrhaphy* (surgical suturing)	suturing of a lung
pneumonotomy (noo-mo-NOT-ah-mee)	*pneumon/o* (air, lung); *-tomy* (cutting operation)	incision into a lung
rhinoplasty (RY-no-plass-tee)	*rhin/o* (nose); *-plasty* (surgical repair)	surgery performed on the nose

(continued)

TERM AND PRONUNCIATION	ANALYSIS	MEANING
rhinotomy (ry-NAW-toh-mee)	*rhin/o* (nose); *-tomy* (cutting operation)	surgical incision into the nose
sinusotomy (sy-nuh-SOT-oh-mee)	*sinus/o* (sinus); *-tomy* (cutting operation)	incision into a sinus
spirometer (spy-ROM-eh-tehr)	from the Latin word *spirare* (breath, blow, live); from the Greek word *metron* (measure)	a device used to measure respiratory gases
thoracentesis (THOH-rah-sen-TEE-sihs)	*thorac/o* (thorax); *-centesis* (surgical puncture)	insertion of a needle into the pleural cavity to withdraw fluid for diagnostic purposes, to drain excess fluid, or to re-expand a collapsed lung
tracheoplasty (TRAY-kee-oh-plass-tee)	*trache/o* (trachea); *-plasty* (surgical repair)	surgical repair of the trachea
tracheostomy (tray-kee-OS-toh-mee)	*trache/o* (trachea); from the Greek *stoma* (mouth)	surgical creation of an opening into the trachea to form an airway or to prepare for the insertion of a tube for ventilation
tracheotomy (tray-kee-AH-toh-mee)	*trache/o* (trachea); *-tomy* (cutting operation)	incision into the trachea for purpose of restoring airflow to the lungs
Practice and Practitioners		
otolaryngologist (oh-to-LAYR-ihn-GAW-loh-jist)	*ot/o* (ear); *laryng/o* (larynx); *-logist* (one who specializes)	physician who specializes in diagnosis and treatment of ear, nose, and throat diseases
otolaryngology (oh-to-LAYR-ihn-GAW-loh-jee)	*ot/o* (ear); *laryng/o* (larynx); *-logy* (study of)	branch of medical study concerned with the ear, nose, and throat and diagnosis and treatment of its diseases
pulmonologist (PULL-muhn-AW-loh-jist)	*pulmon/o* (lung); *-logist* (one who specializes)	physician who specializes in diagnosing and treating respiratory disorders
pulmonology (PULL-muhn-AW-loh-jee)	*pulmon/o* (lung); *-logy* (study of)	medical specialty of diagnosing and treating respiratory disorders
respiratory therapist	from the Latin word *respirare* (breathe, blow back, blow again) + therapist	allied health care professional who specializes in airway management, mechanical ventilation, and blood acid–base balance

EXERCISES

 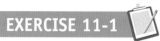 FIGURE LABELING: THE RESPIRATORY SYSTEM

alveolar duct
alveoli
capillaries
diaphragm
epiglottis

esophagus
laryngopharynx
larynx (vocal cords)
left lung
mediastinum

nares
nasal cavity
nasopharynx
oropharynx
pharynx

right bronchus
right lung
terminal bronchiole
trachea

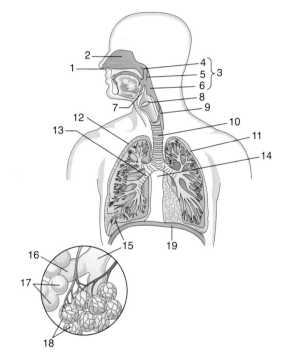

1. _____

2. _____

3. _____

4. _____

5. _____

6. _____

7. _____

8. _____

9 _____

10. _____

11. _____

12. _____

13. _____

14. _____

15. _____

16. _____

17. _____

18. _____

19. _____

EXERCISE 11-2 CASE STUDY

MEDICAL RECORD

Analyze the following medical record and answer the questions below.

HISTORY: A 30-year-old female who c/o a nonproductive cough, dyspnea, and a fever of 3 days; patient has a negative history for smoking and has otherwise been in good health.

PHYSICAL EXAM: T 102°F, BP 104/65, R 26, P 108

Tachypnea is accompanied by mild cyanosis, and inspiratory rales are noted during a stethoscope exam. WBC is elevated, CXR shows diffuse infiltrates at the bases of both lungs. An ABG taken while the patient was breathing room air was abnormal and showed the patient had low oxygen content in the blood. A sputum specimen contained WBCs.

DIAGNOSIS: Pneumonia of unknown etiology.

TREATMENT PLAN: Admit patient to the ICU. Administer antibiotics and oxygen by face mask and monitor patient's status.

1. What are the findings on physical examination? Circle the answer.
   A. Fast breathing, blue skin, and crackles heard in the lungs as the patient inhales
   B. Slow breathing, blue skin, and rales heard in the lungs as the patient holds her breath
   C. Slow breathing, blue skin, and rhonchi heard in the lungs as the patient exhales
   D. Fast heart rate, blue skin, and rales heard in the lungs as the patient inhales
   E. Fast breathing, blue skin, and wheezing heard in the lungs as the patient inhales

2. What is the patient's chief complaint? Circle the answer.
   A. Cannot breathe, fever, and coughing up material from lungs
   B. Dry cough and difficulty breathing
   C. Fever, coughing up sputum, and breathing fast
   D. Hoarse throat, dry cough, and fever
   E. Fever with a dry cough and difficulty breathing

3. Do you know what c/o means? Did you guess that it may mean "complains of," given its context in the sentence, or maybe having seen it somewhere else? The only standard meaning for this abbreviation is "in care of" or simply "care of." It's a longstanding postal abbreviation that has no place at all in a medical report. Guesswork, at least of this kind, should not be part of anyone's job in the medical professions.

4. The entire report appears to have been written by someone with no regard for the well-being of this patient. Analyze each sentence for grammatical errors. Rewrite the report and then get together with your classmates to compare individual versions. The science of grammar and principles of composition determine the message. Faulty grammar produces wrong results, just as does any other faulty science.

EXERCISE 11-3 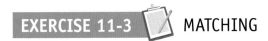 MATCHING

Match the term in Column A with the correct definition in Column B.

COLUMN A

1. _____ alveoli

2. _____ diaphragm

3. _____ pulmonary

4. _____ trachea

5. _____ epiglottis

6. _____ pneumonia, pneumonitis

7. _____ larynx

8. _____ bronchioles

9. _____ asthma

10. _____ pharynx

11. _____ emphysema

12. _____ bronchitis

13. _____ dyspnea

14. _____ tracheotomy

15. _____ bronchiostenosis

16. _____ apnea

17. _____ visceral pleura

18. _____ bronchoscopy

COLUMN B

A. the lid or flap that helps prevent food and drink from entering the trachea

B. the "voice box"

C. indicating something in or associated with the lungs

D. the major muscle of the respiratory system

E. tiny "sacs" in the lungs that receive oxygen from the bronchioles and transfer it to the capillaries

F. the "windpipe"; air flows through it to the bronchi

G. inflammation of a lung, caused by infection, chemical inhalation, or trauma

H. incision into the trachea

I. inner lining of the lung

J. the smallest extensions of the bronchi, which pass air directly to the alveoli

K. a lung disease characterized by reversible inflammation and constriction

L. throat

M. narrowing of a bronchial tube

N. inflammation of the mucous membrane of the bronchial tubes

O. difficult breathing

P. inspection using a bronchoscope

Q. absence of breathing

R. condition in which the alveoli are inefficient due to distension

EXERCISE 11-4 DEFINITIONS

Write the medical term for each definition.

1. the process of breathing in   _____

2. spitting up of blood   _____

3. any disease of the chest   _____

4. inflammation of sinus   _____

5. difficulty in speaking   _____

6. air in the pleural cavity   _____

7. incision into the pleura   _____

8. pain in the pleural region   _____

9. herniation of lung tissue or pleura   _____

EXERCISE 11-5 WORD BUILDING

Use *bronch/o* or *bronchi/o* to build the following terms:

1. inflammation of the bronchi   _____

2. chronic dilation of the bronchioles   _____

Use the suffix *-itis* to build the following terms:

3. inflammation of the larynx   _____

4. inflammation of a sinus   _____

5. inflammation of the epiglottis   _____

Use the suffix *-pnea* to build the following terms:

6. rapid breathing   _____

7. slow breathing   _____

8. painful or difficult breathing   _____

9. difficulty breathing while lying down _____

EXERCISE 11-6   CASE STUDY

An 88-year-old female is seen in the physician's office complaining of SOB, dizziness, orthopnea, elevated temperature, and a cough. She was referred to the hospital for evaluation. Bubbling rales are heard upon inspiration over the R bronchi. RUL congestion is seen on an X-ray exam. Vital signs are as follows: temperature, 102; pulse, 100; and rapid respirations, 24 and labored. She was placed on antibiotic treatment and was released to her family with medications after 3 days of hospitalization.

1. Define:

   A. Bubbling rales   _____

   B. Orthopnea   _____

EXERCISE 11-7   FILL IN THE BLANKS WITH MEANINGS OF ABBREVIATIONS

1. R   _____

2. CXR   _____

3. T&A   _____

4. ERV   _____

5. TV   _____

6. CF   _____

7. SOB   _____

8. TB   _____

9. ABG   _____

10. COPD   _____

11. CO_2 _____

12. IRV   _____

13. O_2 _____

14. PFT   _____

15. RV   _____

16. TLC   _____

EXERCISE 11-8 CROSSWORD PUZZLE: THE RESPIRATORY SYSTEM

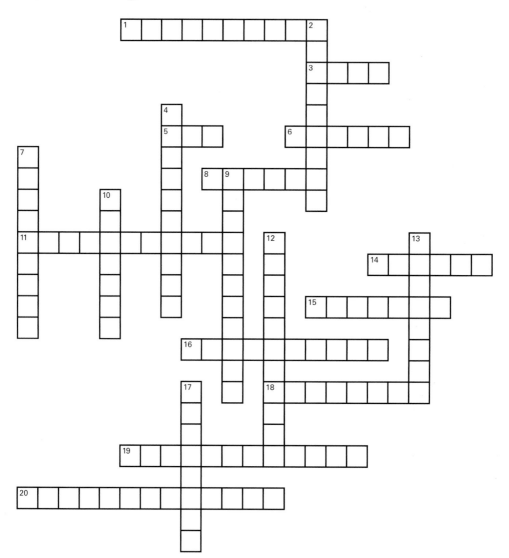

ACROSS

1. small bronchi
3. suffix meaning "breathing"
5. abbreviation for arterial blood gas
6. disease characterized by wheezing and inflammation of the bronchi
8. mucus expectorated from the mouth
11. area between lungs
14. vocal cords are found here
15. throat
16. inflammation of the bronchi
18. terminal end of the bronchial tree
19. instrument used to visualize inside the bronchi
20. needle inserted into the pleural space

DOWN

2. type of COPD with overexpansion of alveoli
4. inflammation of the voice box
7. same as pneumonitis
9. study of the lungs
10. windpipe
12. collapsed lung
13. singular form for bronchi
17. inflammation of the inner lining of the nose

CHAPTER 11 QUIZ

Multiple Choice

1. Pertussis is the medical term for:
   a. strep throat
   b. diphtheria
   c. whooping cough
   d. Lyme disease

2. Expectoration of blood is called:
   a. hematemesis
   b. hemoptysis
   c. anosmia
   d. dysphonia

3. What is the uppermost part of the pharynx?
   a. oropharynx
   b. laryngopharynx
   c. nasopharynx
   d. hypopharynx

4. What is the serous membrane that lines the walls of the pulmonary cavity?
   a. visceral pleura
   b. parietal pleura
   c. visceral peritoneum
   d. parietal peritoneum

5. What is the term for slow breathing?
   a. bradyphasia
   b. tachypnea
   c. bradypnea
   d. tachyphasia

6. Which procedure involves making an opening in the trachea to facilitate breathing?
   a. intubation
   b. tracheocentesis
   c. tracheoplasty
   d. tracheostomy

7. Which of the following would probably cause dysphonia?
   a. rhinitis
   b. laryngitis
   c. otitis
   d. ophthalmodynia

8. What is surgical puncture of the lungs?
   a. pneumoconiosis
   b. pneumocentesis
   c. pneumomelanosis
   d. pneumogenesis

9. What is pleurisy (pleuritis)?
   a. effusion of fluid into the air/tissue of the lungs
   b. softening of the lungs
   c. engorgement of the pulmonary vessels with fluid
   d. inflammation of the membrane that surrounds the lungs and lines the walls of the chest cavity

10. Which of the following is the same as pharyngitis?
    a. sore throat
    b. inflammation of the pharynx
    c. examination of the throat
    d. a fungal condition of the pharynx

11. What is the membrane that surrounds the lungs?
    a. pharynx
    b. palate
    c. pleura
    d. polyp

12. What is the term for difficult breathing while lying down?
    a. dysphonia
    b. hyperpnea
    c. dyspnea
    d. orthopnea

13. Which term means the drawing of air into the lungs?
    a. respiration
    b. orthopnea
    c. inspiration
    d. hypoxia

14. What is another term for *pneumonia*?
    a. pleuropneumonia
    b. pneumonitis
    c. pulmonary edema
    d. pulmonary insufficiency

15. What is chronic dilation of the bronchi?
    a. bronchiectasis
    b. bronchopathy
    c. bronchiolitis
    d. bronchoscopy

16. What is a collapse of part of a lung or alveoli called?
    a. asthma
    b. atelectasis
    c. SIDS
    d. cystic fibrosis

17. A thin watery discharge from the nose is known as?
    a. hemoptysis
    b. rhinitis
    c. rhinorrhea
    d. rhinolithiasis

18. What is a lobectomy?
    a. incision of the lung
    b. excision of a lung
    c. excision of a lobe of an organ
    d. bilateral incision of the skull

19. What condition describes alternating periods of apnea and dyspnea?
    a. Kussmaul breathing
    b. Cheyne-Stokes respirations
    c. atelectasis
    d. rales

12 *The Digestive System*

INTRODUCTION

The digestive system is composed of a continuous tract beginning with the oral cavity and ending at the anus (Fig. 12-1). This tract, called the **alimentary canal** or the **gastrointestinal (GI) tract**, is complemented by accessory organs that convert food and fluids into a form that permits the body to absorb nutrients. The GI tract is divided into two sections: the **upper GI tract**, which consists of the **oral cavity** (mouth), **esophagus**, and **stomach**, and the **lower GI tract**, which consists of the **intestines**. The three main functions of the digestive system are digestion, absorption, and elimination.

Apart from the specialists who treat the oral cavity and other shared organs of other systems, the specialists concerned with the digestive system are **gastroenterologists** and **proctologists**. The specialties are **gastroenterology** and **proctology**, respectively.

Many of the word elements related to the digestive system are listed in Table 12-1. After studying the table carefully, complete Exercise 12-1, and then check your answers in Appendix A.

STRUCTURE AND FUNCTION

The food we eat needs to be converted into a form our bodies can use and that conversion is the job performed by the digestive tract and associated organs.

The Upper Gastrointestinal Tract

Digestion begins in the oral cavity where food is broken apart by **mastication**, which is a technical term for chewing. **Saliva** produced by the **salivary glands** moistens the food, which helps form a **bolus**, a technical term for a small ball of masticated food that is then pushed back and downward with the tongue.

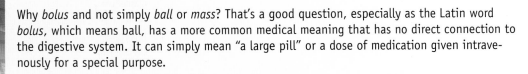

Why *bolus* and not simply *ball* or *mass*? That's a good question, especially as the Latin word *bolus*, which means ball, has a more common medical meaning that has no direct connection to the digestive system. It can simply mean "a large pill" or a dose of medication given intravenously for a special purpose.

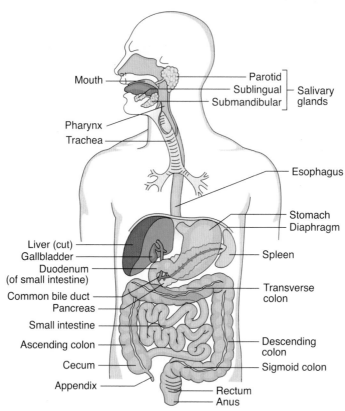

FIGURE 12-1 **Digestive system.** Some of the divisions of the large and small intestines are shown. The accessory organs are the salivary glands, liver, gallbladder, and pancreas. *From Cohen BJ. Medical Terminology: An Illustrated Guide. 5th ed. Philadelphia, PA: Lippincott Williams & Wilkins; 2007.*

TABLE 12-1	WORD ELEMENTS COMMONLY FOUND IN DIGESTIVE SYSTEM TERMS	
Element	**Type**	**Definition**
abdomin/o	root	abdomen
bucc/o	root	cheek
cheil/o	root	lip
chol/e, chol/o	root	bile, gall
cholangi/o	root	bile duct
cholecyst/o	root	gallbladder
choledoch/o	root	common bile duct
col/o, colon/o	root	colon
dent/i, dent/o	root	teeth
duoden/o	root	duodenum
-emesis	suffix	vomit
enter/o	root	intestine
esophag/o	root	esophagus
gastr/o	root	stomach
gingiv/o	root	gums
gloss/o	root	tongue
hepat/o	root	liver

Element	Type	Definition
ile/o	root	ileum
jejun/o	root	jejunum
lapar/o	root	abdomen
-lith	suffix	stone
pancreat/o	root	pancreas
-pepsia	suffix	digestion
phag/o	root	eating, swallowing
-phagia	suffix	eat or swallow
proct/o	root	anus and rectum
pylor/o	root	pylorus
rect/o	root	rectum
-scope	suffix	device for visual examination
-scopy	suffix	visual examination
sial/o	root	salivary glands
sigmoid/o	root	sigmoid colon
stomat/o	root	mouth

Word Elements Exercise DEFINING WORD ELEMENTS

Write the definition of each word element in the blank space to the right.

1. -phagia _____

2. choledoch/o _____

3. stomat/o _____

4. sigmoid/o _____

5. abdomin/o _____

6. enter/o _____

7. lapar/o _____

8. rect/o _____

9. -lith _____

10. sial/o _____

11. hepat/o _____

12. pylor/o _____

13. chol/e, chol/o _____

(continued)

14. cholangi/o _____

15. esophag/o _____

16. -emesis _____

17. -scope _____

18. gloss/o _____

19. jejun/o _____

20. gastr/o _____

21. cheil/o _____

22. ile/o _____

23. pancreat/o _____

24. bucc/o _____

25. cholecyst/o _____

26. -pepsia _____

27. col/o, colon/o _____

28. dent/i, dent/o _____

29. phag/o _____

30. duoden/o _____

31. proct/o _____

32. gingiv/o _____

33. -scopy _____

Next, the bolus enters the pharynx, which as you know from Chapter 11 is also part of the respiratory tract. From the pharynx, the bolus passes into the **esophagus** where it is lubricated with mucus before being carried into the stomach by wavelike muscular contractions called **peristalsis**. The **cardiac sphincter** is a ringlike muscle that controls the flow from the esophagus into the stomach.

The stomach is the center of the system, both physically and functionally. Its first job is to act as a temporary storage place for the food while it does its second job: secreting acid and enzymes to help break down proteins, fats, and carbohydrates. Digestion thus includes not only mechanical changes, such as the reduction of particle size and liquefaction (converting solids to liquids), but also the chemical changes needed to produce fuel for the body's cells. After 3 or 4 hours, the stomach's contents, which by this stage consist of a liquid called **chyme** (pronounced kyme), begin to enter the small intestine. Chyme passes through the **pyloric sphincter**, a muscle at the distal end of the stomach, and into the **duodenum**. Figure 12-2 illustrates the pathway of food through the GI tract.

The Lower Gastrointestinal Tract

The lower GI tract begins with the small intestine, which extends from the pyloric sphincter to the first part of the large intestine. Although it is about 20 feet in length, it is known as the small intestine because it is smaller in diameter than the large intestine. The small intestine is divided into three parts: the **duodenum**, **jejunum**, and **ileum** (Fig. 12-3). From the duodenum, chyme moves into the jejunum and from there into the ileum. The **ileocecal sphincter** controls the flow from the ileum into the **cecum**, the first part of the large intestine.

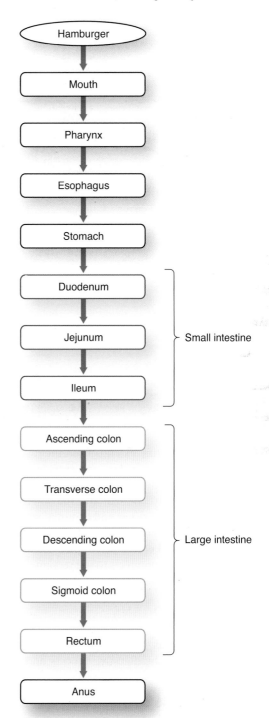

FIGURE 12-2 Pathway of food through the gastrointestinal tract.

Isn't the ileum also the name of one of the three bones making up the hip? No, that's the ilium. Although both words are pronounced the same, they have one letter that is different. If you remember that hip and ilium both have an "i" in the middle, you will be able to distinguish these two terms, which have different roots.

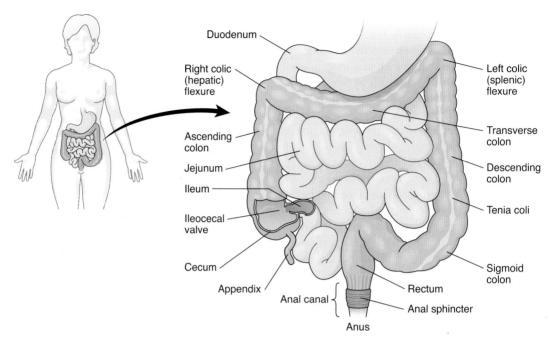

FIGURE 12-3   The small and large intestines. The small intestine, illustrated in *light pink*, is made up of the duodenum, jejunum, and ileum. The large intestine, illustrated in *darker pink*, can be divided into the ascending colon, transverse colon, and the descending colon. The intestinal tract terminates at the anus. *From Cohen BJ, Wood DL. Memmler's The Human Body in Health and Disease. 10th ed. Baltimore, MD: Lippincott Williams & Wilkins; 2004.*

The large intestine extends from the distal portion of the ileum to the anus. It is divided into three parts: the **cecum**, **colon**, and **rectum**. The cecum is the beginning part of the large intestine. Attached to the cecum is a blind tube called the **vermiform appendix**. Vermiform, which means wormlike, is usually omitted, and the single word *appendix* is the preferred term. The appendix consists of lymphatic tissue and is, functionally speaking, part of the lymphatic system.

The colon is subdivided into four parts: the **ascending colon**, **transverse colon**, **descending colon**, and **sigmoid colon** (see Fig. 12-3). The last part, the sigmoid colon, continues from the descending colon and connects to the rectum. The rectum takes up approximately the last 6 inches of the large intestine and terminates at the anus, through which waste products are eliminated.

ACCESSORY ORGANS

The **salivary glands**, **liver**, **gallbladder**, and **pancreas**, although not part of the alimentary canal, play a key role in the digestive process and are referred to as **accessory organs** of the digestive system (Fig. 12-4).

Salivary Glands

The senses of taste and smell stimulate the salivary glands to secrete **saliva**, a watery liquid that contains enzymes that begin the digestive process. Saliva also helps eliminate bacteria in the mouth and keeps the teeth and tongue clean. Figure 12-1 shows the location of the salivary glands.

Liver

The liver, located in the upper right quadrant of the abdomen under the dome of the diaphragm, plays many important roles in digestion, metabolism, and detoxification of harmful substances. One of its main digestive functions is the manufacture and secretion of **bile**. Our bodies need bile

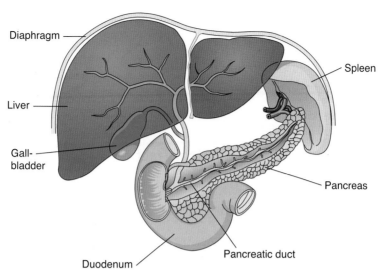

FIGURE 12-4 **Some of the accessory organs of digestion.** *Modified from Cohen BJ. Medical Terminology: An Illustrated Guide. 5th ed. Philadelphia, PA: Lippincott Williams & Wilkins; 2007.*

to process fats before they are released into the bloodstream. Once bile is produced in the liver, it travels down the **common bile duct** to the gallbladder for storage. The liver is an important organ whose functions are integrated into many of the body's systems.

Gallbladder

Although the liver produces and recycles bile, the **gallbladder**, which is located in a depression under the liver, stores, condenses, and delivers the bile to the small intestine. The gallbladder is also sometimes referred to as the **cholecystis** or **cholecyst**, from the root *cholecyst/o* (see Fig. 12-4).

Pancreas

The pancreas is an elongated feather-shaped organ that lies posterior to the stomach. It has both digestive and endocrine functions. It produces digestive enzymes that aid in processing carbohydrates and fats in foods as well as secreting hormones directly into the bloodstream.

DISORDERS AND TREATMENTS

Disorders of the Upper Gastrointestinal Tract

Disorders of the upper GI tract may involve infections, such as **stomatitis** and **gingivitis** in the oral cavity. **Parotiditis** (also known as parotitis) is an inflammation of the parotid gland. (See Fig. 12-1

 Quick Check: Key Terms

Fill in the blanks.

1. Cholecyst and cholecystis are other names for the _____.

2. The stomach has two main jobs. The first is the temporary storage of food. What is the other one? _____.

3. Name the three divisions of the small intestine. _____, _____, and _____.

for location of the parotid gland.) Other abnormal conditions such as **dental caries** or cavities and **bruxism** (an involuntary clenching or grinding of teeth) can occur in the mouth.

A few common disorders of the upper digestive tract include the following:

- **Dysphagia**: difficulty in swallowing
- **Esophagitis**: inflammation of the esophagus
- **Hiatus** (also **hiatal**) **hernia**: stomach protruding into the thoracic cavity (Fig. 12-5)
- **Gastroesophageal reflux disease**: upward flow of stomach acid into the esophagus
- **Gastritis**: inflamed gastric mucosa

Disorders of the Lower Gastrointestinal Tract

Disorders of the lower GI tract include obstructions, inflammation, or structural abnormalities. These conditions are listed below.

- **Crohn's disease**: inflammation in the mucosal lining of the intestine (usually the small intestine)
- **Appendicitis**: a common acute inflammatory disease. The appendix can become abscessed and may rupture, causing **peritonitis** (an inflammation of the peritoneum, which is the sac that lines the abdominal cavity).
- **Diverticula**: abnormal pouches in the intestinal wall that form as increased pressure pushes the wall of the colon outward at weakened points.
- **Diverticulosis**: abnormal pouches in the colon
- **Diverticulitis**: inflammation of the diverticula

Hiatal Hernia

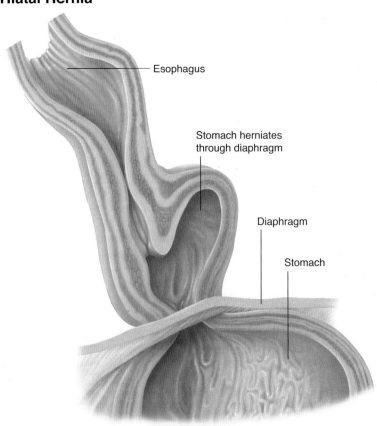

Esophagus

Stomach herniates through diaphragm

Diaphragm

Stomach

FIGURE 12-5   Hiatal hernia.

- **Intestinal obstruction**: refers to a lack of movement of the intestinal contents through the intestine
- **Intussusception**: a telescoping of a section of bowel inside an adjacent section
- **Volvulus**: a twisting of the bowel
- **Inguinal hernia**: protrusion of a small loop of intestine through a weak spot in the lower abdominal wall or groin

Disorders of the Accessory Organs of the Digestive System

Many of the conditions that affect the digestive system accessory organs are obstructions caused by stones, tumors, or inflammatory processes. A few of these are described below.

- **Cholelithiasis**: a condition in which calculi or stones reside in the gallbladder or bile ducts
- **Cholecystitis**: inflammation of the gallbladder
- **Cholangiolitis**: inflammation of a bile duct
- **Choledocholithiasis**: obstruction of the biliary tract by gallstones
- **Hepatitis:** inflammation of the liver
- **Jaundice** (also called **icterus**): a symptom of hepatitis characterized by a yellow appearance of skin or eyes
- **Cirrhosis** of the liver: chronic liver disease

Additional conditions, symptoms, and disorders of the digestive system include **anorexia** (loss of appetite), **bulimia** (binge eating followed by self-induced vomiting and misuse of laxatives), **eructation** (belching or burping gas), **hyperemesis** (excessive vomiting), **dyspepsia** (indigestion), and **hemorrhoids** (enlarged veins in or near the anus).

Abbreviation Table	THE DIGESTIVE SYSTEM
ABBREVIATION	**MEANING**
BE	barium enema
BM	bowel movement
EGD	esophagogastroduodenoscopy
GB	gallbladder
GBS	gallbladder X-ray series
GERD	gastroesophageal reflux disease
GI	gastrointestinal
HCl	hydrochloric acid
IBS	irritable bowel syndrome
LES	lower esophageal sphincter
NGT	nasogastric tube
NPO	nothing by mouth
PO	per os, or by mouth
TPN	total parenteral nutrition
UGI	upper gastrointestinal

Study Table THE DIGESTIVE SYSTEM

TERM AND PRONUNCIATION	ANALYSIS	MEANING
Structure and Function		
alimentary canal (al-ih-MEN-tah-ree)	from the Latin word *alimentarius* (pertaining to food) + canal	the digestive tract, the gastrointestinal (GI) tract
antibody (AN-tih-body)	*anti-* (against) + body	antibodies contained in saliva that act as antibacterial agents
bilirubin (BIHL-ee-ROO-bin)	from the Latin *bilus* (bile) and *ruber* (red)	waste produced by worn out red blood cells breaking down
cardiac sphincter (KAR-dee-ak sfink-ter)	*cardi/o* (heart); *-ac* (adjective suffix); from the Greek word *sphingein* (to bind tight)	the ringlike muscle between the esophagus and stomach that controls food flow
colon (KOH-luhn); also called the *large intestine*	from the Greek word *kolon* (large intestine)	the large intestine, divisible into the ascending, transverse, descending, and sigmoid colons
common bile duct	common English words	tube that transports bile from the liver to the gallbladder
deglutition (dee-glu-TISH-uhn)	from the Latin word *deglutire* (to swallow, overwhelm, abolish)	swallowing
duodenal (doo-oh-DEE-nuhl)	from the Greek word *dodekadaktylon* (literally "12 fingers long"; named by Greek physician Herophilus) + *-al* (adjective suffix)	adjective form of duodenum used in the terms naming some digestive system disorders
duodenum (doo-oh-DEE-num)	from the Greek *dodekadaktylon* (12 fingers long)	segment of the small intestine connecting with the stomach
esophagus (ee-SOF-ah-guhs)	from the Greek *oisophagos* (gullet, literally "what carries and eats")	the part of the digestive tract between the pharynx and stomach
fundus (FUN-duhs)	a Latin word meaning "bottom"	the part of the stomach lying above the cardia notch
gallbladder	from Old English *galla* (to shine, yellow); from Old English *bledre* (to blast, blow up, swell up)	small pear-shaped organ that stores bile
gastric (GAS-trik)	*gastr/o* (stomach); *-ic* (adjective suffix)	adjective form of stomach
gastrointestinal tract (GAS-troh-in-TES-tin-ahl)	*gastr/o* (stomach); from Latin *intestina*, plural of *intestinus* (internal, inward, intestine) + tract	the alimentary canal; also, simply, the GI tract

TERM AND PRONUNCIATION	ANALYSIS	MEANING
ileocecal sphincter (EEL-ee-oh-see-kal)	*ile/o* (ileum); from the Latin *caecum* (blind); *-al* (adjective suffix); sphincter (from the Greek word *sphingein*: to bind tight)	muscular ring that separates the distal portion of the ileum and the beginning of the cecum (large intestine)
ileum (ILL-ee-uhm)	a Latin word meaning "flank," "groin"	the longest segment of the small intestine, which leads into the large intestine
intestine (ihn-TESS-tin); the term includes the small intestine and the large intestine, also called the *colon*	from Latin *intestina*, plural of *intestinus* (internal, inward, intestine)	the small intestine is divisible into the duodenum, jejunum, and ileum; the large intestine comprises the cecum, colon, rectum, and anus
jejunum (jeh-JOO-nuhm)	from the Latin word *jejunus* (empty, fasting, abstinent, hungry)	eight-foot-long segment of the small intestine between the duodenum and the ileum
pancreas (PAN-kree-as)	from the Greek words *pan* (all) and *kreas* (flesh, meat)	organ of the digestive system that has both exocrine and endocrine functions; secretes enzymes that aid in digestion
pancreatic (pan-kree-AT-ik)	*pancreat/o* (pancreas); *-ic* (adjective suffix)	adjective for pancreas
peristalsis (pear-ih-STAL-sis)	from the Greek word *peristaltiko* (clasping and compressing)	wavelike muscular contractions that move food along in the digestive tract
pharynx (FAYR-inx)	from the Greek word *pharunx* (throat)	passageway just below the nasal cavity and mouth
pyloric sphincter (pye-LOHR-ik sfink-ter)	*pylor/o* (pylorus); *-ic* (adjective suffix); sphincter (from the Greek word *sphingein*: to bind tight)	ring muscle between the stomach and duodenum
salivary glands (SAL-ih-vahr-ee)	from the Latin word *salivarius* (slimy, clammy) + gland from the Latin word *glans* (acorn)	collectively, the parotid, sublingual, and submandibular salivary glands
stoma (STOH-mah)	a Greek word meaning "mouth," "opening"	an artificial opening
stomach (STUM-uhk)	stomach	digestive organ composed of four parts: the fundus, the cardia, the body, and the antrum
Common Disorders		
anorexia (an-orh-ECKS-ee-ah)	from the Greek *an* (without) + *orexis* (appetite, desire)	loss of appetite
appendicitis (ay-PEN-dih-SY-tis)	from the Latin word *appendix* (something attached); *-itis* (inflammation)	inflammation of the appendix

(continued)

TERM AND PRONUNCIATION	ANALYSIS	MEANING
ascites (ay-SYTE-ees)	from the Greek word *askos* (bag)	abnormal accumulation of fluid in the peritoneal cavity
bruxism (BRUKS-ism)	from the Greek word *ebryxa*, root from *brykein* infinitive of the verb; *ebryxa* (to gnash the teeth) + *-ism* (condition)	involuntary grinding of the teeth that usually occurs during sleep
bulimia (bull-EE-mee-ah)	from the Greek word *boulemia* (hunger)	eating disorder characterized by episodes of binge eating followed by self-induced vomiting and misuse of laxatives
cholangiolitis (KOH-lan-GY-oh-LY-tis)	*cholangi/o* (bile, duct); *-itis* (inflammation)	inflammation of the bile ducts
cholecystitis (KOH-lee-siss-TY-tiss) cholecyst (KOH-leh-sihst)	*cholecyst/o* (gallbladder); *-itis* (inflammation)	inflammation of the gallbladder
cholecystopathy (KOH-lee-siss-TOP-ah-thee)	*cholecyst/o* (gallbladder); *-pathy* (disease)	any disease of the gallbladder
choledocholithiasis (KOH-le-DOKO-lith-EYE-ah-sis)	*choledoch/o* (common bile duct); *-lithiasis* (condition of having stones)	inflammation of the bile duct caused by gall stones
cholelithiasis (KOH-lee-lih-THYE-ah-sis)	*chol/e* (bile, gall); *-lithiasis* (condition of having stones)	formation or presence of stones in the gallbladder or common bile duct
cirrhosis (sir-OH-sis)	from the Greek word *kirrhos* (tawny), named for the orange-yellow appearance of a diseased liver	chronic disease of the liver
colitis (ko-LY-tihs)	*col/o* (colon); *-itis* (inflammation)	inflammation of the colon
constipation (kon-stih-PAY-shun)	from the Latin word *constipare* (to press or crowd together)	decrease in the frequency of bowel movements; difficulty in passing stools; and/or hard, dry stools
Crohn's disease	named after American B.B. Crohn (1884–1983), one of the team that described it in 1932	chronic inflammation of part(s) of the intestinal tract
dental caries (kayr-eez)	*dent/i* (tooth); *-al* (adjective suffix) + *caries*, a Latin word meaning "rot," "rottenness," "corruption"	tooth decay
diverticulitis (dye-ver-tik-yoo-LYE-tis)	from the Latin word *diverticulum* (a side road); *-itis* (inflammation)	inflammation of a diverticulum or sac in the intestinal tract
duodenitis (doo-odd-eh-NY-tihs)	*duoden/o* (duodenum); *-itis* (inflammation)	inflammation of the duodenum

TERM AND PRONUNCIATION	ANALYSIS	MEANING
dyspepsia (dis-PEP-see-ah)	from the Greek word *dyspeptos* (hard to digest); *-ia* (condition of)	impairment of digestion
dysphagia (dis-FA-jee-ah)	*dys-* (difficulty); *phag/o* (eating, swallowing); *-ia* (condition of)	difficulty swallowing
enteritis (ehn-teh-RY-tihs)	*enter/o* (intestine); *-itis* (inflammation)	inflammation of the intestine
enterohepatitis (EN-teh-roh- hep-ah-TI-tihs)	*enter/o* (intestine); *hepat/o* (liver); *-itis* (inflammation)	inflammation of the intestine and liver
enteropathy (en-tehr-OP-ah-thee)	*enter/o* (intestine); *-pathy* (disease)	any intestinal disease
eructation (ee-RUK-tay-shun)	from the Latin verb *eructo* (belch)	act of belching or burping gas up from the stomach
gastric ulcers (GAS-trik)	*gastr/o* (stomach); *-ic* (adjective suffix) + ulcer, from the Latin *ulcus*, related to the Greek word *helkos* (wound, sore)	erosion of the gastric mucosa
gastritis (gas-TRY-tihs)	*gastr/o* (stomach); *-itis* (inflammation)	inflammation of the stomach
gastrocele (GAS-troh-seel)	*gastr/o* (stomach); *-cele* (hernia)	hernia of the stomach
gastroduodenitis (GAS-troh-doo-oh-deh-NY-tihs)	*gastr/o* (stomach); *duoden/o* (duodenum); *-itis* (inflammation)	inflammation of the stomach and duodenum
gastroenteritis (GAS-troh-en-teh-RY-tihs)	*gastr/o* (stomach); *enter/o* (intestine); *-itis* (inflammation)	inflammation of the stomach and intestine
gastroesophageal reflux disease (GAS-troh-ee-sof-a-JEE-al) (GERD)	*gastr/o* (stomach); *esophag/o* (esophagus); *-al* (adjective suffix); + reflux disease	upward flow of stomach acid into the esophagus
gingivitis (JIN-jeh-vye-tis)	*gingiv/o* (gums); *-itis* (inflammation)	inflammation of the gums
hemorrhoids (hem-ROYDs)	from the Greek word *haimorrhoides* derived from *haima* (blood); and *rhoos* (a flowing)	enlarged veins in or near the anus that may cause pain or bleeding
hepatitis (hep-ah-TY-tihs)	*hepat/o* (liver); *-itis* (inflammation)	inflammation of the liver
hepatogenic (heh-pah-toh-JEN-ik)	*hepat/o* (liver); *-genic* (originating)	originating in the liver
hepatomegaly (heh-PAH-to-MEG-ah-lee)	*hepat/o* (liver); *-megaly* (enlargement)	enlarged liver

(continued)

TERM AND PRONUNCIATION	ANALYSIS	MEANING
hiatal hernia (HYE-ay-tahl HER-nee-ah)	from the Latin word *hiatus* (gaping, opening); *-al* (adjective suffix) + the Latin word *hernia* (rupture)	protrusion of the stomach through the diaphragm into the thoracic cavity
hyperemesis (hy-per-EM-ih-sis)	*hyper-* (excessive); *-emesis* (vomit)	excessive vomiting
inguinal hernia (ING-gwi-nahl HER-nee-ah)	from the Latin word *inguinalis* (of the groin) + the Latin word *hernia* (rupture)	outpouching of intestines into the inguinal or groin region
intussusception (in-tuh-suh-SEP-shun)	from the Latin word *intus* (within); from the Latin word *suscipere* (undertake; support, accept)	one part of the intestine slipping or telescoping over another
jaundice (JAWN-dis) or icterus (IK-tehr-us)	from Middle French word *jaunisse* (yellow)	yellowish cast to the skin, sclera (white part of the eye), and mucous membranes caused by bile deposits
jejunitis (jeh-joo-NY-tihs)	*jejun/o* (jejunum); *-itis* (inflammation)	inflammation of the jejunum
melena (MEL-in-nah)	from the Greek word *melas* (black)	blood in the stool
pancreatitis (PAN-kree-ah-TY-tihs)	*pancreat/o* (pancreas); *-itis* (inflammation)	inflammation of the pancreas
pancreatopathy (PAN-kree-ah-TOP-ah-thee)	*pancreat/o* (pancreas); *-pathy* (disease)	any disease of the pancreas
parotiditis (pah-RAH-ti-DYE-tis)	parotid from the Greek words *para-* (beside) and *otos* (ear); *-itis* (inflammation)	inflammation of the parotid salivary glands
peritonitis (PAYR-ih-toh-NYE-tis)	from the Greek words *peri-* (around) and *teinein* (to stretch); *-itis* (inflammation)	inflammation of the peritoneal cavity
polyp (PAHL-ip)	from the Latin word *polypus* (cuttlefish)	growth protruding from a stalk in the digestive tract
sialoadenitis (SY-ah-loh-ah-deh-NY-tihs)	*sial/o* (saliva, salivary gland); *aden/o* (gland); *-itis* (inflammation)	inflammation of a salivary gland
sialoangiitis (SY-ah-loh-an-jee-EYE-tihs)	*sial/o* (saliva, salivary gland); *angi/o* (vessel); *-itis* (inflammation)	inflammation of a salivary duct
sialorrhea (SY-ah-loh-REE-ah)	*sial/o* (saliva, salivary gland); *-rrhea* (discharge)	excessive production of saliva
sialostenosis (SY-ah-loh-steh-NO-sihs)	*sial/o* (saliva, salivary gland); *-stenosis* (narrowed, blocked)	narrowing of a salivary duct
stomatitis (STOH-mah-tye-tis)	*stomat/o* (mouth); *-itis* (inflammation)	inflammation of the mouth

TERM AND PRONUNCIATION	ANALYSIS	MEANING
Diagnosis and Treatment		
antacids (ant-AS-ids)	from *anti-* (against) + acids	medications used to neutralize acid production
antidiarrheal (an-ty-DYE-ah-REE-al)	*anti-* (against); from the Greek *dia-* (through) + *-rrhea* (discharge); *-al* (adjective suffix)	drugs that relieve diarrhea by absorbing the excess fluid or by decreasing intestinal motility
antiemetic (an-ty-EE-meh-tik)	*anti-* (against); *-emesis* (vomit); *-ic* (adjective suffix)	drugs used to relieve vomiting
antiflatulence (an-ty-FLAT-yoo-lens)	*anti-* (against); from the Latin word *flatus* (a blowing, a breaking wind)	drugs taken to relieve gas or flatus
colonoscope (ko-LAWN-uh-skope)	*colon/o* (colon); *-scope* (instrument for viewing)	device used in colonoscopy
colonoscopy (ko-luh-NAW-skuh-pee)	*colon/o* (colon); *-scopy* (viewing)	visual examination of the colon with a colonoscope
duodenoscopy (doo-oh-deh-NOS-kuh-pee)	*duoden/o* (duodenum); *-scopy* (viewing)	visual examination of the duodenum with the aid of an endoscope
emetic (ee-MET-ik)	*emesis* (vomit); *-ic* (adjective suffix)	drugs that stimulate or induce vomiting; frequently used in poisoning cases
enteroscope (en-TEHR-oh-skope)	*enter/o* (intestine); *-scope* (instrument for viewing)	lighted instrument for visually examining the intestines
enteroscopy (en-tehr-OS-koh-pee)	*enter/o* (intestine); *-scopy* (viewing)	visual examination of the intestines
gastroscope (GAS-troh-scope)	*gastr/o* (stomach); *-scope* (instrument for viewing)	lighted instrument for visually examining the stomach
gastroscopy (gas-TRAH-scoh-pee)	*gastr/o* (stomach); *-scopy* (viewing)	visual examination of the stomach with a lighted instrument
H2 blockers or H2-receptor antagonists	H2 (or histamine2), a common chemical in the body, signals the stomach to make acid; H2 blockers oppose histamine's action and reduce the amount of acid the stomach produces; + blocker, a common English word	drugs that block the release of gastric acid; used to treat gastroesophageal reflux disease
hepatoscopy (he-pah-TOSS-kuh-pee)	*hepat/o* (liver); *-scopy* (viewing)	visual examination of the liver
sialography (sy-ah-LOG-rah-fee)	*sial/o* (saliva, salivary gland); *-graphy* (the process of recording)	radiography of salivary glands and ducts

(continued)

TERM AND PRONUNCIATION	ANALYSIS	MEANING
Practice and Practitioners		
gastroenterologist (GAS-troh-en-tehr-OL-oh-jist)	*gastr/o* (stomach); *enter/o* (intestine); *-logist* (one who studies a certain field)	a specialist in the diagnosis and treatment of digestive system disorders
gastroenterology (GAS-troh-en-tehr-OL-oh-jee)	*gastr/o* (stomach); *enter/o* (intestine); *-logy* (the study of)	the specialty concerned with the digestive system
internal medicine	two common English words	specialty in the diagnosis and nonsurgical treatment of serious and/or chronic illnesses; the phrase is quite commonly used in North America (but not necessarily elsewhere); it also covers subspecialties in specific organs, such as the liver, kidneys, etc.
internist (IN-tur-nist)	internal (English adjective meaning "inside") + *-ist* (practitioner)	a specialist in internal medicine
proctologist (prok-TAH-lo-jist)	*proct/o* (anus and rectum); *-logist* (one who studies a certain field)	a specialist in the diagnosis and treatment of rectal and anal disorders
proctology	*proct/o* (anus and rectum); *-logy* (study of)	study of the rectum and anus
Surgical Procedures		
anastomosis (ah-NAS-tah-MOH-sis)	from the Greek word *anastomoein* (to bring to a mouth)	creation of an opening between two hollow organs
cholecystectomy (KOH-lee-siss-TEK-toh-mee)	*cholecyst/o* (gallbladder); *-ectomy* (surgical removal)	excision of the gallbladder
cholecystotomy (KOH-lee-siss-TOT-oh-mee)	*cholecyst/o* (gallbladder); *-tomy* (incision)	incision into the gallbladder
colectomy (ko-LEK-toh-mee)	*col/o* (colon); *-ectomy* (surgical removal)	excision of all or part of the colon
colopexy (KOH-loh-pehk-see)	*col/o* (colon); *-pexy* (surgical fixation)	fixation of the colon
colostomy (koh-LOSS-tuh-mee)	*col/o* (colon); *-stomy* (permanent opening)	surgical establishment of an opening into the colon
colotomy (ko-LOT-uh-mee)	*col/o* (colon); *-tomy* (incision)	incision into the colon
duodenectomy (doo-oh-deh-NEK-toh-mee)	*duoden/o* (duodenum); *-ectomy* (surgical removal)	excision of the duodenum
duodenostomy (doo-oh-deh-NOS-toh-mee)	*duoden/o* (duodenum); *-stomy* (permanent opening)	surgical establishment of an opening in the duodenum
gastrectomy (gas-TREK-toh-mee)	*gastr/o* (stomach); *-ectomy* (surgical removal)	excision of part of the stomach
hepatopexy (HEH-pah-to-pek-see)	*hepat/o* (liver); *-pexy* (surgical fixation)	fixation of the liver

TERM AND PRONUNCIATION	ANALYSIS	MEANING
jejunectomy (jeh-joo-NEK-toh-mee)	*jejun/o* (jejunum); *-ectomy* (surgical removal)	excision of all or part of the jejunum
jejunoplasty (jeh-JOON-oh-plass-tee)	*jejun/o* (jejunum); *-plasty* (surgical repair)	surgical repair of the jejunum
jejunotomy (jeh-joo-NOT-oh-mee)	*jejun/o* (jejunum); *-tomy* (incision)	incision into the jejunum
pancreatotomy (PAN-kree-ah-TOT-ah-mee)	*pancreat/o* (pancreas); *-tomy* (incision)	incision into the pancreas
sialoadenectomy (SY-al-oh-ah-deh-NEK-tah-mee)	*sial/o* (saliva, salivary gland); *aden/o* (gland); *-ectomy* (surgical removal)	excision of a salivary gland
sialoadenotomy (SY-al-oh-ah-deh-NOT-ah-mee)	*sial/o* (saliva, salivary gland); *aden/o* (gland); *-tomy* (incision)	incision of a salivary gland

EXERCISES

 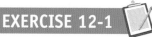 FIGURE LABELING: THE DIGESTIVE SYSTEM

anus
ascending colon
cecum
descending colon
duodenum
esophagus
gallbladder

liver
mouth
pancreas
parotid gland
pharynx
rectum
sigmoid colon

small intestine
stomach
sublingual gland
submandibular gland
transverse colon

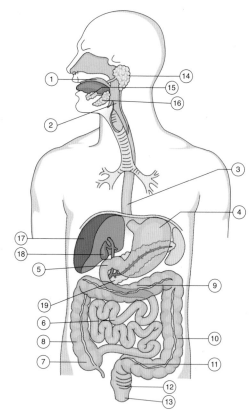

1. _____
2. _____
3. _____
4. _____
5. _____
6. _____
7. _____
8. _____
9. _____
10. _____

11. _____
12. _____
13. _____
14. _____
15. _____
16. _____
17. _____
18. _____
19. _____

EXERCISE 12-2   CASE STUDY

Reggie V., a middle-aged man, began feeling pain in his upper abdomen about a month ago. He described the pain as a burning sensation that at first disappeared after he took over-the-counter antacids. In the last 10 days or so, however, he has noticed that these measures have become less and less helpful.

His pain is not accompanied by SOB, nausea, or chest pains, and his appetite remains normal. His BP was slightly elevated also, and he reported that based on a family history of HTN, his GP advised him to stop smoking cigarettes and restrict caffeinated drinks to one or two a day.

This patient's WBC count was normal. Endoscopy revealed a 1-cm gastric ulcer.

1. What does the abbreviation SOB stand for?

   _____

2. What does the abbreviation BP stand for?

   _____

3. Does the abbreviation HTN have anything to do with the first two abbreviations? Explain how each may relate to the other two.

   _____

   _____

4. What does WBC stand for?

   _____

5. What word elements make up the word "endoscopy" in the case study? What does the term *endoscopy* mean?

   _____

EXERCISE 12-3   WORD BUILDING

To build the term, use the combining form that is provided and add an appropriate suffix.

COMBINING FORM	BODY PART	CREATE A TERM
1. or/o	mouth	adjective form for oral cavity
		_____
2. stomat/o	mouth	inflammation of mouth
		_____
3. bucc/o	cheek	adjective form for cheek
		_____
4. cheil/o	lip	condition of the lip
		_____
5. gingiv/o	gum	removal of gum tissue (mouth)
		_____
6. gloss/o	tongue	incision into the tongue
		_____
7. lingu/o	tongue	adjective form for tongue
		_____
8. gastr/o	stomach	stomach pain
		_____
9. pharyng/o	throat	adjective form for pharynx
		_____
10. enter/o	intestine	inflammation of the small intestine
		_____
11. duoden/o	duodenum	adjective form for duodenum
		_____

12. jejun/o   jejunum   adjective form of jejunum

    _____

13. ile/o   ileum   inflammation of the ileum

    _____

14. col/o   colon   removal of the colon

    _____

15. rect/o   rectum   a herniation of the rectum

    _____

16. an/o   anus   adjective form for anus

    _____

17. proct/o   anus/rectum   one whose medical specialty is the
                                   anus and rectum

    _____

18. hepat/o   liver   an enlarged liver

    _____

19. bil   bile   a bile pigment that is formed from the
                                  destruction of red blood cells

    _____

20. cholecyst/o   gallbladder   removal of the gallbladder

    _____

EXERCISE 12-4 ABBREVIATIONS AND ACRONYMS

Write the expansion for each abbreviation or acronym.

1. BE   _____

2. BM   _____

3. GI   _____

4. IBS   _____

5. GERD   _____

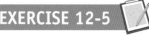

EXERCISE 12-5   CROSSWORD PUZZLE: THE DIGESTIVE SYSTEM

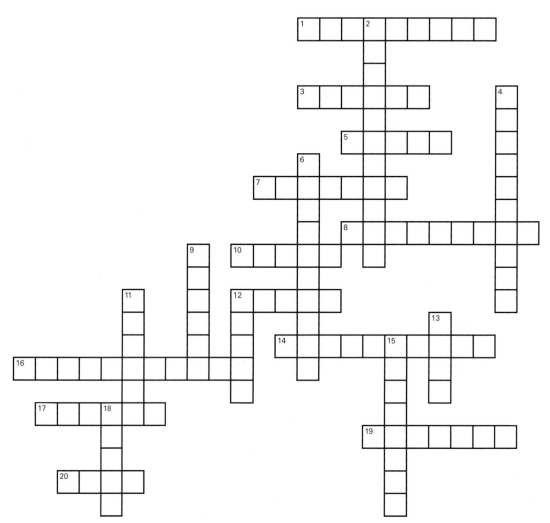

ACROSS

1. difficulty swallowing
3. liquid secreted from salivary gland
5. growth from a stalk found in intestines
7. binge eating
8. chronic liver disease
10. erosion of intestinal mucosa
12. root for stomach
14. burping
16. excessive vomiting
17. pertaining to the cheek
19. second portion of small intestine
20. distal end of the GI tract

DOWN

2. inflammation of the peritoneum
4. inflammation of the mouth
6. gastrointestinal tract
9. gas
11. blood in the stool
12. root for tongue
13. root for salivary gland
15. loss of appetite
18. first part of large intestine

CHAPTER 12 QUIZ

Matching

Match the term in Column A with the correct definition in Column B.

COLUMN A

1. _____ buccal

2. _____ dentalgia

3. _____ esophagitis

4. _____ duodenum

5. _____ enteric

6. _____ emesis

7. _____ jaundice

8. _____ ascites

9. _____ esophagostenosis

10. _____ diarrhea

COLUMN B

A. abnormal fluid accumulation in the abdomen

B. cheek

C. narrowing of the esophagus

D. vomiting

E. yellow

F. toothache

G. first part of small intestine

H. adjective referring to intestine(s)

I. inflammation of esophagus

J. watery discharge from the rectum; liquid stools

Multiple Choice

11. Dysphagia is difficulty with:
    a. talking
    b. swallowing
    c. elimination
    d. digestion

12. Anorexia is:
    a. difficulty in digestion
    b. hyperemesis
    c. loss of appetite
    d. a small ulcer

13. Gas in the stomach or intestines is:
    a. gavage
    b. icterus
    c. flatus
    d. dysentery

14. Diverticulitis is an inflammation of:
    a. small pouches in the intestine
    b. the vermiform appendix
    c. the hypopharynx
    d. descending colon

15. Movement of the bowels by which their contents are propelled toward the rectum is:
    a. pyloroplasty
    b. volvulus
    c. peristalsis
    d. gastroenteric

16. The buccal mucosa is in the:
    a. nostril
    b. stomach and intestines
    c. mouth, inside the cheek
    d. greater curvature of the stomach

17. Belching is called:
    a. volvulus
    b. eructation
    c. gastroenteric
    d. halitosis

18. Vomiting blood is called:
    a. hematitis
    b. indigestion
    c. mastication
    d. hematemesis

19. Telescoping of the intestines into themselves is called:
    a. gastrojejunostomy
    b. intussusception
    c. volvulus
    d. sphincter

20. A colonoscopy is:
    a. an endoscopic study of the colon
    b. an upper endoscopy with biopsy
    c. a type of barium enema
    d. an endoscopic study of the small intestine

13 *The Urinary System*

Upon completion of this chapter, you should be able to:

- Identify and define the word elements of the urinary system.
- Build, spell, and pronounce medical terms that relate to the urinary system.
- Interpret abbreviations relating to the urinary system.
- Define the terms naming the major parts of the urinary system.
- Define terms naming disorders, treatments, and procedures related to the urinary system.
- Label a diagram of the urinary system.

INTRODUCTION

The urinary system is composed of the **kidneys**, **ureters**, **urinary bladder**, and **urethra**. Figure 13-1 illustrates the location of each of these structures. The primary function of the urinary system is to remove wastes and toxins from the body. The process starts with the kidneys, which remove wastes from the bloodstream. The kidneys then convert the waste to urine (water that contains other substances in solution) and transport it to the bladder via the ureters. The urine is then eliminated through the urethra. This process regulates the amount of water in the body and maintains the proper balance of acids and electrolytes, such as salts, and is a necessary function for human survival. The flow chart illustrates this fundamental process.

A physician who specializes in the diagnosis and treatment of urinary disorders is called a **urologist**, and the specialty practice is **urology**. A physician who treats the kidney and kidney disorders is called a **nephrologist**. This area of specialty is named **nephrology**.

Table 13-1 lists most of the word elements used in forming urinary system terms. The root cyst/o is used to form terms having to do with the urinary bladder. However, that root and the terms formed from it may be used in reference to the gallbladder. Therefore, **cystalgia**, **cystectomy**, and **cystopexy** can mean, respectively, pain in, excision of, and surgical fixation of either the urinary bladder or the gallbladder. The term *cystectomy* can also mean excision of a cyst, a word that refers to an abnormal sac that has nothing to do with either the urinary bladder or the gallbladder.

All of these terms come from the Greek word *kystis*, which means "bladder," and careful professionals refer specifically to the gallbladder by coupling the Greek word *chole* (which means "bile") with cyst/o. This distinction yields the terms *cholecystalgia, cholecystectomy, cholecystopexy*, and so on.

Study the word elements listed in Table 13-1, and then test your etymological skills by completing the Word Elements Exercise without referring to the table. Check your answers against those listed in Appendix A.

STRUCTURE AND FUNCTION

The kidneys are bean-shaped organs (hence the source for the name of the kidney bean) and are about the size of a man's fist; they lie at the back of the abdominopelvic cavity, along each side of the spinal column. Each kidney is covered by a thin membrane called the **renal capsule**. A thicker layer of fatty tissue, called the **perirenal fat**, surrounds the renal capsule and thus provides protection for this vital organ. Finally, a thin layer of connective tissue, called the **renal fascia**, forms each kidney's outer covering. The **hilum** is the indented and narrowest part of the kidney, where blood vessels and nerves enter. Figure 13-2 shows the structure of the kidneys.

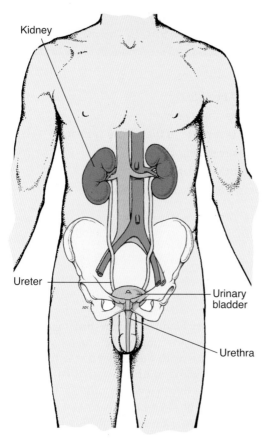

FIGURE 13-1 Primary structures of the urinary system. Anterior view of the kidneys, ureters, bladder, and urethra (male). *From Stedman's Medical Dictionary. 27th ed. Baltimore, MD: Lippincott Williams & Wilkins; 2000.*

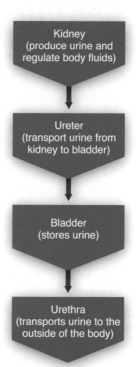

Flow chart illustrating the process of urine formation and excretion. The process of urine formation begins in the kidneys. The kidneys filter waste products from the blood and convert them to urine. The urine is transported from the kidneys by the ureters to the bladder, where it is stored until it is expelled through the urethra via the process of urination.

TABLE 13-1	URINARY SYSTEM WORD ELEMENTS	
Element	**Type**	**Definition**
cyst/o	root	bladder
glomerul/o	root	glomerulus
-iasis	suffix	suffix meaning "condition" or "state"
lith/o	root	stone
nephr/o, ren/o	root	kidney
noct/o	root	night
olig/o	root	little, few
poly-	prefix	prefix meaning "much" or "many"
py/o	root	pus
pyel/o	root	pelvis
ur/o, urin/o	root	urine
ureter/o	root	ureter
urethr/o	root	urethra

Word Elements Exercise   FILL IN THE BLANKS

Write the meaning of each word element in its adjacent blank space.

1. ur/o, urin/o   _____

2. noct/o   _____

3. olig/o   _____

4. -iasis   _____

5. glomerul/o   _____

6. nephr/o, ren/o   _____

7. urethr/o   _____

8. lith/o   _____

9. poly-   _____

10. py/o   _____

11. pyel/o   _____

12. ureter/o   _____

13. cyst/o   _____

✔ Quick Check: A Few Key Points

Fill in the blanks.

1. The urinary system is composed of the _____,
   _____, _____ _____,
   and _____.

2. Although the root cyst/o may be used to refer to either the urinary bladder or the gallbladder, careful speakers and writers use the root _____ in referring to the gallbladder.

3. The indented (narrowest) part of the kidney, where blood vessels and nerves enter, is called the _____.

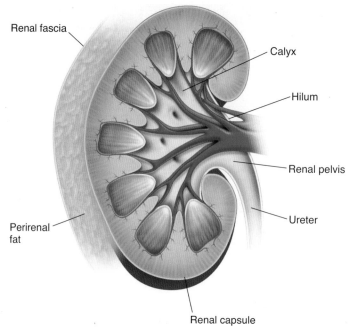

Renal fascia

Calyx

Hilum

Renal pelvis

Ureter

Renal capsule

Perirenal fat

FIGURE 13-2 **Kidney.** Sagittal view of the kidney and internal structures. *From Collins CE.* A Short Course in Medical Terminology. *1st ed. Philadelphia, PA: Lippincott Williams & Wilkins; 2006:210.*

The kidneys produce urine and remove two natural products of metabolism, **urea** and **uric acid**, along with other waste products from the blood. The kidneys also filter, reabsorb, and secrete nonwaste products back into the system.

Filtration and the urine production process begin in the **nephrons**, which are the functional units of the kidneys. Each kidney has approximately 1 million nephrons, and each nephron contains a tiny filtration unit called the **glomerulus**, which consists of a cluster of capillaries. Blood travels through the capillaries, which permit waste products within the **urine** to enter the **ureter**, where it is carried to and stored in the **urinary bladder**.

The bladder collects the urine until the volume triggers the urge to **urinate**, an event known as the **micturition reflex**. Urination is regulated by two **sphincters**, the circular muscles that surround the urethra. They are the internal urethral sphincter, which is located at the entrance to the urethra and is involuntarily controlled, and the external urethral sphincter, which is located at the distal end of the urethra and is under conscious control.

DISORDERS AND TREATMENT

Disorders of the urinary system can encompass any of the urinary structures. Some of these disorders are listed and defined in the following:

- **Dysuria**: painful, difficult urination
- **Incontinence**: the loss of urinary control
- **Retention**: the inability to empty the bladder
- **Urinary tract infections**: infection of the urinary tract (includes the following)
  - **Cystitis**: infection of the lower urinary tract, commonly called a bladder infection
  - **Urethritis**: also an infection of the lower urinary tract, and also called a bladder infection
  - **Pyelonephritis**: infection of the upper urinary tract (pelvis and kidneys)
  - **Nephritis**: infection of the upper urinary tract (kidneys)
  - **Glomerulonephritis**: can involve one or both kidneys
  - **Renal failure**: kidneys cease urine production

What's the difference between the roots nephr/o and ren/o? Both may be used to refer to the kidneys. However, nephr/o is used in the names of most, but not all, kidney disorders and treatments. Applying standard suffixes yields nephritis, nephralgia, nephrectomy, nephrorrhaphy, nephrotomy, and nephromegaly. In general, the term *nephrology* is also more common than renology, but the adjective renal is far more common than its counterpart, nephric.

Abbreviation Table THE URINARY SYSTEM

ABBREVIATION	MEANING
BPH	benign prostatic hypertrophy; enlarged prostate
BUN	blood urea nitrogen; a blood test to measure kidney function by the level of nitrogenous waste and urea that is in the blood
CAPD	continuous ambulatory peritoneal dialysis
ESRD	end-stage renal disease
GFR	glomerular filtration rate
IVP	intravenous pyelogram; contrast is injected into a vein and is excreted by the kidney to show the urinary system
KUB	kidneys, ureter, and bladder; also a reference to an X-ray of the kidneys, ureters, and bladder taken as a flat plate of the abdomen
PSA	prostate-specific antigen
UA	urinalysis
UTI	urinary tract infection

Study Table THE URINARY SYSTEM

TERM AND PRONUNCIATION	ANALYSIS	MEANING
Structure and Function		
electrolyte (ee-LEK-troh-lyte)	from the Greek words *electron* (electron) and *lytos* (soluble)	electricity-conducting compound in solution
glomerulus (gloh-MER-yu-luhs)	a Latin word meaning "small ball," "round knot"	capillary network found inside each nephron
hilum (HY-luhm)	a Latin word meaning "a small thing," "a trifle"	narrow part of the kidney where blood vessels and nerves enter
kidney (KID-nee)	originally *kidenere*, perhaps a compound of Old English *cwið* "womb" + *ey* "egg," in reference to the shape of the organ	organ that excretes urine
nephron (NEFF-ron)	from the Greek word *nephros* (kidney)	tiny structure within the kidney in which the urine-production process begins

(continued)

TERM AND PRONUNCIATION	ANALYSIS	MEANING
perirenal fat (PERH-ih-REE-nahl)	*peri-* (around); *ren/o* (kidney) *-al* (adjective suffix)	fatty tissue surrounding the renal capsule
renal fascia (REE-nahl FASH-ee-ah)	*ren/o* (kidney); *-al* (adjective suffix) + *fascia*, a Latin word meaning "band," "sash"	protective outer covering of the kidney
retroperitoneal (reh-troh-pehr-ih-toh-NEE-al)	*retro-* (backward, behind); from the Greek word *peritenein* (to stretch over)	space between the parietal peritoneum and the muscles and bones of the peritoneum
sphincters (SFINK-tehrs)	from the Greek word *sphincter* (band, anything that binds tight)	circular muscle that surrounds a tube such as the urethra and constricts the tube when it contracts
urea (yu-REE-ah)	from the French word *uree* (urine)	natural waste product of metabolism that is excreted in urine
ureters (yu-REE-tehrs; also YUR-eh-tehrs)	from the Greek word *oureter*, from *ourein* (to urinate)	two tubes that transfer urine from the kidneys to the urinary bladder
urethra (yu-REE-thrah)	from the Greek word *ourethra*, from *ourein* (to urinate)	tube that conducts urine away from the bladder for expulsion
uric acid (YUR-ik)	*ur/o* (urine); *-ic* (adjective suffix) + acid, common English Word	natural waste product of metabolism that is excreted in urine
urinary bladder (YUR-ihn-ayr-ee BLAD-dehr)	from the Greek word *ouron* (urine) + Anglo-Saxon, *blaedre* (bladder)	temporary storage receptacle for urine
urinate (YUR-ihn-ayt)	*urin/o* (urine) + *-ate* (verb suffix)	passing of urine
urine (YUR-ihn)	from the Greek word *ouron* (urine)	water and soluble substances excreted by the kidneys
void (voyd)	from Old French *voide* (empty, hollow, waste)	to urinate

Common Disorders and Symptoms

albuminuria (al-byu-mihn-YUR-ee-ah)	from the vulgar Latin *albumen* (egg white) + *ur/o* (urine); *-ia* (condition)	presence of protein in urine
anuria (an-YUR-ee-ah)	*an-* (without); *ur/o* (urine); *-ia* (condition)	absence of urine formation
calculus (KAL-kyu-luhs); plural: calculi (KAL-kyu-lye)	a Latin word meaning "stone"	a kidney stone (in the context of this body system)
cystalgia (sihs-TAL-jee-ah)	*cyst/o* (bladder); *-algia* (pain)	pain in a bladder, most often used to signify the urinary bladder

TERM AND PRONUNCIATION	ANALYSIS	MEANING
cystitis (sihs-TY-tihs)	cyst/o (bladder); -itis (inflammation)	inflammation of the bladder
cystocele (SIHS-toh-seel)	cyst/o (bladder); -cele (hernia)	hernia of the bladder
cystolith (SIS-toh-lith)	cyst/o (bladder); -lith (stone)	bladder stone
diuretic (dy-yu-REHT-ik)	from the Greek dia- (through) + ourein (urine)	drug that promotes the excretion of urine
dysuria (dihs-YUR-ee-ah)	dys- (difficult); ur/o (urine); -ia (condition)	difficult or painful urination
enuresis (ahn-your-REE-sis)	from Greek enourein (to urinate in)	bedwetting
glomerulonephritis (glom-MER-yu-lo-neh-FRY-tihs)	glomerul/o (glomerulus); nephr/o (kidney); -itis (inflammation)	renal disease characterized by inflammation of glomeruli (not the result of kidney infection)
glycosuria (gly-kohs-YUR-ee-ah)	glycos- (sugar); ur/o (urine); -ia (condition)	urinary excretion of carbohydrates
hematuria (he-mat-YUR-ee-ah)	hemat/o (blood); ur/o (urine); -ia (adjective suffix)	urinary excretion of blood
incontinence (in-KON-tih-nents)	from the Latin word incontinentia (inability to retain)	inability to control urine
nephralgia (neh-FRAL-jee-ah)	nephr/o (kidney); -algia (pain)	pain in the kidneys
nephritis (neh-FRY-tihs)	nephr/o (kidney); -itis (inflammation)	inflammation of the kidney
nephrolithiasis (NEFF-ro-lih-THY-ah-sihs)	nephr/o (kidney); lith/o (stone); -iasis (condition)	the presence of renal calculi
nephromegaly (neh-fro-MEG-ah-lee)	nephr/o (kidney); -megaly (enlargement)	enlargement of one or both kidneys; renomegaly
nephropathy (neh-FROP-ah-thee)	nephr/o (kidney); -pathy (disease)	any disease of the kidney
nephroptosis (neh-FROP-toh-sis)	nephr/o (kidney); -ptosis (falling downward, prolapse)	prolapse of the kidney
nocturia (noc-TUR-ee-ah)	noct/o (night); ur/o (urine); -ia (condition)	excessive urination at night
oliguria (oh-lih-GUR-ee-ah)	olig/o (few); ur/o (urine); -ia (condition)	diminished urine production
polyuria (pol-ee-YUR-ee-ah)	poly- (much, many); ur/o (urine); -ia (condition)	excessive urine production
pyelonephritis (PY-loh-NEH-FRY-tihs)	pyel/o (pelvis); nephr/o (kidney); -itis (inflammation)	inflammation of the renal or kidney pelvis due to local bacteria infection
pyuria (pu-YOUR-ee-ah)	py/o (pus); ur/o (urine); -ia (condition)	pus in the urine

(continued)

TERM AND PRONUNCIATION	ANALYSIS	MEANING
renal calculus (REE-nahl KAL-ku-luhs)	*ren/o* (kidney); *calculus*, a Latin word meaning "stone"	a kidney stone
renal failure (REE-nahl)	*ren/o* (kidney); *-al* (adjective suffix) + failure, common English word	impairment of renal function, either acute or chronic, with retention of urea, creatinine, and other waste products
renal hypoplasia (REE-nahl HY-poh-PLAYZ-ee-ah)	*ren/o* (kidney); *hypo-* (below normal); *-plasia* (formation, development)	an underdeveloped kidney
retention (ree-TEN-shun)	from the Latin word *retentio* (a retaining, a holding back)	the inability to empty the bladder
uremia (yu-REE-mee-ah) or azotemia (ays-oh-TEAM-ee-ah)	*ur/o* (urine); *-emia* (blood condition)	an excess of urea in the blood
ureteritis (yu-ree-teh-RY-tihs)	*ureter/o* (ureter); *-itis* (inflammation)	inflammation of a ureter
urethralgia (yu-ree-THRAL-jee-ah)	*urethr/o* (urethra); *-algia* (pain)	pain in the urethra (sometimes also called *urethrodynia*)
urethritis (yu-ree-THRY-tihs)	*urethr/o* (urethra); *-itis* (inflammation)	inflammation of the urethra
urethrostenosis (yu-REE-throh-steh-NO-sihs)	*urethr/o* (urethra); *sten/o* (narrow); *-sis* (condition)	narrowing of the urethra
urinary tract infection (yur-ihn-ARY)	*urin/o* (urine); *-ary* (adjective suffix); + tract + infection	microbial infection of any part of the urinary tract

Practice and Practitioners

nephrologist (neh-FROL-oh-jist)	*nephr/o* (kidney); *-logist* (one who studies a special field)	a medical specialist who diagnoses and treats disorders of the kidney
nephrology (neh-FROL-oh-jee)	*nephr/o* (kidney); *-logy* (study of)	medical specialty dealing with the kidneys
urologist (yu-ROL-oh-jist)	*ur/o* (urine); *-logist* (one who studies a special field)	a medical specialist who diagnoses and treats disorders of the urinary system
urology (yu-ROL-oh-jee)	*ur/o* (urine); *-logy* (study of)	the medical specialty dealing with the urinary system

Diagnosis, Treatment, and Procedures

catheter (CATH-eh-tehr)	from the Greek word *kathienai* (to let down, thrust in)	a flexible tube that enables passage of fluid from or into a body cavity
cystectomy (sihs-TEK-toh-mee)	*cyst/o* (bladder); *-ectomy* (excision)	excision of the urinary bladder

TERM AND PRONUNCIATION	ANALYSIS	MEANING
cystopexy (SIHS-toh-pek-see)	*cyst/o* (bladder); *-pexy* (fixation)	surgical fixation of the urinary bladder
cystoscopy (sihs-TOS-ko-pee)	*cyst/o* (bladder); *-scopy* (use of an instrument for viewing)	visual inspection of the bladder by means of an instrument called a cystoscope
dialysis (dy-AL-ih-sihs)	a Greek word meaning "dissolution," "separation"	filtration to remove colloidal particles from a fluid; a method of artificial kidney function
diuretic (dy-yu-REHT-ik)	from the Greek *dia-* (through) + *ourein* (urine)	a drug that promotes the excretion of urine
hemodialysis (HEE-mo-dy-AL-ih-sihs)	*hemo-* (blood) + *dialysis*, a Greek word meaning "dissolution," "separation"	removal of unwanted substances from the blood by passage through a semipermeable membrane
lithotripsy (LITH-oh-trip-see)	*lith/o* (stone); *-tripsy* (crushing)	treatment in which a stone in the kidney, urethra, or bladder is broken up into small particles
nephrectomy (neh-FREK-toh-mee)	*nephr/o* (kidney); *-ectomy* (removal)	removal of a kidney
nephrolithotomy (NEH-froh-lih-THOT-oh-mee)	*nephr/o* (kidney); *lith/o* (stone); *-tomy* (incision into)	incision into the kidney to remove a calculus (kidney stone)
ureteroplasty (yu-REE-tehr-oh-plass-tee)	*ureter/o* (ureter); *-plasty* (surgical repair)	surgical repair of a ureter
ureterorrhaphy (yu-REE-tehr-OR-rah-fee)	*ureter/o* (ureter); *-rrhaphy* (surgical suturing)	suture of a ureter
ureteroscope (yu-REE-tehr-oh-skohp)	*ureter/o* (ureter); *-scope* (instrument for viewing)	instrument used to visually examine the ureter
urinalysis (yur-ih-NAL-ih-sihs)	*urin/o* (urine); *-alysis* from the English word analysis	analysis of urine

EXERCISES

EXERCISE 13-1   FIGURE LABELING: THE URINARY SYSTEM

| left kidney | right kidney | urethra |
| left ureter | right ureter | urinary bladder |

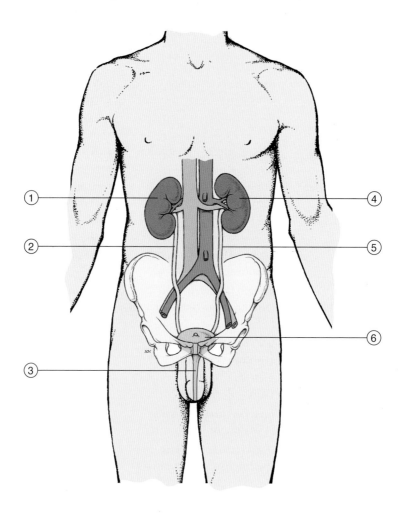

1. _____   4. _____

2. _____   5. _____

3. _____   6. _____

EXERCISE 13-2   CASE STUDY

CASE STUDY
Read the following case study. There are 11 phrases that can be reworded with a medical term that was introduced in this chapter. Determine what the term is and write your answers in the space provided.

Heather is a 40-year-old female who saw (1) <u>a specialist who treats disorders of the urinary system</u> for complaints of urinary frequency, (2) <u>painful urination</u>, (3) <u>blood in her urine</u>, and low abdominal pain. She also was experiencing a low-grade fever and general fatigue. The doctor ordered a (4) <u>laboratory reading of her urine</u> and an (5) <u>X-ray of her kidneys, ureters, and bladder</u>. The laboratory results showed red blood cells in the urine, and the urine was cloudy with an odor. Tests indicated multiple (6) <u>small, round, calcified objects</u> in the (7) <u>urine reservoir</u>. Heather was diagnosed with a (8) <u>condition of having bacteria in the urinary tract</u> and also (9) <u>stones</u> in her bladder. The doctor ordered a(n) (10) <u>drug used to kill bacteria</u>, and he told Heather that she needed to have a (11) <u>procedure in which a scope is inserted into the bladder</u> to remove the stones. Heather's symptoms improved, and she returned to have the procedure. Her recovery was uneventful.

1. _____   7. _____

2. _____   8. _____

3. _____   9. _____

4. _____   10. _____

5. _____   11. _____

6. _____

EXERCISE 13-3   DEFINITIONS

Define the following terms and abbreviations:

1. nephrotomy   _____

2. nephrolithiasis   _____

3. dialysis   _____

4. CAPD   _____

5. pyuria   _____

6. ureteroplasty   _____

7. UTI   _____

8. ureterorrhaphy   _____

9. periurethral   _____

10. nephromegaly   _____

EXERCISE 13-4 MATCHING TERMS WITH DEFINITIONS

Match the terms in Column 1 with the correct definitions in Column 2.

TERM	DEFINITION
1. _____ nephron	A. capillary network found inside each nephron
2. _____ urethra	B. urination
3. _____ renal calculus	C. pain in the bladder
4. _____ glomerulus	D. tube that conducts urine away from the bladder for excretion
5. _____ micturition	E. electricity-conducting compound in solution
6. _____ uric acid	F. narrow part of the kidney where blood vessels and nerves enter
7. _____ ureters	G. functional unit of the kidney
8. _____ hilum	H. two tubes that transfer urine from the kidneys to the urinary bladder
9. _____ electrolyte	I. X-ray of the ureter
10. _____ UA	J. natural waste product of metabolism excreted in the urine
11. _____ nephralgia	K. a kidney stone
12. _____ nephritis	L. excision of a kidney, ureter, and at least part of the urinary bladder
13. _____ urethrostenosis	M. inflammation of the kidney
14. _____ nephrolithotomy	N. narrowing of the urethra
15. _____ nephroureterocystectomy	O. any disease of the kidney
16. _____ ureterography	P. pain in the kidneys
17. _____ cystalgia	Q. incision into the kidney to remove a calculus (kidney stone)
18. _____ nephropathy	R. urinalysis

EXERCISE 13-5 WORD BUILDING

Use the root *nephr/o* to build the following terms:

1. inflammation of the kidney   _____

2. inflammation of the kidney and the renal pelvis   _____

3. condition of having stones in the kidney   _____

4. incision into the kidney   _____

Use the root *ur* or *urin* to build the following terms:

5. a urinary stone   _____

6. urinary waste products in the blood   _____

7. examination of a urine sample   _____

8. excessive urination   _____

9. blood in the urine   _____

10. no urine production from the kidney   _____

EXERCISE 13-6 TRUE OR FALSE

Put an X in the True or False column next to each statement. If False, write the correct answer in the Correction column for any statements you identify as false.

STATEMENT	TRUE	FALSE	CORRECTION, IF FALSE
1. Diuretics are medications that promote urination.	____	____	_____
2. Renal fascia is the fatty tissue surrounding the renal capsule.	____	____	_____
3. The two tubes that transfer urine from the kidneys to the urinary bladder are the urethritis.	____	____	_____
4. A natural waste product of metabolism that is excreted in urine is called urea.	____	____	_____
5. The urinary bladder serves as a temporary storage receptacle for urine.	____	____	_____

6. Narrowing of the urethra is referred to as urethrostenosis.   ____ ____ _____

7. The word element -*logist* in urologist means "study."   ____ ____ _____

8. An incision into the kidney to remove a kidney stone is called a nephrectomy.   ____ ____ _____

9. An incision into the ureter is called a ureteroplasty.   ____ ____ _____

10. Inflammation of the bladder is called cystodynia.   ____ ____ _____

EXERCISE 13-7   FILL IN THE BLANKS WITH THE APPROPRIATE ABBREVIATIONS

MEANING	ABBREVIATION
1. intravenous pyelogram; contrast is injected into a vein and is excreted by the kidney to show the urinary system	_____
2. kidneys, ureter, and bladder; also a reference to an X-ray of the kidneys, ureters, and bladder taken as a flat plate of the abdomen	_____
3. continuous ambulatory peritoneal dialysis	_____
4. blood urea nitrogen; a blood test to measure kidney function by the level of nitrogenous waste and urea that is in the blood	_____
5. glomerular filtration rate	_____
6. end-stage renal disease	_____
7. prostate-specific antigen	_____
8. urinalysis	_____
9. urinary tract infection	_____
10. benign prostatic hypertrophy; enlarged prostate	_____

EXERCISE 13-8 CROSSWORD PUZZLE: THE URINARY SYSTEM

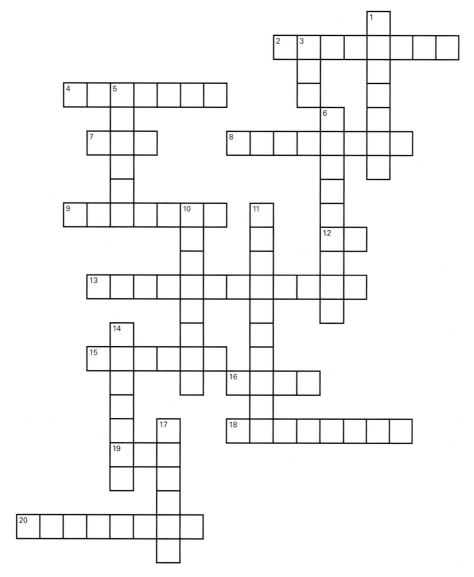

ACROSS

2. artificial kidney function
4. functional unit of the kidney
7. abbreviation for blood urea nitrogen
8. drug that promotes urination
9. urine reservoir
12. abbreviation for urinalysis
13. drooping kidney
15. urea in the blood
16. urinate
18. inflammation of the bladder
19. root for kidney
20. urinating at night

DOWN

1. painful urination
3. intravenous pyelogram
5. pus in the urine
6. blood in the urine
10. bedwetting
11. removal of the bladder
14. tube from the kidney to bladder
17. no urine production

◀ CHAPTER 13 QUIZ

Using the knowledge gained from previous chapters and the terms introduced in this chapter and in the study table, place the proper term in the sentences below.

cystoscopy	dysuria	IVP	nephrolithiasis	nephropexy
nephropyelitis	pyelolithotomy	renal transplant	ureterectomy	

1. Tom suffered from chronic renal failure. His sister donated one of her normal kidneys to him and he had a(n) _____.

2. Cindy had a floating kidney that required surgical fixation. Her urologist performed a surgical procedure known as a(n) _____.

3. The surgeons operated on Robert to remove a calculus from his renal pelvis. The name of this surgery is _____.

4. Judy had to have one of her ureters removed due to a stricture. This procedure is called _____.

5. The physician had to examine Joshua's bladder for blood. They used a special instrument. This procedure is called a(n) _____.

Define the following terms:

6. antibiotic _____

7. antispasmodic _____

8. BUN _____

9. enuresis _____

10. renal hyperplasia _____

Multiple Choice

11. The _____ carry the urine from the kidney pelvis down to the urinary bladder.
    a. urethra   c. cortex
    b. meatus   d. ureters

12. The inability to hold urine is called:
    a. polyuria   c. hematuria
    b. incontinence   d. enuresis

13. Excretion of urine from the bladder is properly termed as:
    a. voiding   c. urination
    b. micturition   d. all of the above

14. The functioning unit of the kidney is the:
    a. nephron
    b. cortex of the kidney
    c. glomeruli
    d. pelvis of the kidney

15. What does anuria mean?
    a. no urine in the bladder
    b. no urine from the kidney
    c. painful urination
    d. pus in the urine

16. What term means destruction of kidney tissue?
    a. nephrolithiasis
    b. neurolysis
    c. nephrolysis
    d. resection

14 *The Reproductive System*

LEARNING OBJECTIVES

Upon completion of this chapter, you should be able to:

- List terms naming the major organs, functions, and disorders of the male and female reproductive systems.
- Recognize the elements that make up terms related to the male and female reproductive systems.
- Identify and interpret selected abbreviations relating to the reproductive system.
- Label diagrams of the male and female reproductive systems.
- Analyze and define the new terms introduced in this chapter.

INTRODUCTION

The primary function of the reproductive system is to perpetuate life. The reproductive process begins with **fertilization**, which occurs when a male **gamete** (also called a **sperm** or **spermatozoon**; plural: **spermatozoa**) fertilizes a female gamete (also called an **ovum**; plural: **ova**). The collective name for any female or male organ that produces a gamete is **gonad**.

The single cell formed at fertilization is called a **zygote**, which contains more than a trillion molecules, despite its diameter of only 0.1 mm. These trillion or so molecules all communicate and work together in the **gestation** process. The term *gestation* refers to the time lapse between the formation of the zygote and birth.

Obstetricians (from *obstetrix*, the Latin word for midwife) are the specialists who provide medical care to pregnant women and deliver babies. **Gynecologists** diagnose and treat disorders of the female reproductive system, and **urologists** diagnose and treat disorders of the urinary and male reproductive systems. Two additional specialists are the **neonatologist**, who specializes in newborns, and the **pediatrician**, who specializes in the diagnosis and treatment of childhood disorders.

STRUCTURE AND FUNCTION

The Male Reproductive System

The male reproductive system includes terms that also refer to the urinary system. The major organs consist of the **testes** (singular: **testis**), **seminal vesicles**, **prostate**, and **bulbourethral glands** (also called the **Cowper's glands**). The supporting structure and accessory organs are the **scrotum** and **penis** (Fig. 14-1).

The primary function of the male reproductive system is to produce sperm. The process, called **spermatogenesis**, involves cell division known as **meiosis**, which reduces the number of chromosomes from 46 to 23.

Spermatogenesis begins in the **testes** and is initiated by the secretion of **androgens**. The most significant of these hormones is **testosterone**. After spermatogenesis is complete, the **spermatozoa** (singular: **spermatozoon**) travel to the **epididymis**, a coil-shaped tube at the upper part of the testicle where the sperm are stored to mature. Once the sperm mature, they leave the epididymis and enter the **ductus deferens**, also called the **vas deferens**, which leads to the ejaculatory duct in the prostate. From there, the sperm travel through the **seminal vesicles**, which are glands located at the base of the urinary bladder. The seminal vesicles produce a fluid that nourishes the sperm

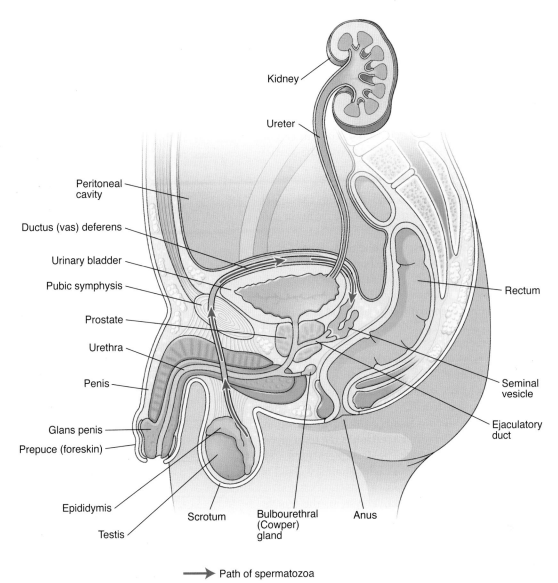

Kidney

Ureter

Peritoneal cavity

Ductus (vas) deferens

Urinary bladder

Pubic symphysis

Prostate

Urethra

Penis

Glans penis

Prepuce (foreskin)

Epididymis

Scrotum

Testis

Bulbourethral (Cowper) gland

Anus

Rectum

Seminal vesicle

Ejaculatory duct

⟶ Path of spermatozoa

FIGURE 14-1   Male reproductive system, sagittal view. A sagittal view of the male reproductive system. The *blue arrows* illustrate the pathway of sperm. Parts of the urinary and digestive systems are also shown. *From Cohen BJ. Medical Terminology: An Illustrated Guide. 5th ed. Philadelphia, PA: Lippincott Williams & Wilkins; 2007.*

and forms much of the volume of the **semen**, which is produced in the prostate gland, located just below the urinary bladder.

The bulbourethral glands are located on either side of the urethra. They produce a mucus-type secretion that joins the semen to become part of the ejaculated fluid. The pathway of sperm from spermatogenesis to ejaculation is shown in Figure 14-2.

The Female Reproductive System

The female organs of reproduction are the **uterus**, two **ovaries**, two **fallopian tubes**, the **vagina**, and the **mammary glands** (Fig. 14-3).

The **uterus** is a pear-shaped organ that has an upper rounded portion called the **fundus** and a lower narrow portion referred to as the **cervix**, which extends into the vagina. The uterus is composed of three layers of tissues: the **perimetrium**, which is the outer surrounding layer; the **myometrium**, which is the middle muscular layer; and the **endometrium**, which is the inner layer. The endometrium reacts to hormonal changes every month, and the result is **menstruation**, which involves a shedding of the endometrial lining.

Two **ovaries** (singular: **ovary**) lie on either side of the uterus in the pelvic cavity. At birth, the ovaries of a female child already contain immature **ova** (ova is plural for **ovum**).

The fallopian tubes extend out from the upper portion of the uterus. Fertilization occurs in the fallopian tube.

The vagina is a muscular tube that extends from the cervix to the outside of the body. The vagina has the following functions:

- Allows for passage outside the body of the monthly **menstrual** flow of blood and tissue
- Acts as a receptacle for semen during sexual intercourse
- Serves as the birth canal during a normal vaginal birth

The mammary glands (breasts) are also an important part of the female reproductive system: They are the milk-producing glands, which provide nourishment for the newborn. **Lactation** is the term given to the production of milk. The dark-pigmented area that surrounds the nipple of each mammary gland is called the **areola**.

Like the male reproductive system, the female reproductive system provides gametes for fertilization, but its function in the process continues by providing an environment for a fertilized egg to develop into to a fully formed baby.

The preparation for the process is accommodated by the **menstrual cycle**, a recurrent periodic change in the ovaries and uterus that occurs approximately every 28 days. Hormonal activity controls the menstrual cycle, which has three phases: **secretory** (secretion of hormones), **proliferative** (preparation of the endometrial lining for implantation if fertilization occurs), and **menses** (the end of one cycle and the beginning of another). If male spermatozoa are present during **ovulation**, the possibility of fertilization exists.

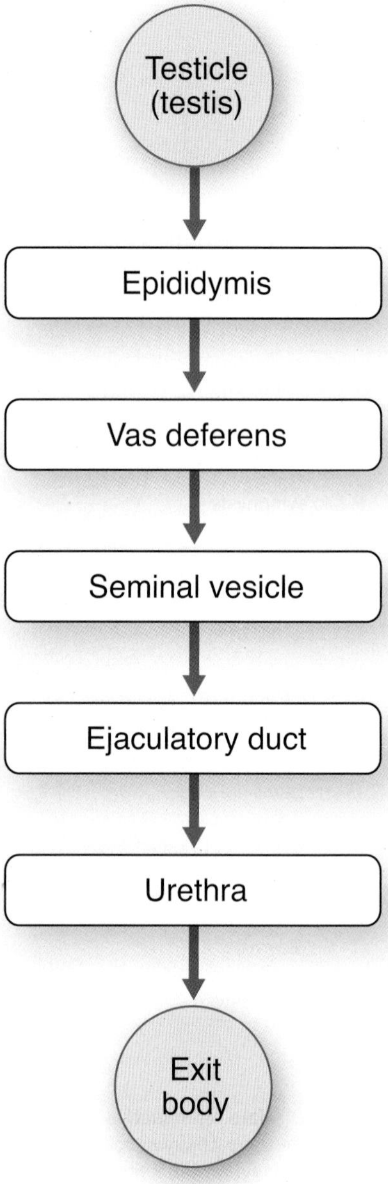

FIGURE 14-2 **Pathway of sperm.**

Terms Associated with Pregnancy

Gestation, which is a synonym for pregnancy, comes from the Latin verb *gesto*, meaning "to bear." When an ovum is penetrated by the male spermatozoon, it travels through the oviduct (fallopian tube) and implants into the uterus. Once implanted, the fertilized egg is called an **embryo** during the first 8 weeks of gestation. Between the 8th week and birth, which under normal circumstances occurs between weeks 38 and 40, the term **fetus** is used. The fetus receives nourishment from the

TABLE 14-1 REPRODUCTIVE SYSTEM WORD ELEMENTS	
Root	**Meaning**
amni/o	amnion; innermost of the extraembryonic membranes enveloping the embryo in utero and containing the amniotic fluid
balan/o	glans penis
cervic/o	cervix
circum/o	around
colp/o, vagin/o	vagina
gonad/o	gonads, sex glands
gynec/o	woman, female
lact/o	milk
mast/o, mamm/o	breast
men/o	menses, menstruation
nat/o	birth
oophor/o, oo	ovary, egg
orch/o, orchi/o, orchid/o, test/o	testes
ovari/o	ovary
prostat/o	prostate gland
salping/o	tube, fallopian tube
spermat/o, sperm/o	sperm
uter/o, hyster/o, metr/o	uterus
vas/o	vessel, vas deferens
vulv/o	vulva

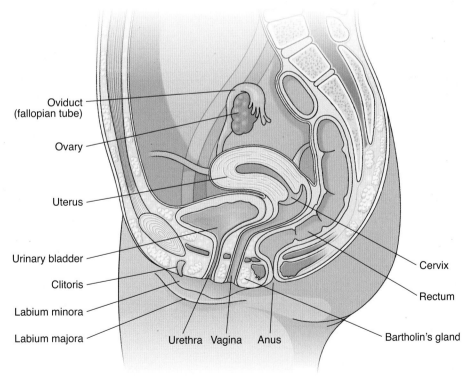

FIGURE 14-3 **The female reproductive system and adjacent structures, sagittal view.** The internal organs of reproduction are the uterus, two ovaries, two fallopian tubes, vagina, and hymen. *From Cohen BJ. Medical Terminology: An Illustrated Guide. 5th ed. Philadelphia, PA: Lippincott Williams & Wilkins; 2007.*

Word Elements Exercise CONVERTING WORDS TO WORD ROOTS

Study Table 14-1 carefully before attempting this exercise. Write out the root that would be used in creation of a term involving each of the words listed below.

ROOT

1. breast _____

2. sperm _____

3. tube, fallopian tube _____

4. vessel, vas deferens _____

5. around _____

6. ovary, egg _____

7. vagina _____

8. prostate gland _____

9. amnion _____

10. birth _____

11. uterus _____

12. vulva _____

13. testes _____

14. cervix _____

15. glans penis _____

16. gonads, sex glands _____

17. woman, female _____

18. milk _____

19. menses, menstruation _____

20. ovary _____

Quick Check: A Few Terms Sometimes Overlooked

Fill in the blanks.

1. The primary function of the male reproductive system is _____ _____.

2. The term used to refer to the production of milk is _____.

3. A synonym for pregnancy is _____.

---

uterine wall through the umbilical cord and the **placenta**. The **amniotic sac**, filled with **amniotic fluid**, contains the fetus until birth (Fig. 14-4).

Diagnostic tests and procedures associated with pregnancy include **amniocentesis** (Fig. 14-5), which is the extraction of amniotic fluid from the **amniotic sac**. The extracted fluid is most commonly used to discover or rule out the presence of a genetic disorder, but it can also help in determining fetal lung maturity, which bears on the safety of an early delivery, indicates whether the mother's immune system is having an adverse effect, and reveals the age and sex of the fetus.

Gravida/para/abortus, or sometimes just **gravida/para**, is a shorthand notation for a woman's history. The number following gravida indicates the number of times a patient has been pregnant regardless of whether these pregnancies were carried to term. A current pregnancy, if any, is included in this count. Para indicates the number of births that occurred after 20 weeks (including viable and nonviable [i.e., stillbirths]). Pregnancies consisting of multiples, such as twins or triplets, count as one birth for the purpose of this notation. Abortus is the number of pregnancies that were lost for any reason, including induced abortions or miscarriages. The abortus term is sometimes dropped when no pregnancies have been lost. Stillbirths are not included.

Therefore, the obstetric history of a woman who has had two pregnancies (both of which resulted in live births) would be noted as G_2P_2. The obstetrical history of a woman who has had four pregnancies, one of which was a miscarriage before 20 weeks, would be noted as $G_4P_3A_1$ (in the United Kingdom, this is written as $G_4P_3+_1$). That of a woman who has had one pregnancy of twins with successful outcomes would be noted as G_1P_1.[1]

DISORDERS AND TREATMENTS

Disorders common to both the male and female reproductive systems are briefly described under the following sections: sexually transmitted diseases, other infections, structural abnormalities, and tumors. Additional conditions are included at the end of this section.

Sexually Transmitted Diseases

Sexually transmitted diseases, which result from sexual contact, include the following: **HIV, gonorrhea, chlamydia, pelvic inflammatory disease (PID), syphilis**, and **human papillomavirus (HPV) infection**.

The HIV attacks the immune system after it is transmitted through blood or other infected body fluids. Gonorrhea is a highly contagious disease caused by bacteria that may also be transmitted to a child during birth. Chlamydia is another common infection spread through sexual contact. This

[1]Hatfield N, Klossner NJ. *Introductory Maternity & Pediatric Nursing*. Hagerstown, MD: Lippincott Williams & Wilkins; 2006.

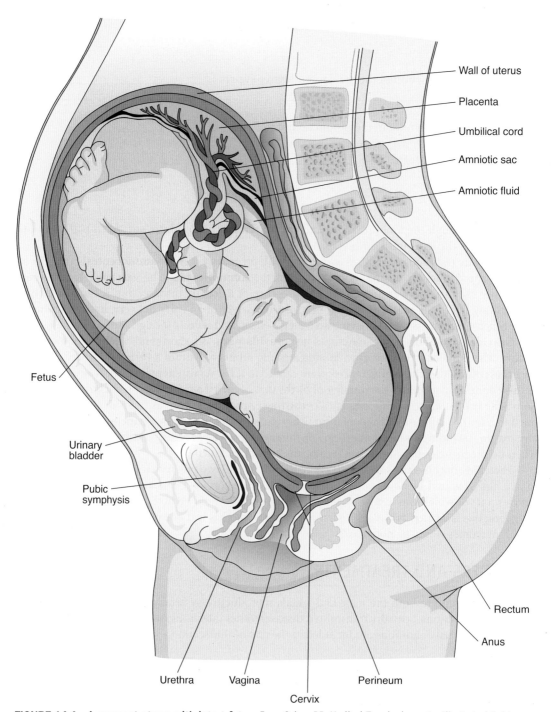

FIGURE 14-4   A pregnant uterus with intact fetus. *From Cohen BJ. Medical Terminology: An Illustrated Guide. 5th ed. Philadelphia, PA: Lippincott Williams & Wilkins; 2007.*

disease may involve the reproductive organs in women. PID, an infection of the uterus, ovaries, and fallopian tubes, can prevent fertilization. If a woman has PID and an egg does become fertilized, the zygote may implant outside the uterus, which is known as an **ectopic** pregnancy (*ektopos* is Greek for "out of place"). An ectopic pregnancy can be life threatening. Syphilis is a highly contagious disease caused by bacteria. HPV is a sexually transmitted virus that can lead to cervical cancer.

Other Infections

Infections of the female reproductive system may result from exposure to bacteria, fungi, or viruses. Many of the conditions are marked by inflammation, the terms for which are indicated by the suffix *-itis*, which you learned in early chapters. They include the following: **mastitis**, **oophoritis**, and **salpingitis**. Salpingitis is a condition that can lead to a closing off of the fallopian tubes, thereby causing infertility.

Male reproductive system infections include **epididymitis**, inflammation of the epididymis; **prostatitis**, inflammation of the prostate; and **balanitis**, inflammation of the head of the penis, which occurs in uncircumcised male infants.

Structural Abnormalities

In adult women, the uterus may be out of position or actually may have a bend in its body. The

FIGURE 14-5 Amniocentesis. A needle is inserted through the abdominal wall into the uterus, and a sample of amniotic fluid is removed from the amniotic sac. *From Cohen BJ*. Medical Terminology: An Illustrated Guide. *5th ed. Philadelphia, PA: Lippincott Williams & Wilkins; 2007.*

following terms name the variant conditions: **anteversion** (Fig. 14-6A) is an abnormal tipping forward of the entire uterus, **anteflexion** (Fig. 14-6B) is an exaggerated forward bend of the uterus,

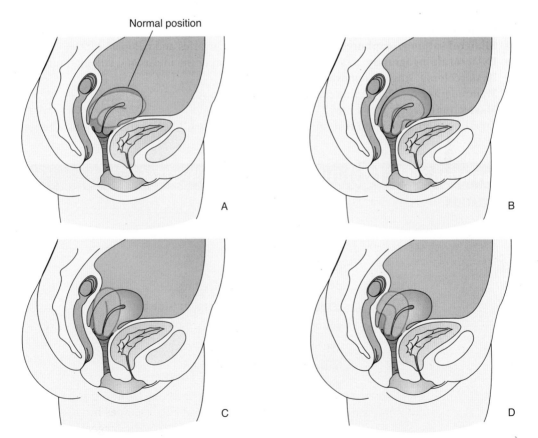

FIGURE 14-6 Uterine flexion and version. The *blue-shaded figure* represents the abnormal positioning of the uterus. **A.** Anteversion. **B.** Anteflexion. **C.** Retroversion. **D.** Retroflexion. *From Pillitteri A.* Maternal and Child Nursing. *4th ed. Philadelphia, PA: Lippincott Williams & Wilkins; 2003.*

retroversion (Fig. 14-6C) is an abnormal tipping of the entire uterus backward, and **retroflexion** (Fig. 14-6D) is an abnormal tipping with the body of the uterus bent back on itself. A **prolapsed uterus** involves the descent of the uterus or cervix into the vaginal canal. Two other conditions involving structural abnormalities of the female reproductive system are a **cystocele**, which is a protrusion of the bladder into the anterior wall of the vagina, and a **rectocele**, which is a protrusion of the rectum into the posterior wall of the vagina.

Tumors

Benign tumors in the female reproductive system are sometimes called **fibroids**. Cysts, which may also be considered a benign tumor, are usually caused by hormonal disturbances.

Cancer of the endometrium is the most common type of cancer in the female reproductive system. A **hysterectomy** is a common treatment. **Endometriosis** is a condition some women have during their childbearing years when estrogen levels are high. It occurs when the endometrial tissue that lines the uterus grows outside the uterus.

Some diagnostic and surgical treatments and procedures of the female reproductive system include the following:

- **Amniocentesis**: amniotic fluid is tested for fetal abnormalities (see Fig. 14-5).
- **Colposcopy**: visual examination of the tissues of the cervix and vagina using a **colposcope**
- **Papanicolaou test** (**Pap smear**): scraping of the cervical tissues to diagnose cervical cancer or other conditions of the cervix and surrounding tissues
- **Dilation and curettage**: dilation of the cervix and scraping of the lining of the uterus
- **Cone biopsy**: surgical removal of a cone-shaped section of the cervix
- **Laparoscopy**: visual examination of the interior of the abdomen by means of a laparoscope
- **Oophorectomy**: removal of one ovary
- **Bilateral oophorectomy**: removal of both ovaries
- **Bilateral salpingo-oophorectomy**: removal of both ovaries and fallopian tubes
- **Hysterosalpingography**: a radiographic examination of the uterus and fallopian tubes
- **Hysterectomy**: surgical removal of the uterus
- **Mammography**: radiographic examination of the breast
- **Mastectomy**: removal of a breast
- **Tubal ligation**: procedure that interrupts the continuity of the uterine or fallopian tubes

Abbreviation Table   THE REPRODUCTIVE SYSTEM

ABBREVIATION	MEANING
BPH	benign prostatic hypertrophy
CS	cesarean section
D&C	dilation and curettage
DUB	dysfunctional uterine bleeding
EDC	estimated date of confinement (due date)
GC	gonorrhea
GYN	gynecology
HRT	hormone replacement therapy
HSG	hysterosalpingogram
HSV	herpes simplex virus
IUD	intrauterine device
IVF	in vitro fertilization
LMP	last menstrual period

ABBREVIATION	MEANING
OB	obstetrics
PID	pelvic inflammatory disease
PMS	premenstrual syndrome
STD	sexually transmitted disease
TAH	total abdominal hysterectomy
TURP	transurethral resection of the prostate
VD	venereal disease

Study Table   THE REPRODUCTIVE SYSTEM

TERM AND PRONUNCIATION	ANALYSIS	MEANING
Structure and Function		
androgens (AN-droh-jehns)	from the Greek words *andros* (man) and *genein* (to produce)	hormones that promote the production of male gametes
cervix (SURV-ihks)	a Latin word meaning "neck" (as in the neck of the uterus)	common term for the uterine cervix
chromosome (KROM-oh-som)	from the Greek word *khroma* (color) and *soma* (body), so called because the structures contain a substance that stains readily with basic dyes	a gene-bearing bundle of DNA found in the nucleus of all cells
embryo (EHM-bree-oh)	from the Greek word *embryon* (young animal, literally, "that which grows")	name change from *zygote* after the first cell division until the eighth week of pregnancy
epididymis (ehp-ih-DIHD-ih-muhs)	from the Greek words *epi* (on) + *didymos* (testicle)	organ in which the male sperm become functional
fallopian (fah-LOH-pee-ahn) tubes; also called uterine (YU-teh-rihn) tubes	named after Gabriello Fallopio (1523–1562), an Italian anatomist who first described them	tubes between the ovaries and the uterus
fertilization (FUR-tih-ly-ZAY-shun)	from the Latin word *fertilis* (fruitful)	the joining of the male and female gametes (in the context of the human reproductive system)
fetus (FEE-tuhs)	a Latin word meaning "the bearing," "bringing forth," or "hatching of young"	name change from *embryo* after the eighth week of pregnancy to birth
gamete (GAH-meet)	a Greek word meaning "a wife"; also *gametes* (a husband), from *gamein* (to take a wife, to marry)	term given to both the female ovum and the male spermatozoon
gestation (jehs-TAY-shun)	from the Latin word *gestare* (to bear, carry, gestate)	development that occurs between the formation of the zygote and birth of the child

(continued)

TERM AND PRONUNCIATION	ANALYSIS	MEANING
gonad (GOH-nad)	from the Greek word *gone* (seed, act of generation, race, family)	gamete-generating organ (ovary or testis)
gravida (GRA-vee-dah)	from the Latin word *gravis* (heavy, profound, important)	a pregnant woman
lactation (lack-TAH-shun)	from the Latin word *lactare* (to suckle, entice, lead on, induce); derived from the Latin word *lac* (milk)	milk production
mammary gland (MAM-mar-ry)	from the Latin word *mamma* (breast) + gland	breasts
menarche (meh-NAR-kee)	from the Greek words *men* (month) and *arkhe* (beginning)	beginning of menses
menopause (MEN-oh-pawz)	from the Latin words *mensis* (month) and *pausis* (a cessation, a pause)	normal stopping of the monthly period or menses
menses (MEN-seez)	plural form of the Latin word *mensis* (month)	end of one uterine cycle and the beginning of another
menstrual cycle (MEN-strew-ahl SY-kl); also called the uterine cycle (YU-tehr-in SY-kl)	from the Latin word *mensis* (month) + cycle	part of the reproductive system process in women, comprising three phases: secretory, proliferative, and menses
mitosis (my-TOH-sihs)	from the Greek word *mitos* (wrap, thread) + *-osis* (process)	process of cell division by which one cell becomes two, both of which contain the maternal and paternal chromosomes
ovary (OH-vah-ree)	from the Latin word *ovum* (egg)	small almond-shaped organ located on either side of the uterus
ovulation (OH-vyu-LAY-shun)	from the Latin word *ovum* (egg) + *atio* (process)	release of a mature ovum from the ovary
ovum (OH-vuhm); ova (OH-vah)	a Latin word meaning "egg"	the female gamete; ovum is singular, ova is plural
para (PAR-ah)	from the Latin verb *pario* (to bring forth, produce, create)	a woman who has given birth to a viable fetus
penis (PEE-nihs)	from the Latin *penis* (tail)	male sex organ that transports the male sperm into the female vagina
placenta (pla-SEN-tah)	a Latin word meaning "cake"	a spongy organ that is attached to the fetus by the umbilical cord and that provides nourishment to the fetus

TERM AND PRONUNCIATION	ANALYSIS	MEANING
pregnancy (PREG-nan-see)	from the prefix *pre-* (before) and the Latin word *gnascor* (to be born)	period of time when the fetus grows inside of the uterus
progestins (pro-JESS-tihns)	from *pro-* (before) and the Latin word *gestare* (to carry); + -*in* (suffix denoting chemical)	female hormones generated in the ovaries
prostate gland (PRAH-stayt)	from the Greek word *prostates* (one standing in front)	male gland that produces and stores prostatic fluid, a fluid medium that is part of semen
reproductive tract	from the Latin prefix *re-* (again) and the Latin word *producere* (to produce) + tract, common English word	in the male reproductive system, the ductwork leading from the epididymis to the outside of the body
scrotum (SKROH-tum)	from the Latin word *scrotum* cognate with Old English *scrud* (garment, source of shroud)	the sac that encloses and protects the testicles
semen (SEE-mehn)	a Latin word meaning "seed"	combination of male gametes, their associated glandular secretions, and prostatic fluid
seminal vesicle (SEH-min-ahl)	from the Latin word *semen* (seed) + vesicle from the Latin word *vesica* (bladder, balloon)	glands at the base of the urinary bladder that secrete a thick substance that nourishes sperm
sperm (spurm); spermatozoon (SPUR-mah-tah-ZOH-on); spermatozoa (SPUR-mah-tah-ZOH-ah)	from the Greek word *sperma* (seed) and *zoion* (animal)	the male gamete; sperm is singular or plural; spermatozoon is singular, spermatozoa is plural
spermatogenesis (SPUR-mah-toh-JEHN-ih-sihs)	*spermat/o* (sperm); -*genesis* (production)	production of sperm
testes (TEHS-teez); singular: testis (TEHS-tihs)	from the Latin word *testiculus* dim. of *testis* (witness) (the organ being evidence of virility)	the organs that produce and store the male gametes
testosterone (tehs-TOSS-teh-rohn)	from the Latin word *testis* (witness); -*sterone* (steroid hormone)	the male reproductive hormone (androgen) prominent in male gamete production
urethra (yu-REETH-rah)	from the Greek word *ourethra* (passage for urine)	male ductwork that acts as a part of both the male urinary and male reproductive systems
uterine cervix (YU-teh-rihn)	*uter/o* (uterus); -*ine* (adjective suffix) + *cervix*, Latin word for neck	the "neck" located at the lower end of the uterus

(continued)

TERM AND PRONUNCIATION	ANALYSIS	MEANING
uterine cycle; also called the menstrual cycle	*uter/o* (uterus); *-ine* (adjective suffix) + cycle, common English word	part of the reproduction system process in women, comprising three phases: secretory, proliferative, and menses
uterine tubes (YU-teh-rihn); also called fallopian (fah-LOH-pee-ahn) tubes	*uter/o* (uterus); *-ine* (adjective suffix) + tubes, common English word	tubes between the ovaries and the uterus
uterus (YU-teh-ruhs)	a Latin word meaning "womb," "belly"	reproductive organ in which the fertilized oocyte is implanted and in which the child develops
vas deferens (vas DEHF-eh rehnz)	from the Latin words *vas* (vessel) and *deferens* (carrying down)	duct leading out of the epididymis (also called the *ductus deferens*)
zygote (ZY-goht)	from the Greek word *zygotos* (yoked)	single cell formed at fertilization
Common Disorders		
amenorrhea (ah-MEN-oh-REE-ah)	*a-* (without); *men/o* (menses); *-rrhea* (flowing, discharge)	absence of menstruation
anorchism (an-OR-kism)	*an-* (without); *orch/o* (testes); *-ism* (condition)	congenital absence of one or both testes
anteflexion (an-tee-FLEX-shun)	*ante-* (something positioned in front of); from the Latin word *flectere* (to bend)	an exaggerated forward bend of the uterus
anteversion (an-tee-VER-shun)	*ante-* (something positioned in front of); from the Latin word *versio* (turning)	abnormal tipping forward of the entire uterus
azoospermia (ay-ZOH-oh-SPER-mee-ah)	from the Greek word *azoos* (lifeless) + *sperm/o* (sperm)	absence of sperm in the semen
balanitis (bal-ah-NIGH-tis)	*balan/o* (glans penis); *-itis* (inflammation)	inflammation of the glans penis
benign prostatic hypertrophy (BPH)	benign (common English word) + *prostat/o* (prostate) + *-ic* (adjective suffix); *hyper-* (above normal); *-trophy* (nourishment or development)	an enlarged, noncancerous prostate; prostatomegaly
cervicitis (sur-vih-SY-tihs); also trachelitis (trak-ih-LY-tihs)	*cervic/o* (cervix); *-itis* (inflammation)	inflammation of the uterine cervix
cryptorchism (kript-OR-kism); also cryptorchidism (kript-OR-kid-izm)	from the Greek word *kryptos* (hidden); *orch/o* (testes); *-ism* (condition)	undescended testicles or when one or both testes fail to descend into the scrotum
cystocele (SIS-toh-seel)	*cyst/o* (bladder); *-cele* (hernia)	protrusion of the bladder into the anterior wall of the vagina

TERM AND PRONUNCIATION	ANALYSIS	MEANING
dysmenorrhea (dis-MEN-oh-REE-ah)	*dys-* (bad, difficult); *men/o* (menses); *-rrhea* (flowing, discharge)	painful menstruation
endometriosis (EN-doh-MEE-tree-OH-sis)	from the Greek words *endo* (within) and *metra* (womb) + *-osis* (condition)	presence of endometrial tissue outside the uterus
epididymitis (ep-ih-did-ih-MY-tis)	from the Greek words *epi* (on) and *didymos* (testicle); *-itis* (inflammation)	inflammation of the epididymis
gonorrhea (gon-oh-REE-ah)	from the Greek *gonos* (offspring); *-rrhea* (discharge, flowing)	highly contagious sexually transmitted disease caused by bacteria
hydrocele (HIGH-droh-seel)	*hydro-* (water); *-cele* (hernia)	hernia filled with fluid in the testes
hysteralgia (HIHS-teh-RAL-jee-ah); also hysterodynia (HIHS-teh-roh-DIHN-ee-ah)	*hyster/o* (womb, uterus); *-algia/-dynia* (pain)	pain in the uterus
hysterectomy (HIS-ter-EK-toh-mee)	*hyster/o* (womb, uterus); *-ectomy* (excision)	removal of the uterus
hysteropathy (hiss-ter-ROP-ah-thee)	*hyster/o* (womb, uterus); *-pathy* (disease)	any disease of the uterus
mastitis (mast-EYE-tis)	*mast/o* (breast); *-itis* (inflammation)	inflammation of the breast
menorrhagia (MEN-oh-RAY-jee-ah)	*men/o* (menses); *-rrhagia* (rapid flow of blood)	increased amount and duration of flow
oligomenorrhea (oh-LIG-oh-MEN-oh-REE-ah)	*olig/o* (having little); *men/o* (menses); *-rrhea* (discharge, flowing)	markedly reduced menstrual flow along with abnormally infrequent menstruation
oligospermia (oh-LIG-oh-SPER-mee-ah)	*olig/o* (having little); *-sperm/o* (sperm); *-ia* (condition)	low sperm count
oophoritis (oo-foh-RY-tihs)	*oophor/o* (ovary); *-itis* (inflammation)	inflammation of an ovary
orchialgia (or-kee-AL-jee-ah)	*orchi/o* (testes); *-algia* (pain)	pain in the testes
orchiopathy (or-kee-OP-ah-thee)	*orchi/o* (testes); *-pathy* (disease)	any disease of the testes
orchitis (or-KY-tihs)	*orchi/o* (testes); *-itis* (inflammation)	inflammation of a testis
ovarialgia (oh-vahr-ee-AL-jee-ah)	*ovari/o* (ovary); *-algia* (pain)	pain in an ovary
ovaritis (ohv-ah-RY-tihs)	*ovari/o* (ovary); *-itis* (inflammation)	inflammation of an ovary (see also *oophoritis*)

(continued)

TERM AND PRONUNCIATION	ANALYSIS	MEANING
pelvic inflammatory disease (PID)	common English words	acute or chronic suppurative inflammation of female pelvic structures (endometrium, uterine tubes, pelvic peritoneum) due to infection by *Neisseria gonorrhoeae*, *Chlamydia trachomatis*, or other organisms
phimosis (fi-MOH-sis)	from the Greek word *phimoo* (to muzzle); *-osis* (condition)	narrowing of the opening of the foreskin so it cannot be retracted or pulled back to expose the glans penis
prolapsed uterus	common English word; *uterus* is a Latin word meaning "womb"	descent of the uterus or cervix into the vagina
prostatitis (PROS-tah-TYE-tis)	*prostat/o* (prostate); *-itis* (inflammation)	inflammation of the prostate
rectocele (REK-toh-seel)	*rect/o* (rectum); *-cele* (hernia)	protrusion of the rectum into the posterior wall of the vagina
retroflexion (re-troh-FLEX-shun)	*retro-* (backward) + flexion, from the Latin word *flectere* (to bend)	abnormal tipping with the body of the uterus bent back on itself
retroversion (re-troh-VER-shun)	*retro-* (backward); from the Latin word *versio* (to turn)	an abnormal tipping of the entire uterus backward
salpingitis (sal-pin-JY-tiss)	*salping/o* (tube, fallopian tube); *-itis* (inflammation)	inflammation of the uterine tube
sexually transmitted disease (STD)	common English words	diseases that are transmitted through sexual intercourse or sexual contact (HIV, syphilis, chlamydia)
syphilis (SIF-ih-lis)	from a poem *Syphilis sive Morbus Gallicus* by Fracastorius, *Syphilus* being a shepherd and principal character	a highly contagious sexually transmitted disease that is caused by a bacterium
vaginitis (VAJ-ih-NIGH-tis)	*vagin/o* (vagina); *-itis* (inflammation)	inflammation of the vaginal tissues that may be infectious or due to several other causes
varicocele (VAR-ih-ko-seel)	*varic/o* (varix, varicose, varicosity); *-cele* (hernia)	a varicose vein of the testes
Practice and Practitioners		
gynecologist (guy-neh-KOL-oh-jist)	*gynec/o* (woman, female); *-logist* (one who studies a certain field)	a specialist of the female reproductive system
gynecology (guy-neh-KOL-oh-jee)	*gynec/o* (woman, female); *-logy* (study of)	the study of the female reproductive system

TERM AND PRONUNCIATION	ANALYSIS	MEANING
neonatology (NEE-oh-nay-TOL-oh-jee)	*neo-* (new); *nat/o* (birth); *-logy* (study of)	the medical specialty dealing with newborns
neonatologist (NEE-oh-nay-TOL-oh-jist)	*neo-* (new); *nat/o* (birth); *-logist* (one who studies a certain field)	the medical specialist dealing with newborns
obstetrician (OB-steh-trish-uhn)	from the Latin word *obstetricis* (midwife), derived from the Latin word *obstare* (to stand opposite to)	a physician who specializes in the medical care of women during pregnancy and childbirth
obstetrics (ob-STET-rihks)	from the Latin word *obstetricis* (midwife), derived from the Latin word *obstare* (to stand opposite to)	medical specialty concerned with the medical care of women during pregnancy and childbirth
pediatrician (pee-dee-a-TRISH-an)	from the Greek *paid-*, stem of *pais* (child) + *-iatr/o* (pertaining to medicine)	medical specialist of children
pediatrics (pee-dee-AT-riks)	from the Greek *paid-*, stem of *pais* (child) + *-iatr/o* (pertaining to medicine)	medical specialty dealing with children
Diagnostic and Surgical Procedures		
amniocentesis (am-nee-oh-sen-TEE-sihs)	*amni/o* (amnion); *-centesis* (surgical puncture for aspiration)	extraction and diagnostic examination of amniotic fluid from the amniotic sac
cervicectomy (surv-ih-SEK-toh-mee); also, rarely, trachelectomy (trak-eh-LEK-toh-mee)	*cervic/o* (cervix); *-ectomy* (excision); from the Greek word *trachelos* (neck)	excision of the uterine cervix
cervicoplasty (SURV-ih-ko-plass-tee); cervicotomy (surv-ih-KOT-oh-mee); also trachelotomy (trak-eh-LOT-oh-mee)	*cervic/o* (cervix); *-plasty* (surgical repair); *-tomy* (incision into); trachelotomy is from the Greek word *trachelos* (neck) + *-tomy* (incision into)	surgical repair of the uterine cervix *or* the neck incision of the uterine cervix; *tracheotomy* is the term used to denote an incision into the neck (trachea), but *trachelotomy* refers to the uterine cervix and is synonymous with cervicotomy
cesarean section (c-section) (seh-SAYR-ee-ahn); other spellings are caesarean and caesarian	etymology uncertain	surgical operation through the abdominal wall and uterus for delivery of the baby
circumcision (SER-kum-SI-shun)	*circum/o* (around); from the Latin word *caedo* (cut)	a surgical procedure to remove the foreskin of the penis
colposcopy (kole-POSS-koh-pee)	*colp/o* (vagina); *-scopy* (use of an instrument for viewing)	using an endoscopic instrument to examine the vagina and cervix

(continued)

TERM AND PRONUNCIATION	ANALYSIS	MEANING
dilation and curettage (D&C)	from the Latin word *dilatare* (to make wider, enlarge) + from the French word *curette* (scoop)	dilation of the cervix and curettage, which involves scraping of the lining of the uterus
hysterectomy (hiss-toh-REK-toh-mee)	*hyster/o* (uterus); *-ectomy* (excision)	surgical removal of the uterus
hysteropexy (HISS-teh-roh-pek-see)	*hyster/o* (uterus); *-pexy* (fixation)	surgical fixation of the uterus
hysteroplasty (HISS-teh-roh-plass-tee)	*hyster/o* (uterus); *-plasty* (surgical repair)	surgical repair of the uterus
hysterotomy (hiss-teh-ROT-oh-mee)	*hyster/o* (uterus); *-tomy* (incision into)	incision of the uterus
laparoscopy (lap-ah-RAH-sko-pee)	*lapar/o* (of or pertaining to the abdominal wall, flank); *-scopy* (use of an instrument for viewing)	direct visualization of the interior of the abdomen with the use of a laparoscope
mammography (mam-OG-rah-fee)	*mamm/o* (breast); *-graphy* (process of recording)	examination of the breast by means of an imaging technique, such as radiography
mastectomy (MAS-tek-toh-mee)	*mast/o* (breast); *-ectomy* (excision)	removal of a breast
oophorectomy (oo-foh-REK-toh-mee)	*oophor/o* (ovary); *-ectomy* (excision)	excision of an ovary; ovariectomy
oophoroplasty (OO-foh-roh-plass-tee)	*oophor/o* (ovary); *-plasty* (surgical repair)	surgical repair of an ovary
oophorotomy (oo-foh-ROT-oh-mee)	*oophor/o* (ovary); *-tomy* (incision into)	incision into an ovary
orchiectomy (or-kee-EK-toh-mee)	*orchi/o* (testes); *-ectomy* (excision)	removal of one or both testes (less commonly, orchechtomy or orchidectomy)
orchioplasty (ORK-ee-oh-plass-tee)	*orchi/o* (testes); *-plasty* (surgical repair)	surgical repair of a testis
orchiotomy (or-kee-OT-ah-mee)	*orchi/o* (testes); *-tomy* (incision into)	incision into a testis
ovariectomy (oh-vahr-ee-EK-toh-mee)	*ovari/o* (ovary); *-ectomy* (excision)	excision of one or both ovaries
ovariotomy (oh-vahr-ee-OT-oh-mee)	*ovari/o* (ovary); *-tomy* (incision into)	incision of an ovary
Pap smear (Papanicolaou)	named after George Papanicolaou, who developed the technique	exfoliative biopsy or a scraping of the cervix to diagnose conditions of the cervix and surrounding tissues
salpingo-oophorectomy	*salping/o* (tube, fallopian tube) + *oophor/o* (ovary); *-ectomy* (excision)	removal of an ovary and fallopian tube

TERM AND PRONUNCIATION	ANALYSIS	MEANING
transurethral resection of the prostate (TURP)	from the Latin *trans* (across) + from the Greek word *ourethra* (urethra); + re- (again) from the Latin *secare* (to cut)	the removal of part or all of the prostate through the urethra
tubal ligation (TOO-ball lie-GAY-shun)	tube + -*al* (adjective suffix) + ligation, from the Latin word *ligare* (to bind)	surgical procedure performed for female sterilization where each fallopian tube is tied off or "ligated" to prevent the ovum from reaching the uterus
uteropexy (YU-teh-roh-pek-see)	*uter/o* (uterus); -*pexy* (fixation)	surgical fixation of the uterus (see also *hysteropexy*)
uteroplasty (YU-teh-roh-plass-tee)	*uter/o* (uterus); -*plasty* (surgical repair)	surgical repair of the uterus (see also *hysteroplasty*)
uterotomy (yu-teh-ROT-oh-mee)	*uter/o* (uterus); -*tomy* (incision into)	incision of the uterus (see also *hysterotomy*)
varicocelectomy (VAR-ee-coh-SEEL-ek-toh-mee)	*varic/o* (varix, varicose, varicosity); -*cele* (hernia); -*ectomy* (excision)	the removal of a portion of an enlarged vein to remove a varicocele
vasovasostomy (vay-soh-vay-ZOS-toh-mee)	*vas/o* (vessel, vas deferens); -*stomy* (creation of an opening)	procedure to restore fertility to a vasectomized male; reconnect the vas deferens

EXERCISES

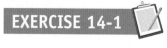

EXERCISE 14-1   FIGURE LABELING: THE MALE REPRODUCTIVE SYSTEM

Label the figure of the male reproductive system.

bulbourethral gland   prepuce (foreskin)   urethra
ejaculatory duct   prostate   urinary bladder
epididymis   scrotum   ductus (vas) deferens
glans penis   seminal vesicle
penis   testis

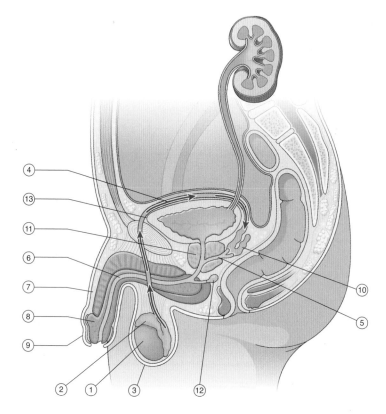

1. _____   8. _____

2. _____   9. _____

3. _____   10. _____

4. _____   11. _____

5. _____   12. _____

6. _____   13. _____

7. _____

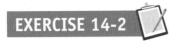

EXERCISE 14-2   FIGURE LABELING: THE FEMALE REPRODUCTIVE SYSTEM

Label the figure of the female reproductive system.

anus	labium majora	urethra
cervix	labium minora	urinary bladder
clitoris	rectum	uterus
fallopian tube	ovary	vagina

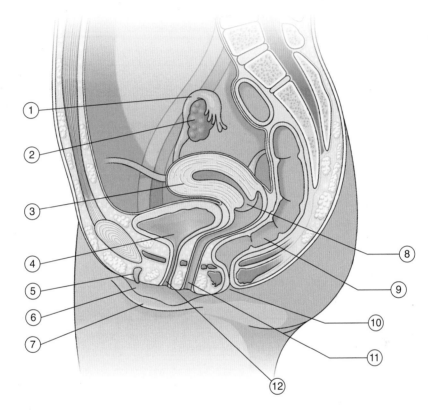

1. _____   7. _____

2. _____   8. _____

3. _____   9. _____

4. _____   10. _____

5. _____   11. _____

6. _____   12. _____

EXERCISE 14-3 DECIPHERING MEDICAL DOCUMENTS

Read the following excerpt from a hospital report, and answer the questions that follow.

A 27-year-old gravida II, para I woman without significant medical history. Blood work was normal before delivery of a stillborn 1-pound, 11-ounce infant during week 21. Although ultrasound studies during week 14 and amniocentesis during week 15 were unremarkable, intrauterine fetal demise had occurred during week 18.

1. Gravida II, para I is a nonstandard way to indicate this classification. What is the standard way? _____

   _____

2. What is amniocentesis? _____

   _____

3. In the final sentence, both "fetal" and "demise" are self-evident terms. Using your knowledge of word elements, define intrauterine.

   _____

4. Does this "medical" report give information that would help one investigating the cause of death?

   _____

5. What does "unremarkable" mean? Does it mean normal? If so, what is considered normal?

   _____

6. Describe the tone of this document in one sentence.

   _____

7. If you were the woman who is discussed in this report, how would you assess the level of care you received?

   _____

8. Reexamine your answer to question 1 and compare it to answers given by your classmates.

   _____

EXERCISE 14-4   BUILDING MEDICAL TERMS

The root *hyster/o* refers to the uterus. Use it to write a term that means:

1. surgical fixation of the uterus   _____

2. removal of the uterus   _____

3. rupture of the uterus   _____

4. suture of the uterus   _____

The root *metr/o* also means uterus. Use it to write a term that means:

5. any uterine disease   _____

6. inflammation of the uterus   _____

7. uterine hemorrhage   _____

The root *vagin/o* means vagina. Use it to write a term that means:

8. relating to the vagina   _____

9. vaginal hernia   _____

10. inflammation of the vagina   _____

11. relating to the vagina and labia   _____

The root *colp/o* also means vagina. Use it to write a term that means:

12. visual examination of the vagina using an instrument   _____

13. suture of the vagina   _____

The root *prostat/o* means prostate gland. Use it to write a term that means:

14. removal of the prostate   _____

15. pertaining to the prostate   _____

16. inflammation of the prostate   _____

The root *vesicul/o* means seminal vesicle. Use it to write a term that means:

17. disease of the seminal vesicle   _____

18. inflammation of the seminal vesicle   _____

The roots *orchid/o*, *orchi/o*, and *orch/o* refer to the testes. Write a term that means:

19. inflammation of the testes   _____

20. disease of the testes   _____

21. testicular pain   _____

EXERCISE 14-5 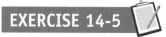 SURGICAL PROCEDURE TERM IDENTIFICATION

Name the anatomical parts operated on in the following procedures.

1. salpingectomy _____

2. hysterectomy _____

3. tubal ligation _____

4. colporrhaphy _____

5. mammoplasty _____

6. oophorectomy _____

7. orchiectomy _____

8. vasectomy _____

9. balanoplasty _____

10. mastectomy _____

EXERCISE 14-6 MATCHING TERMS WITH DEFINITIONS

Match the terms in Column 1 with the correct definitions in Column 2.

TERM	DEFINITION
1. _____ vas deferens	A. combination of sperm and associated liquids that nourish the sperm
2. _____ prostate gland	B. pain in the ovary
3. _____ spermatogenesis	C. organs that produce and store male gametes
4. _____ epididymis	D. duct leading out of the epididymis
5. _____ semen	E. production of sperm
6. _____ orchialgia	F. inflammation of an ovary
7. _____ testes	G. pain in the testes
8. _____ hysterectomy and bilateral oophorectomy	H. release of the female gamete from the ovary

9. _____ ovarialgia

10. _____ hysteropexy

11. _____ period of gestation

12. _____ oophoritis

13. _____ ovulation

14. _____ ovum

15. _____ cervicectomy

I. organ in which the male sperm become functional; lies on top of the testes

J. excision of the uterine cervix

K. surgical fixation of the uterus

L. the female gamete

M. surgical removal of the uterus and right and left ovaries

N. time lapse between zygote formation and birth

O. gland that surrounds the urethra; secretes alkaline fluid that assists in sperm motility

EXERCISE 14-7　THE MEANINGS OF ABBREVIATIONS

1. STD _____

2. DUB _____

3. IVF _____

4. VD _____

5. LMP _____

6. HSG _____

7. TURP _____

8. EDC _____

9. D&C _____

10. HRT _____

11. IUD _____

12. GC _____

13. HSV _____

14. OB _____

15. PID _____

16. BPH _____

17. PMS _____

18. CS _____

19. TAH _____

20. GYN _____

EXERCISE 14-8 CROSSWORD PUZZLE: THE REPRODUCTIVE SYSTEM

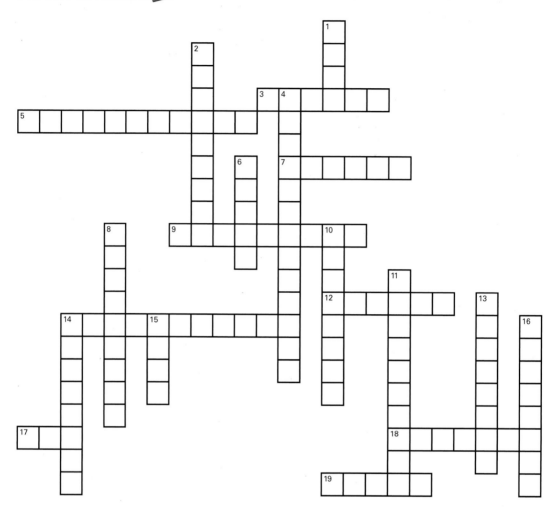

ACROSS

3. neck of the uterus
5. endoscopic examination of the abdomen
7. root word for ovary
9. cutting and sealing vas deferens, male sterilization
12. dark pigmented area around nipple
14. inflammation of the prostate
17. root word for vas deferens and vessel
18. another term for fallopian tube
19. root word for woman

DOWN

1. root word for vulva
2. GC
4. growth of endometrial tissue outside of the uterus
6. tissue that partially covers the entrance to vagina
8. herniation of urinary bladder into vaginal wall
10. beginning of menstruation
11. instrument used to examine the vagina and cervix
13. area between the external vulva to the anus
14. narrowing of the opening of the prepuce so foreskin cannot be retracted
15. abbreviation for transurethral resection of the prostate
16. inflammation of the testis

CHAPTER 14 QUIZ

Multiple Choice

1. The surgical removal of testes is called:
   a. orchidectomy
   b. vasectomy
   c. circumcision
   d. cauterization

2. A prolapsed uterus means that the uterus is:
   a. bent backward on itself
   b. descended down into the vagina
   c. tipped forward
   d. tipped backward

3. Menarche is:
   a. the beginning of menstruation
   b. the end of menopause
   c. part of the first trimester
   d. another name for gestation

4. Cryptorchidism is:
   a. underdeveloped testicles
   b. small ovaries
   c. ruptured ovaries
   d. undescended testicles

5. Removal of fluid from the area around the fetus to analyze is called:
   a. cervicentesis
   b. amniocentesis
   c. intrauterine analysis
   d. none of the above

6. The surgical procedure that removes the prostate gland is called a:
   a. vasectomy
   b. prostatectomy
   c. vasoligation
   d. circumcision

7. A Papanicolaou test is done to detect:
   a. fibroids
   b. metritis
   c. cancer of the cervix
   d. ovarian cancer

8. A difficult or painful monthly blood flow is termed:
   a. dysmenorrhea
   b. menorrhea
   c. dysmetrorrhagia
   d. menometrorrhagia

9. A colposcope is used to visualize the:
   a. testis
   b. epididymis
   c. cervix
   d. vagina

True or False

Place an X in the "True" or "False" column next to each statement. Write the correct answer in the "Correction, if False" column for any statements you identify as false.

STATEMENT	TRUE	FALSE	CORRECTION, IF FALSE
10. Fertilization is the development that occurs between the formation of the zygote and birth of the child.	____	____	_____
11. The tubes between the ovaries and the uterus are called the fallopian tubes.	____	____	_____
12. The joining of the male and female gametes is called ovulation.	____	____	_____
13. IVF is an abbreviation for intravenous filtration.	____	____	_____
14. The term for the release of the female gamete is *proliferation*.	____	____	_____
15. The male ductwork that acts as a part of both the male urinary and male reproductive systems is called the urethra.	____	____	_____
16. Hysteralgia is pain in the uterus.	____	____	_____
17. Obstetrician is the medical specialty concerned with the medical care of women during pregnancy and childbirth.	____	____	_____
18. Endometriosis is difficult or painful menses.	____	____	_____
19. Mammography is examination of cells from a mucosal surface, especially the uterine cervix.	____	____	_____

15 *The Special Senses of Sight and Hearing*

LEARNING OBJECTIVES

Upon completion of this chapter, you should be able to:

- List terms naming the major organs, functions, and disorders of the eyes and ears.
- Recognize and define the elements that make up terms related to the eyes and ears.
- Interpret selected abbreviations relating to the eyes and ears.
- Define terms naming disorders of the eyes and ears.
- Label diagrams showing major components of the eyes and ears.
- Analyze and define the new terms introduced in this chapter.

INTRODUCTION

We get the English words *sense* and *sentience* from the Latin verb *sentire*, which refers to the human ability to perceive our surroundings and thus to attain wisdom. Issuing from those two words, the phrase *special senses* refers to the five avenues along which perception travels, namely, the senses of touch, taste, smell, sight, and hearing. Sight and hearing are treated in a single chapter because, unlike smell, taste, and touch, which rely on chemical responses, sight and hearing include terminology associated with bodily organs that process electromagnetic energy (sight) and mechanical energy (hearing). Each will, however, be treated separately in a section of its own.

THE EYES

Table 15-1 lists most of the elements that make up terms related to the eyes. Some suffixes and prefixes already learned may also be listed.

Carefully study Table 15-1 before attempting to complete the Word Elements Exercise.

Structure and Function of the Eyes

Light waves are part of the electromagnetic spectrum, and our eyes work like a motion picture camera, taking continuous pictures and transmitting them instantaneously to the brain, which converts them to images in motion. Although light energy and brain waves are both part of the electromagnetic spectrum, brain waves have much lower frequencies and, therefore, much longer wavelengths than those of light. So, our eyes must also convert detected light frequencies so that the brain can enable us to "see" objects and their motions.

The main external structures of the eye include the **orbit**, the eyelids, the **conjunctiva**, and the **lacrimal** apparatus, also called **tear ducts**. The orbit, also known as the eye socket, is a cavity formed by several bones that contain the eyeball. Each eye has a pair of eyelids (an **upper palpebra** and a **lower palpebra**) that protect the eyeball from dust, foreign particles, light, and impact. The edges of the eyelids have eyelashes and sebaceous glands that secrete an oily substance onto the inner side of the eyelids for lubrication. The **canthi** (singular of **canthus**) are the corners of the eye where the upper and lower **palpebrae** (plural of palpebra) join together. See Figure 15-1 for the protective structures of the eye.

The **conjunctiva** is the mucous membrane lining on the underside of the eyelid. This membrane acts as a protective covering for the exposed surface of the eyeball. The **lacrimal glands** produce and store tears, which cleanse the eye. They are located above the outer corner of each

TABLE 15-1	WORD ELEMENTS RELATED TO THE EYES
Word Element	**Refers to**
blephar/o	eyelid
conjunctiv/o	conjunctiva (plural: conjunctivae)
corne/o	cornea
dacry/o	tears, lacrima
dacryocyst/o	tears or lacrimal sac
dipl/o	two, double
irid/o, ir-, irit/o	iris
kerat/o	hard, cornea
lacrim/o	tear, lacrimal apparatus
ocul/o	eye
ophthalm/o	eye
-opia	suffix for eye vision
-opsia	suffix for vision
opt/o	light, eye, vision
phak/o, phac/o	lens
presby/o	old age
pupil/o	pupil
retin/o	retina
scler/o	sclera (also means hard)
uve/o	middle layer of the eye containing muscles and blood vessels

Word Elements Exercise — DEFINING WORD ELEMENTS RELATED TO THE EYE

Write the definition of each of the elements given.

1. retin/o _____

2. dacryocyst/o _____

3. -opsia _____

4. opt/o _____

5. ocul/o _____

6. uve/o _____

7. dipl/o _____

8. dacry/o _____

9. lacrim/o _____

10. -opia _____

11. irid/o, ir-, irit/o _____

12. ophthalm/o _____

13. phak/o, phac/o _____

14. presby/o _____

15. blephar/o _____

16. conjunctiv/o _____

17. pupil/o _____

18. corne/o _____

19. scler/o _____

20. kerat/o _____

eye and secrete tears, which are also called **lacrimal fluid**. These glands help maintain moisture on the eyeball. The **lacrimal sac** is also known as a tear sac or **dacryocyst**. Figure 15-2 illustrates the lacrimal gland and associated structures.

The eyeball is made up of three layers: the **sclera**, the **uveal tract** (contains the **choroid**, **iris**, and **ciliary body**), and the **retina** (Fig. 15-3). The sclera, also known as the white of the eye, helps maintain the shape of the eyeball and gives protection to it. The **cornea**, an extension of the sclera, is the transparent portion that provides most of the optical power of the eye through its ability to bend light rays to focus on the surface of the retina.

The **iris** is the pigmented muscular ring that surrounds and controls the size of the pupil, through which light enters the eye. The **ciliary body** is located within the choroid and consists of a group of muscles that suspend the lens and adjust it to direct the light entering the eye. The lens is responsible for focusing images on the **retina**. It is held in place by the ligaments of the ciliary body. These muscles control the shape of the lens to allow for far and near vision, a process called **accommodation** (Fig. 15-4). The choroid is the opaque layer of the eyeball that contains vessels that provide the blood supply to the eye.

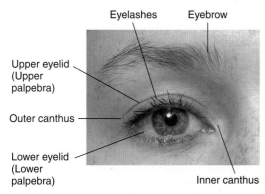

FIGURE 15-1 The protective structures of the eye.
From Cohen BJ. Medical Terminology: An Illustrated Guide. *5th ed. Philadelphia, PA: Lippincott Williams & Wilkins; 2007.*

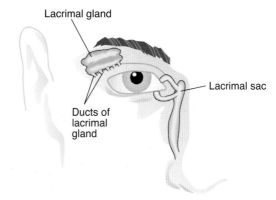

FIGURE 15-2 Lacrimal glands. The right lacrimal gland and associated structures are shown. *From Cohen BJ*. Medical Terminology: An Illustrated Guide. *5th ed. Philadelphia, PA: Lippincott Williams & Wilkins; 2007.*

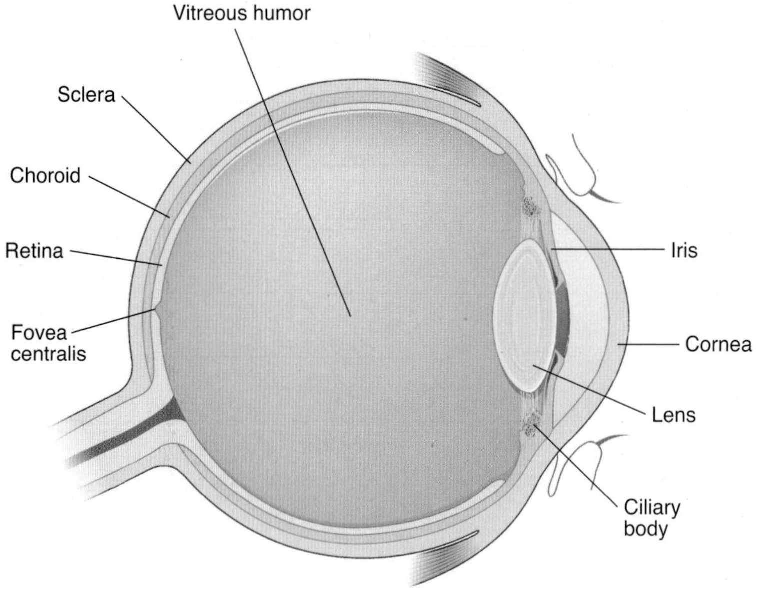

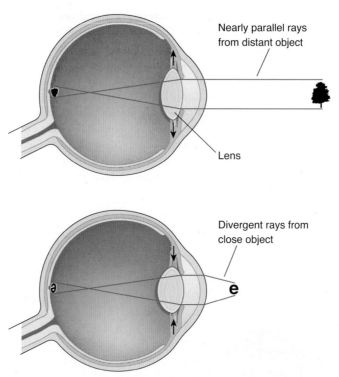

FIGURE 15-3 **Structures of the eyeball.** The innermost layer of the retina contains specialized cells called rods and cones. The rods have black and white receptors that respond to dim light. The cones have color receptors. *Modified from Cohen BJ. Medical Terminology: An Illustrated Guide. 5th ed. Philadelphia, PA: Lippincott Williams & Wilkins; 2007.*

FIGURE 15-4 **Accommodation.** The muscles control the shape of the lens to allow for far and near vision. The top figure has an elongated lens allowing distant vision. The lower figure has a shortened lens, allowing the eye to focus on near objects. *From Cohen BJ. Medical Terminology: An Illustrated Guide. 5th ed. Philadelphia, PA: Lippincott Williams & Wilkins; 2007.*

✔ *Quick Check: A Few Key Synonyms*

Fill in the blanks.

1. The main external structures of the eye include the _____,
   the _____, the _____, and the
   _____ apparatus.

2. Each eye has a pair of _____ to protect the eye from foreign particles,
   light, and impact.

3. The common word for lacrimal fluid is _____.

The innermost layer, the **retina**, is the sensitive layer of the eye that contains the specialized light-sensitive cells called **rods** (black and white receptors that respond to dim light) and **cones** (color receptors that provide high visual acuity). These photosensitive cells receive the light waves that come in through the cornea and convert them into nerve impulses. The **fovea centralis** is a pit in the middle of the retina that is saturated with cone cells that permit the best possible color vision.

The interior spaces of the eyeball contain fluid. The space between the cornea and the lens is filled with a watery fluid called the **aqueous humor**, and the large open space between the lens and retina contains a semi-gelatinous liquid, the **vitreous humor**.

Disorders and Treatments of the Eye

Errors in refraction, infections, and disorders of the eyelids are common. Refractive errors can be corrected with glasses, contact lenses, or surgical techniques that include the reshaping of the cornea. Some eye conditions are treated with medications and, in some cases, surgery.

Refractive Errors

Some people suffer from farsightedness, which gives us two terms: the first is **presbyopia**, which is farsightedness caused by aging. The other term, **hyperopia**, occurs when the eyeball loses its shape slightly for any reason, causing images to fall behind the retina. When images fall in front of the retina, the condition is called nearsightedness or **myopia** (Fig. 15-5). Another error of refraction is called **astigmatism**, which means the light coming into the eye does not focus on a single point; this condition is caused by an irregularity of the curve of the cornea that distorts light entering the eye. Corrective lenses can usually compensate for any refractive error.

Infections

Conjunctivitis, commonly known as pinkeye, is an inflammation of the transparent membrane (conjunctiva) that lines the eyelid and part of the eyeball. The inflammation causes small blood vessels in the conjunctiva to become more prominent, which gives a pink or red cast to the sclera or whites of the eyes. **Keratitis** is an inflammation of the cornea that occurs when the cornea has been scratched or otherwise damaged. An inflamed tear sac is called **dacryocystitis**.

Disorders of the Eyelids

Blepharoptosis is a condition that features the drooping of the upper eyelid. **Ectropion** is the turning outward (eversion) of the edge of the eyelid. **Entropion** is the opposite, a condition that causes the eyelid to turn inward. A **hordeolum** is commonly called a **sty**, which is caused by an infection of the glands near the eyelid.

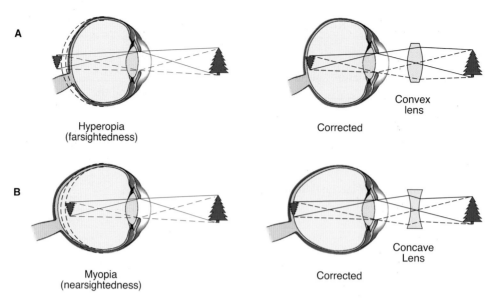

FIGURE 15-5 **Errors of refraction. A.** Hyperopia or farsightedness. The image falls behind the retina, making it difficult to see up close. The corrective lens places the image properly on the retina. **B.** Myopia or nearsightedness. The image falls in front of the retina, making it difficult to see far. The corrective lens places the image properly on the retina. *From Cohen BJ. Medical Terminology: An Illustrated Guide. 5th ed. Philadelphia, PA: Lippincott Williams & Wilkins; 2007.*

Other Disorders of the Eye

Xerophthalmia, also known as dry eyes, occurs when the surface of the eye becomes dry, often from wearing contact lenses or from a diminished flow of tears.

Glaucoma is a disease characterized by an increase in intraocular pressure that causes damage to the optic nerve. If left untreated, it can result in permanent blindness. Symptoms frequently go unnoticed by the patient until the optic nerve has been damaged.

A cloudiness or opacity of the lens is called a **cataract** (Fig. 15-6). Cataracts may be caused by disease, injury, chemicals, or exposure to various physical elements. Surgery to replace the clouded lens with an artificial intraocular lens is a common treatment for cataracts.

Practice and Practitioners: The Eyes

An ophthalmologist provides eye care ranging from examining eyes and prescribing corrective lenses to performing surgery. Such a wide range of activities and responsibilities requires ophthalmologists to have completed an undergraduate college degree, a doctorate in medicine, a 1-year internship, and 3 or more additional years of specialized clinical training in the field of ophthalmology. An **optometrist** is a health care professional who examines eyes and prescribes corrective lenses. In the United States, optometrists are doctors of optometry, which requires an undergraduate college degree and an additional 4 years of training at an accredited school of optometry. The technicians who fill eyeglass prescriptions and dispense eyewear are called **opticians**. This occupation requires a high school diploma and successful completion of an accredited optician program, which consists about 1 year of study.

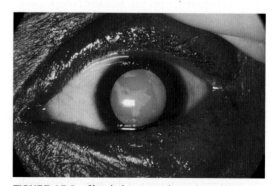

FIGURE 15-6 **Clouded cataract lens.** *From Cohen BJ. Medical Terminology: An Illustrated Guide. 5th ed. Philadelphia, PA: Lippincott Williams & Wilkins; 2007.*

TABLE 15-2	WORD ELEMENTS RELATED TO THE EAR	
Word Element	**Refers to**
acous/o, acus/o, acoust/o	hearing
audi/o	sound
aur/o	ear
auricul/o	ear
myring/o	tympanic membrane (eardrum)
ot/o	ear
staped/o	stapes
tympan/o	eardrum

WORD ELEMENTS RELATED TO THE EAR

Before beginning this section, study Table 15-2 carefully and complete the Word Elements Exercise.

Structure and Function of the Ears

The ear serves a dual purpose: provision of hearing and equilibrium. The outer ear is specially designed to bring sound waves into the inner parts of the ear, where they are converted to electrical signals the brain can process. The ear is divided into three sections: the external ear, middle ear, and internal ear. The external ear, located along the sides of the head, is called the **pinna** or **auricle**. Its purpose is to funnel sound waves into the **auditory canal**. Numerous glands line the auditory canal and secrete **cerumen**, better known as *earwax*. Cerumen protects the ear by preventing dust, insects, and some bacteria from entering the middle ear.

Word Elements Exercise	DEFINING WORD ELEMENTS RELATED TO THE EAR

Write the definition of each of the elements given.

1. audi/o _____

2. ot/o _____

3. acous/o, acus/o, acoust/o _____

4. myring/o _____

5. tympan/o _____

6. aur/o _____

7. staped/o _____

8. auricul/o _____

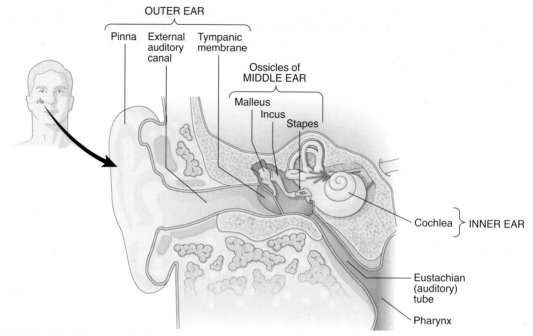

FIGURE 15-7   The ear and its internal structures. *From Cohen BJ. Medical Terminology: An Illustrated Guide. 5th ed. Philadelphia, PA: Lippincott Williams & Wilkins; 2007.*

Sound waves entering the ear vibrate the **tympanic membrane** (Fig. 15-7). Just beyond the tympanic membrane is the middle ear. A tiny cavity in the skull houses three small bones (**ossicles**) called the **malleus, incus**, and **stapes** (Fig. 15-8). These are also sometimes referred to as the hammer, anvil, and stirrup because of their shapes. Sound waves affect these tiny bones and cause them to transmit sound vibrations to the inner ear. Also found inside of the middle of each ear is the **eustachian tube** (also called the **auditory tube**), which reaches from the middle ear to the nasopharynx to help equalize pressure in the ear with outside atmospheric pressure.

The inner ear is called a **labyrinth** or maze because of its complicated construction. It contains the sensory receptors for hearing and balance. One of the major structures in the labyrinth is the **cochlea**. Receptors in the cochlea change sound waves into electrical signals that the brain can process.

Disorders of the Ear

Hearing loss may range from a partial loss of hearing that includes only a certain range of frequencies to complete **deafness**. A **conductive** hearing loss is defined as one in which the outer or middle ear cannot conduct sound vibrations to the inner ear. A **sensorineural** hearing loss involves nerve deafness. **Presbycusis** is a progressive hearing loss that may occur as one ages. **Anacusis** is total deafness.

Ear disorders can occur in any of the three parts of the ear, namely, the outer, middle, or inner ear. **Impacted cerumen**, which is an accumulation of **cerumen** (earwax) in the external auditory canal, may cause a hearing loss. An earache, termed **otalgia** or **otodynia**, may be

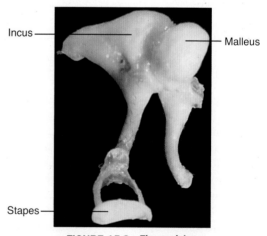

FIGURE 15-8   The ossicles.

Quick Check: A Few Key Synonyms

Fill in the blanks.

1. What are the formal names of the ossicles, sometimes referred to as the hammer, anvil, and stirrup? The _____, the _____, and the _____ apparatus.

2. What is another name for the auditory tube? _____.

3. A major structure in the labyrinth changes sound waves into electrical signals. What is it called? _____.

caused by trauma or infections. **Otitis** is any inflammation of the ear, but the term **otitis media** is used to name an inflammation in the middle ear.

Other inflammations are **myringitis**; **mastoiditis**, which is an inflammation of the mastoid process; and **labyrinthitis**, which is an inflammation of the labyrinth.

Two other disorders of the ear include **otosclerosis** (sound is unable to travel from the outer to the inner ear) and **Ménière's syndrome**, a chronic disease of the inner ear characterized by vertigo, tinnitus, and periodic hearing loss. **Vertigo** is dizziness and/or a loss of balance sometimes associated with Ménière's syndrome. **Tinnitus is** a ringing, buzzing, or roaring sound in the ears.

Some disorders of the ear are treated by surgical intervention. Some of these procedures include the following:

- **Otoplasty**: surgical repair of the pinna of the ear
- **Mastoidectomy**: surgical removal of the mastoid process
- **Myringectomy** or **tympanectomy**: surgical removal of all or part of the tympanic membrane
- **Myringotomy**: surgical incision of the eardrum to create an opening for placement of ventilating or drainage tubes
- **Tympanoplasty**: surgical correction of a damaged tympanic membrane
- **Stapedectomy**: surgical removal of the stapes
- **Labyrinthotomy**: a surgical incision into the labyrinth

ABBREVIATIONS

The following table lists common abbreviations relating to the eyes and ears. The Latin words *dexter* and *sinister* mean, respectively, "right" and "left." These two Latin words give us a lot of English words, such as ambidextrous (able to use either hand equally well), dextrous (good with one's hands), sinister (odd or spooky—probably because 83% of the population is right-handed), etc. The first letter of each of these two words, namely, D and S, have also found their way into abbreviations for the eyes and ears. AD means right ear because *A* refers to audi/o "the ear," and *D* refers to *dexter* "the right side." Likewise, AS refers to the left ear. The root ocul/o refers to the eye, and thus OD is the right eye, and OS is the left eye.

Are abbreviations good or bad? The good thing about abbreviations is that they save time. The bad thing about them is that time saved seldom equals accuracy lost. Looking up the abbreviation AU will get you 49 answers, one of which is "both ears" and another of which is "aortic stenosis." Heart surgery is not going to help someone who is suffering hearing loss in both ears. By the way, neither of those meanings has a connection with Australia, which is also among the 49 meanings given for the AU abbreviation.

Abbreviation Table SIGHT AND HEARING

ABBREVIATION	MEANING
AD	right ear
AS	left ear
ASL	American Sign Language
AU	both ears
dB	decibel
ECCE	extracapsular cataract extraction
EOM	extraocular movement
ERG	electroretinography
ICCE	intracapsular cataract extraction
IOP	intraocular pressure
OD	right eye
OM	otitis media
OS	left eye
OU	both eyes
PVD	posterior vitreous detachment (referring to the vitreous body)

Word Elements Exercise ABBREVIATIONS

Fill in the blanks with the meaning of each of the following as it might be used in connection with the eyes or ears.

ABBREVIATION	MEANING
1. ICCE	_____
2. AU	_____
3. OM	_____
4. dB	_____
5. PVD	_____
6. AD	_____
7. OD	_____
8. OS	_____
9. ASL	_____

10. AS	_____
11. ECCE	_____
12. EOM	_____
13. ERG	_____
14. IOP	_____
15. OU	_____

Study Table — SIGHT AND HEARING

TERM AND PRONUNCIATION	ANALYSIS	MEANING
Structure and Function: Eye		
accommodation (ah-KOM-moh-DAY-shun)	common English word	the process that allows the shape of the lens to change for near and far vision
aqueous humor (A-kwee-us HUE-mor)	from the Latin word *aqua* (water) + humor, from the Latin word *umor* (body fluid)	thick watery substance filling the space between the lens and the cornea
canthus (KAN-thus)	from the Greek word *kanthus* (corner of the eye)	angle where the upper and lower eyelids meet
choroid (KOH-royd)	derived from the Greek words *chorion* (skin, leather; a spot or plot of ground) and *eidos* (form, likeness, appearance, resemblance)	opaque middle layer of the eyeball
ciliary body (SIL-ee-her-ee)	from the Latin word *ciliaris* (pertaining to eyelashes) + body	set of muscles and suspensory ligaments that adjust the lens
cones	from the Greek word *konos* (cone)	color receptors on the retina that have high visual acuity
conjunctiva (kon-JUNK-tih-vuh); plural: conjunctivae (kon-JUNK-tih-vay)	from the Latin words *con* (with) and *jungere* (to join)	the mucous membrane covering the anterior of the eyeball and inner eyelid
cornea (KOR-nee-uh)	from the Latin word *cornus* (horn)	transparent shield of tissue forming the outer wall of the eyeball
dacryocyst (DACK-ree-oh-sist)	from the Greek words *dakryon* (tear) and *kytis* (bag)	tear sac, lacrimal sac
extraocular (EX-trah-AWK-yu-lahr)	*extra-* (outside); *ocul/o* (eye); *-ar* (adjective suffix)	situated outside the eye

(continued)

TERM AND PRONUNCIATION	ANALYSIS	MEANING
fovea centralis (FOH-avee-ah sen-TRAH-lis)	*fovea*, a Latin word meaning "small pit" + *centralis*, a Latin word meaning "central"	a pit in the middle of the retina that is the area of sharpest vision
iris (EYE-rihs); plural: irides (IHR-ih-deez)	a Greek word meaning "lily," "iris of the eye," originally "messenger of the gods," personified as the rainbow	the anterior part of the vascular tunic; it is the colored part of the eye
lacrimal apparatus (LAK-rih-mahl app-ah-RAT-uhs)	from the Latin words *lacrima* (tear) + *ad* (toward) and *parare* (to make ready)	collectively: the lacrimal gland, lake, canaliculi (small canals), and sac, along with the nasolacrimal duct
lens (lenz)	common English word	the refractive structure of the eye, lying between the iris and the vitreous body
ocular (OK-yoo-lahr)	*ocul/o* (eye); *-ar* (adjective suffix)	adjective referring to the eye
optic nerve (OP-tik nuhrv)	*opt/o* (light, eye, vision); *-ic* (adjective suffix) + nerve	the cranial nerve responsible for vision
orbit (OR-biht)	from the Latin word *orbita* (wheel track, course, orbit)	bony depression in the skull that houses the eyeball
palpebra (pal-PEE-brah)	a Latin word meaning "eyelid"	eyelid
photoreceptors (FOH-toh-ree-SEPP-tohrs)	from the Greek word *phos* (light) and the Latin word *recipere* (to receive)	retinal cones and rods
pupil (PYOO-pihl)	from the Latin word *pupilla* (little girl-doll) so called from the tiny image one sees of oneself reflected in the eye of another	the dark part in the center of the iris through which light enters the eye
retina (RETT-ih-nah)	from Medieval Latin *retina* probably from the Latin word *rete* (net)	light-sensitive membrane forming the innermost layer of the eyeball
rods	a common English word	black and white receptors on the retina that respond to dim light
sclera (SKLER-ah); plural: sclerae (SKLER-ay)	from the Greek word *skleros* (hard)	the outer surface of the eye; part of the fibrous tunic
uvea (YOO-vee-ah)	from the Latin word *uva* (grape)	vascular layer of the eye
vitreous body (VIH-tree-uhs BOD-ee)	from the Latin word *vitreus* (of glass, glassy) + body	a transparent jellylike substance filling the interior of the eyeball
vitreous humor (VIH-tree-uhs HYU-mohr)	from the Latin word *umor* (body fluid)	the fluid component of the vitreous body

TERM AND PRONUNCIATION	ANALYSIS	MEANING
Common Disorders: Eye		
amblyopia (am-blee-OH-pee-ah)	from the Greek word *ambly* (dim); *-opia* (eye, vision)	condition that occurs when visual acuity is not the same in both eyes; also called "lazy eye"
astigmatism (ah-STIG-mah-tizm)	*a-* (without) + from the Greek word *stigmatos* gen. of *stigma* (a mark, spot, puncture)	fuzzy vision caused by the irregular shape of one or both eyeballs
blepharitis (bleff-ah-RY-tiss)	*blephar/o* (eyelid); *-itis* (inflammation)	inflammation of the eyelid
blepharoconjunctivitis (BLEFF-ah-roh-kon-junk-tih-VY-tiss)	*blephar/o* (eyelid); *conjunctiv/o* (mucous membrane covering the anterior surface of the eyeball and inner eyelid); *-itis* (inflammation)	inflammation of the palpebral conjunctiva, the inner lining of the eyelids
blepharoplegia (BLEFF-ah-roh-pleej-ee-uh)	*blephar/o* (eyelid); *-plegia* (paralysis)	paralysis of an eyelid
blepharoptosis (BLEFF-ahr-opp-TOH-sis)	*blephar/o* (eyelid); *-ptosis* (falling, downward placement, prolapse)	drooping eyelid
blepharospasm (BLEFF-ahr-oh-SPAZ-um)	*blephar/o* (eyelid); from the Greek *spasmos* (spasm, convulsion)	involuntary contraction of the eyelid
cataract (KAT-ah-rakt)	from the Latin word *cataracta* (waterfall)	complete or partial opacity of the ocular lens
conjunctivitis (kon-junk-tih-VY-tiss)	*conjunctiv/o* (mucous membrane covering the anterior surface of the eyeball); *-itis* (inflammation)	inflammation of the conjunctiva; pinkeye
dacryocele (DAKK-ree-oh-seel)	*dacry/o* (tears); *-cele* (hernia)	herniated lacrimal sac (filled with fluid); often called a *dacryocystocele* because *dacryocyst* is a synonym for *lacrimal sac*
dacryocystitis (DAKK-ree-oh-SIST-it is)	*dacryocyst/o* (tear sac); *-itis* (inflammation)	inflammation of the tear sac
dacryolith (DAKK-ree-oh-lith)	*dacry/o* (tears); *-lith* (stone)	a "stone" in the lacrimal apparatus
dacryorrhea (DAK-ree-uh-REE-yuh)	*dacry/o* (tears); *-rrhea* (discharge)	excessive discharge of tears
glaucoma (glaw-KOH-mah)	from the Greek word *glaucoma* (cataract, opacity of the lens) (note: cataracts and glaucoma not distinguished until around 1705)	disease of the eye characterized by increased intraocular pressure and atrophy of the optic nerve

(continued)

TERM AND PRONUNCIATION	ANALYSIS	MEANING
hordeolum (hor-DEE-oh-lum)	from the Latin word *hordeum* (barley)	a sty on the eyelid; a sty is an infection of a gland in the eye
hyperopia (hy-pur-OH-pee-ya) or presbyopia (pres-be-OH-pee-ah)	*hyper-* (above normal); *-opia* (eye, vision)	farsightedness
iridomalacia (IHR-ih-doh-muh-LAY-shee-uh)	*irid/o* (iris); *-malacia* (softening)	softening of the iris
iritis (eye-RY-tiss)	*ir/o* (iris); *-itis* (inflammation)	inflammation of the iris
keratitis (ker-ah-TYE-tis)	*kerat/o* (hard, cornea); *-itis* (inflammation)	inflammation of the cornea
lacrimal (LAK-rih-muhl)	*lacrim/o* (tear, lacrimal apparatus); *-al* (adjective suffix)	referring to or related to tears or the tear ducts and glands
lacrimation (LAK-rih-MAY-shun)	*lacrim/o* (tear, lacrimal apparatus); *-ation* (noun suffix)	excessive tearing; synonym for *dacryorrhea*
myopia (my-OHP-ee-ah)	from the Greek word *myops* (nearsighted)	nearsightedness
oculodynia (AWK-yu-loh-DIN-ee-ah)	*ocul/o* (eye); *-dynia* (pain)	pain in the eyeball
oculopathy (AWK-yu-loh-path-ee)	*ocul/o* (eye); *-pathy* (disease)	generic term for eye disease; synonym for *ophthalmopathy*
ophthalmolith (off-THAL-moh-lith)	*ophthalm/o* (eye); *-lith* (stone)	a stone in the lacrimal apparatus; synonym for *dacryolith*
ophthalmomalacia (off-THAL-moh-muh-LAY-shee-uh)	*ophthalm/o* (eye); *-malacia* (softening)	softening of the eyeball
ophthalmopathy (off-THAL-moh-path-ee)	*ophthalm/o* (eye); *-pathy* (disease)	generic term for eye disease; synonym for oculopathy
presbyopia (prez-bee-OH-pee-ah)	from the Greek word *presbys* (old man); *-opia* (eye, vision)	farsightedness resulting from loss of elasticity of the lens due to aging
retinitis (rett-ih-NY-tiss)	*retin/o* (retina); *-itis* (inflammation)	inflammation of the retina
retinopathy (rett-ihn-AWP-uh-thee)	*retin/o* (retina); *-pathy* (disease)	disease of the retina
scleroiritis (skler-oh-EYE-RY-tiss)	*sclera/o* (sclera); *ir/o* (iris); *-itis* (inflammation)	inflammation of the sclera and iris
strabismus (stra-BIZ-muhs)	from the Greek word *strabismos*, from *strabos* (squinting, squint-eyed)	lack of parallelism in the visual axes; crossed eyes
xerophthalmia (zee-roh-OFF-thal-mee-ah)	from the Greek word *xeros* (dry); *ophthalm/o* (eye); *-ia* (condition)	dry eyes

TERM AND PRONUNCIATION	ANALYSIS	MEANING
Practice and Practitioners: Eye		
ophthalmologist (off-thul-MAWL-uh-jist)	*ophthalm/o* (eye); *-logist* (one who studies a specific field)	physician whose specialty is the diagnosis and treatment of eye disorders
ophthalmology (off-thul-MAWL-uh-jee)	*ophthalm/o* (eye); *-logy* (study of)	medical specialty dealing with the eye
optician (opp-TISH-ihn)	*opt/o* (light, eye, vision)	a maker of lenses
optometrist (opp-TOM-uh-trist)	*opt/o* (light, eye, vision); *-metrist* (one who measures)	one trained in examining the eyes and prescribing corrective lenses
optometry (opp-TOM-uh-tree)	*opt/o* (light, eye, vision); *-metry* (measurement)	science of examining eyes for impaired vision and other disorders
Diagnosis and Treatment: Eye		
ophthalmoscope (OFF-THAL-moh-skope)	*ophthalm/o* (eye); *-scope* (instrument for viewing)	device for examining the interior of the eyeball by looking through the pupil
ophthalmoscopy (OFF-thal-MAW-skuh-pee)	*ophthalm/o* (eye); *-scopy* (use of instrument for viewing	examination of the eye with an ophthalmoscope
refraction (re-FRAK-shun)	from the Latin wod *refractus*, pp of *refringere* (to break up)	deflection of a ray of light into the eye for accommodation or correction of vision as it passes from one medium to another of different density
Surgical Procedures: Eye		
blepharectomy (bleff-ah-REK-tuh-mee)	*blephar/o* (eyelid); *-ectomy* (excision)	surgical removal of part or all of an eyelid
blepharoplasty (BLEFF-ah-roh-plass-tee)	*blephar/o* (eyelid); *-plasty* (surgical repair)	surgery to correct a defective eyelid
blepharotomy (BLEFF-uh-rot-uh-mee)	*blephar/o* (eyelid); *-tomy* (incision into)	surgical incision of an eyelid
conjunctivoplasty (kon-JUNK-tih-voh-plass-tee)	*conjunctiv/o* (conjunctiva); *-plasty* (surgical repair)	surgery on the conjunctiva
dacryocystectomy (dakk-ree-oh-sist-EKK-toh-mee)	*dacryocyst/o* (tear sac); *-ectomy* (excision)	surgical removal of the lacrimal sac
dacryocystotomy (dakk-ree-oh-sist-AW-toh-mee)	*dacryocyst/o* (tear sac); *-tomy* (incision into)	incision into the lacrimal sac
lacrimotomy (lakk-rih-MAW-toh-mee) (uncommon)	*lacrim/o* (tear, lacrimal apparatus); *-tomy* (incision into)	incision into the lacrimal sac; rarely used synonym for dacryocystotomy

(continued)

TERM AND PRONUNCIATION	ANALYSIS	MEANING
phacolysis (fah-KAWL-ih-sis)	*phac/o* (lens); *-lysis* (destruction)	operative removal of the lens in pieces
retinectomy (ret-ihn-EK-tuh-mee)	*retin/o* (retina); *-ectomy* (excision)	surgical removal of part of the retina
retinopexy (RETT-ihn-oh-pexx-ee)	*retin/o* (retina); *-pexy* (surgical fixation)	surgical fixation of a detached retina
retinotomy (rett-ihn-AW-tuh-mee)	*retin/o* (retina); *-tomy* (incision into)	incision through the retina
Structure and Function: Ear		
auricle (AW-rik-uhl)	*auri-* (ear)	one of the two parts of the external ear (the other part is the auditory canal)
cerumen (seh-ROO-men)	from the Latin word *cera* (wax)	waxlike secretion occurring in the external auditory canal
cochlea (KOK-lee-uh)	a Latin word meaning "snail shell"	part of the bony labyrinth
eustachian tube (yu-STAY-shun)	named after Bartolomeo Eustachia (died 1574), who discovered the passages from the ears to the throat	the auditory tube that connects the middle ear to the pharynx
external auditory canal (ODD-ih-tor-ee)	from the Latin word *auditorius* (pertaining to hearing)	one of the two parts of the external ear (the other part is the auricle)
incus (INK-uhs)	a Latin word meaning "anvil"	one of the auditory ossicles (the anvil)
labyrinth (LAB-uh-rinth)	from the Greek word *labyrinthos* (maze, large building with intricate passages)	canals of the inner ear
malleus (MAL-ee-uhs)	a Latin word meaning "hammer"	one of the auditory ossicles (the hammer)
ossicles (OSS-ih-kulz)	from the Latin word *ossiculum* (a small bone)	three small bones in the middle ear: the malleus (hammer), the incus (anvil), and the stapes (stirrup)
pinna (PIN-ah)	a Latin word meaning "feather," "wing," "fin," "lobe"	another term for *auricle*
stapes (STAY-peez)	a Modern Latin word meaning "stirrup"	one of the auditory ossicles (the stirrup)
tympanic cavity (tim-PAN-ik)	*tympan/o* (eardrum); *-ic* (adjective suffix) + cavity	the middle ear
tympanic membrane (tim-PAN-ik MEM-brayn)	*tympan/o* (eardrum); *-ic* (adjective suffix)	the eardrum

TERM AND PRONUNCIATION	ANALYSIS	MEANING
Common Disorders: Ear		
anacusis (ann-ah-KU-sis)	*a-* (without); cusis, from the Greek word *akousis* (hearing)	total deafness
conductive hearing loss (kon-DUK-tihv)	common English words	hearing loss caused by interference with sound transmission in the external auditory canal, middle ear, or ossicles
labyrinthitis (lab-ih-rin-THIGH-tis)	*labyrinth/o* (internal ear); *-itis* (inflammation)	inflammation of the labyrinth
mastoiditis (mas-toy-DYE-tis)	mastoid (mastoid process); *-itis* (inflammation)	inflammation of any part of the mastoid process
Ménière's (men-YEHRS) syndrome	named for Prosper Ménière, the French physician who first described the illness in 1861	chronic disease of the inner ear characterized by vertigo, tinnitus, and periodic hearing loss
myringitis (mir-in-JIGH-tis)	*myring/o* (tympanic membrane); *-itis* (inflammation)	inflammation of the tympanic membrane
otalgia (oh-TAHL-jee-ah)	*ot/o* (ear); *-algia* (pain)	pain in the ear
otitis (oh-TY-tihs)	*ot/o* (ear); *-itis* (inflammation)	inflammation of the ear (otitis externa = the outer ear; otitis media = the middle ear; otitis interna = the inner ear)
otodynia (oh-toh-DIN-ee-uh)	*ot/o* (ear); *-dynia* (pain)	earache
otopathy (oh-TOP-ahth-ee)	*ot/o* (ear); *-pathy* (disease)	any disease of the ear
otoplasty (oh-toh-PLAS-tee)	*ot/o* (ear); *-plasty* (surgical repair)	surgical repair of the pinna of the ear
otorrhea (oh-toh-REE-uh)	*ot/o* (ear); *-rrhea* (discharge)	fluid discharge from the ear
otosclerosis (OH-toh-skler-OH-sihs)	*ot/o* (ear); *scler/o* (hardening); *-osis* (abnormal condition)	formation of spongy bone in the inner ear producing hearing loss
presbycusis (PREZ-be-KOO-sihs)	*presby-* (old); cusis, from the Greek word *akousis* (hearing)	hearing loss that occurs with aging
sensorineural hearing loss (SENTZ-oh-rih-NOO-rahl)	*sensor-* (sensory); *neur/o* (nervous system); *-al* (adjective suffix)	hearing loss caused by a neural condition
tinnitus (TIN-nih-tuhs)	from the Latin word *tinnire* (to ring)	sensation of noises (such as ringing) in the ears
vertigo (VUR-tih-go)	a Latin word meaning "dizziness"	sensation of spinning or whirling; can be caused by infection or other disorder in the inner ear

(continued)

TERM AND PRONUNCIATION	ANALYSIS	MEANING
Practice and Practitioners: Ear		
audiologist (awd-ee-AWL-oh-jist)	*audi/o* (sound, hearing); *-logist* (one who studies a certain field)	specialist who measures hearing efficiency and treats hearing impairment
audiology (awd-ee-AWL-oh-jee)	*audi/o* (sound, hearing); *-logy* (the study of a certain field)	specialty dealing with hearing and hearing disorders
otologist (oh-TOL-oh-jist)	*ot/o* (ear); *-logist* (one who studies a certain field)	specialist in otology, the branch of medical science concerned with the study, diagnosis, and treatment of diseases of the ear and its related structures
otology (oh-TOL-oh-jee)	*ot/o* (ear); *-logy* (the study of a certain field)	branch of medical science concerned with the study, diagnosis, and treatment of diseases of the ear and its related structures
otorhinolaryngologist (oh-TOH-REYE-no-lair-in-GOL-oh-jist)	*ot/o* (ear); *rhin/o* (nose); *g/o* (throat); *-logist* (one who studies a certain field)	physician who specializes in the diagnosis and treatment of ear, nose, and throat disorders
Diagnosis and Treatment: Ear		
audiogram (AW-dee-oh-gram)	*audi/o* (sound, hearing); *-gram* (record or picture)	automatically recorded results of a hearing test with an audiometer
audiometer (aw-dee-AWM-ih-tehr)	*audi/o* (sound, hearing); *-meter* (measurement)	electrical device for measuring hearing
audiometry (aw-dee-AWM-ih-tree)	*audi/o* (sound, hearing); *-metry* (process of measuring)	measuring hearing with an audiometer
cochlear implant (KOK-lee-ahr IM-plant)	from the Latin word *cochlea* (snail shell); *-ar* (adjective suffix) + implant	surgically implanted hearing aid in the cochlea
otoscope (OH-toh-skope)	*ot/o* (ear); *-scope* (instrument for viewing)	device for looking into the ear
otoscopy (oh-TOSS-kuh-pee)	*ot/o* (ear); *-scopy* (use of an instrument for viewing)	looking into the ear with an otoscope
Rinne test (rihn-eh)	named after Heinrich A. Rinne, German otologist (1819–1868)	hearing test using a tuning fork; checks for differences in bone conduction and air conduction
tuning fork (TOO-ning)	common English words	an instrument that vibrates when struck
Weber test (VAY-behr)	named after Wilhelm Edward Weber, German physicist (1804–1891)	hearing test using a tuning fork; distinguishes between conductive and sensorineural hearing loss

TERM AND PRONUNCIATION	ANALYSIS	MEANING
Surgical Procedures: Ear		
labyrinthotomy (lab-ih-rin-THAH-toh-mee)	*labyrinth/o* (internal ear); *-tomy* (incision into)	a surgical incision into the labyrinth
mastoidectomy (mas-toy-DECK-toh-mee)	mastoid (mastoid process) + *-ectomy* (excision)	surgical removal of the mastoid process
myringectomy (mir-ini-JECK-toh-mee) or tympanectomy	*myring/o* (tympanic membrane); *-ectomy* (excision)	surgical removal of all or part of the tympanic membrane
myringoplasty (mih-RIN-go-PLASS-tee)	*myring/o* (tympanic membrane); *-plasty* (surgical repair)	surgical repair of the tympanic membrane (eardrum)
myringotomy (mih-rin-GOT-uh-mee)	*myring/o* (tympanic membrane); *-tomy* (incision into)	incision or surgical puncture of the eardrum
otoplasty (OH-toh-plass-tee)	*ot/o* (ear); *-plasty* (surgical repair)	surgical repair of the pinna of the ear
stapedectomy (stay-peh-DECK-toh-mee)	*staped/o* (stapes); *-ectomy* (excision)	surgical removal of the stapes
tympanectomy (TIM-puh-NEK-tuh-mee)	*tympan/o* (eardrum); *-tomy* (incision into)	surgical removal of the eardrum
tympanocentesis (TIM-puh-noh-senn-TEE-sihs)	*tympan/o* (eardrum); *-centesis* (surgical puncture for aspiration)	puncture of the tympanic membrane with a needle to aspirate middle ear fluid
tympanoplasty (TIM-puh-no-plass-tee)	*tympan/o* (eardrum); *-plasty* (surgical repair)	surgery performed on the eardrum
tympanotomy (TIM-puh-NOT-oh-mee)	*tympan/o* (eardrum); *-tomy* (incision)	synonym for *myringotomy*

EXERCISES

EXERCISE 15-1   FIGURE LABELING: THE EYE

Use the following terms to label the diagram:

choroid	fovea centralis	retina
ciliary body	iris	sclera
cornea	lens	vitreous humor

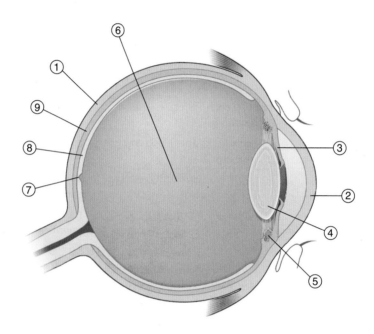

1. _____   6. _____

2. _____   7. _____

3. _____   8. _____

4. _____   9. _____

5. _____

EXERCISE 15-2 OPERATIVE REPORT

Read the following report and define the italicized terminology in the spaces.

PREOPERATIVE DIAGNOSIS: Chronic (1) *otitis media*

OPERATIVE PROCEDURE: Bilateral (2) *myringotomy* and placement of tubes

INDICATIONS: Recurrent ear infections with persistent fluid buildup despite prolonged medical treatment

PROCEDURE: The patient was brought to the operating suite and placed under general mask anesthesia. The ear canals were cleaned of dry (3) *cerumen* and crust. Myringotomies were placed bilaterally. Cultures were taken of the fluid present in the middle ear spaces. Ear tubes were placed in the myringotomy sites bilaterally. (4) *Antibiotic* drops and cotton balls were placed in the ear canal. The patient tolerated the procedure well and was taken to the recovery room.

1. _____

2. _____

3. _____

4. _____

EXERCISE 15-3 MATCHING TERMS WITH DEFINITIONS: EYE

Match the terms in Column 1 with the correct definitions in Column 2.

TERM	DEFINITION
1. _____ ophthalmology	A. transparent shield of tissue covering the iris
2. _____ vitreous humor	B. adjective associated with tears
3. _____ pupil	C. sensitive inner nerve layer of the eye that contains the rods and cones
4. _____ iris	D. the "colored" part of the eye
5. _____ sclera	E. the dark part in the very center of the eye
6. _____ cornea	F. mucous membrane that covers the anterior surface of the eyeball and lines the underside of each eyelid
7. _____ conjunctiva	G. gelatinous liquid between the lens and retina

8. _____ ophthalmoscope

H. part of the outermost layer of the eye, which is white in color

9. _____ retina

I. a device for examining the interior of the eyeball by looking through the pupil

10. _____ lacrimal

J. name of the medical specialty dealing with the eye

EXERCISE 15-4 MATCHING TERMS WITH DEFINITIONS: EAR

Match the terms in Column 1 with the correct definitions in Column 2.

TERM	DEFINITION
1. _____ audiologist	A. the eardrum
2. _____ cerumen	B. mazelike portion of the inner ear
3. _____ otoscope	C. specialist treating abnormal hearing
4. _____ tympanoplasty	D. device for looking in the ear
5. _____ labyrinth	E. inflammation of the middle ear
6. _____ auditory ossicles	F. part of the bony labyrinth (inner ear)
7. _____ otitis media	G. waxlike secretion in the external auditory canal
8. _____ tympanic membrane	H. auditory tube that connects the middle ear to the nasopharynx
9. _____ eustachian tube	I. surgical repair on the tympanic membrane
10. _____ cochlea	J. three small bones in the middle ear: the malleus, incus, and stapes

EXERCISE 15-5 FILL IN THE BLANK

Select a term from the list and complete the statements. Note that not all terms will be used.

antiemetic	cycloplegic	keratitis	otalgia	presbyopia
astigmatism	diplopia	labyrinthitis	otosclerosis	tinnitus
audiometry	glaucoma	Ménière disease	pinna	vertigo
blepharoptosis	hordeolum	OD	presbycusis	xerophthalmia
cataract				

1. A cloudiness or opacity of the lens is called _____.

2. Difficulty hearing due to the aging process is termed _____.

3. The medical term for double vision is _____.

4. Another name for dizziness due to an inner ear disturbance is _____.

5. _____ is a ringing or buzzing of the ears.

6. The external ear component is called the auricle or _____.

7. Another name for a sty is _____.

8. _____ means pain in the ear or an earache.

9. An irregularity of the curve of the cornea that distorts the light entering the eye is called _____.

10. An inflammation of the cornea is called _____.

11. The medical term for "dry eyes" is _____.

12. The drug classification that is prescribed for nausea and vomiting is _____.

13. An ankylosis (fixation) of the bones of the middle ear resulting in a conductive hearing loss is called _____.

14. _____ is the proper term for a drooping eyelid.

15. The measurement of hearing is called _____.

EXERCISE 15-6   CROSSWORD PUZZLE: EYE AND EAR

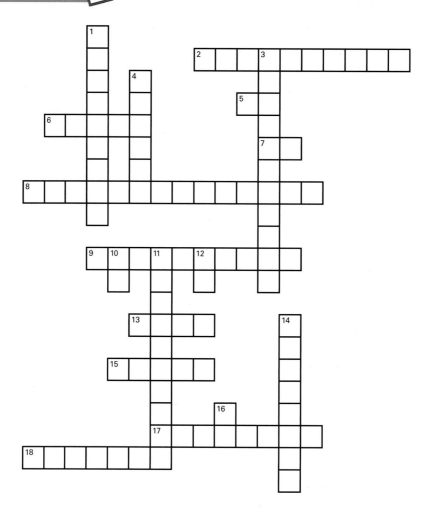

ACROSS

2. deviation of the visual lines of the eye so that the eyes are not directed at the same object
5. abbreviation for right eye
6. root of cornea
7. abbreviation for left eye
8. instrument used to examine the eye
9. tear sac
13. colored muscular ring that surrounds the pupil
15. lay term for ossicle is anvil
17. root for eye
18. earwax

DOWN

1. inner ear mazelike structure
3. health care professional that measures hearing, treats hearing disorder
4. innermost layer of the eye, actual visual receptor
10. abbreviation for left ear
11. bending of light rays
12. abbreviation for both eyes
14. small bones in the ear
16. root for ear

◀ CHAPTER 15 QUIZ

Multiple Choice

1. The medical specialist who treats ear disorders is called a(n):
   a. ophthalmologist
   b. otologist
   c. audiologist
   d. optometrist

2. A term for eardrum is:
   a. tympanic membrane
   b. malleus
   c. oval window
   d. none of the above

3. The function(s) of the ear include:
   a. equilibrium
   b. hearing
   c. sound vibrations
   d. both A and B

4. The ability of the eye to adjust to variations in distance is:
   a. eversion
   b. strabismus
   c. accommodation
   d. presbycusis

5. An inflammation of the tear sac is:
   a. dacryocystitis
   b. scleritis
   c. blepharitis
   d. keratitis

6. The layer of the eye that contains the rods and cones is the:
   a. sclera
   b. choroid
   c. uvea
   d. retina

7. Hearing loss that is due to nerve damage is a:
   a. conductive loss
   b. sensorineural loss
   c. tympanitis
   d. tinnitus

8. The cornea is the transparent part of the eye and is an extension of the:
   a. choroid
   b. iris
   c. sclera
   d. both A and C

9. The ciliary body is:
   a. a group of muscles that suspends the lens
   b. the curved portion of the eye that refracts light
   c. the area between the lens and retina
   d. the protective layer of the eye

10. Farsightedness is called:
    a. myopia
    b. hyperopia
    c. presbyopia
    d. both B and C

Fill in the blank with the correct term.

11. The root word for *stapes* is _____.

12. _____ is an inflammation of the tympanic membrane.

13. _____ is a disease characterized by an increase in intraocular pressure.

14. The tube that goes from the middle ear to the nasopharynx is the _____.

15. The abbreviation for right eye is _____.

16. An inflammation of the mastoid process is _____.

17. A _____ hearing loss is one in which the outer or middle ear cannot conduct the sound vibrations to the inner ear.

18. A surgical incision into the labyrinth is called a _____.

19. The abbreviation for left ear is _____.

20. The _____ contains the sensory receptors for hearing.

APPENDIX A

Answers to Chapter Exercises and Quizzes

CHAPTER 1

EXERCISE 1-1   DEFINING TERMS

1. cardiology
2. gerontology
3. hematology
4. dermatology
5. neurology
6. psychology, psychiatry

EXERCISE 1-2   ANALYZING TERMS

TERM	ROOT	SUFFIX	WORD TYPE AND DEFINITION
1. neuropathy	neuro	-pathy	noun; disease of the nerves
2. psychology	psycho	-logy	noun; the study and science of mental processes and behavior
3. pathogenic	patho	-genic	adjective; causing disease
4. neuralgia	neur	-algia	noun; pain in one or more nerves
5. systemic	system	-ic	adjective: relating to a body system or systems
6. psychiatrist	psych iatr	-ist	noun; a medical doctor who specializes in the diagnosis and treatment of mental and emotional disorders
7. pediatrician	ped iatr	-ician	noun; a physician who deals with the care and treatment of babies and children
8. iatrogenic	iatro	-genic	adjective; refers to ailments caused by a doctor or other medical personnel
9. cardialgia	cardi	-algia	noun; pain in the heart (or stomach)
10. neuritis	neur	-itis	noun; inflammation of a nerve or nerves

CHAPTER 1 QUIZ

1. around
2. study of
3. skin
4. roots, suffix
5. logos, word
6. inflammation, tendon
7. before
8. pain, -dynia
9. -itis
10. psychology

CHAPTER 2

EXERCISE 2-1   COMBINING ROOTS AND SUFFIXES THAT SIGNIFY MEDICAL CONDITIONS

1. card/i/o
   a. cardiocele; herniation of the heart
   b. cardiodynia; heart pain
   c. cardiectasia; dilation of the heart
   d. carditis; inflammation of the heart
   e. cardiomalacia; softening of the heart
   f. cardiomegaly; enlargement of the heart
   g. cardioptosis; drooping of the heart
   h. cardioplegia; paralysis of the heart
   i. cardiorrhexis; rupture of the heart wall
   j. cardiospasm; spasm of the heart
2. dermat/o
   a. dermatitis; inflammation of the skin
   b. dermatoma; tumor of the skin
   c. dermatomegaly; enlargement of the skin
   d. dermatosis; abnormal condition of the skin
3. hem/o, hemat/o
   a. hemolysis; destruction of the blood cells
   b. hematogenesis; produced by the blood
   c. hematoma; localized mass of blood
   d. hematosis; abnormal condition of the blood

4. neur/o
   a. neuralgia; nerve pain
   b. neurectasis; dilation of a nerve
   c. neuritis; inflammation of a nerve
   d. neuroma; tumor of a nerve
5. oste/o
   a. osteodynia; bone pain
   b. osteoma; bone tumor
   c. osteomalacia; softening of the bone
   d. osteopenia; decreased bone density
   e. osteoporosis; decreased bone mass
   f. osteitis; inflammation of the bone
6. psych/o
   a. psychosis; severe mental and behavioral disorder

EXERCISE 2-2   COMBINING ROOTS AND SUFFIXES THAT SIGNIFY DIAGNOSTIC TERMS, TEST INFORMATION, OR SURGICAL PROCEDURES

1. card/i/o
   a. cardiogenic; originating in the heart
   b. cardiogram; graphic record of the heart
   c. cardiograph; machine that produces a cardiogram
   d. cardiography; process of electrically measuring heart function
   e. cardiopathy; heart disease
   f. cardiorrhaphy; suture of the wall of the heart
2. dermat/o
   a. dermatoplasty; surgical repair of the skin
3. hemat/o
   a. hematogenesis; originating with or in the blood
   b. hematometry; examination of blood
4. neur/o
   a. neurectomy; removal of a nerve or part of a nerve
   b. neurogenic; adjectival form of *neurogenesis*
   c. neurogenesis; originating in the nervous system

5. oste/o
   a. osteorrhaphy; suturing broken bone together
   b. osteoplasty; surgical repair of the bone
   c. osteogenesis; formation of bone
   d. ostectomy; excision of bone
   e. osteotomy; cutting of bone
6. path/o
   a. pathogen; a disease-causing agent
   b. pathogenic; adjectival form of *pathogen*
   c. pathogenesis; development of a disease
7. psych/o
   a. psychogenic; adjectival form of *psychogenesis*
   b. psychogenesis; mental development
   c. psychometry; mental testing
   d. psychopathy; mental illness or disorder

EXERCISE 2-3   COMBINING ROOTS AND SUFFIXES ASSOCIATED WITH A MEDICAL SPECIALIST OR SPECIALTY

1. card/i/o
   a. cardiology; medical specialty that diagnoses and treats heart diseases
   b. cardiologist; heart specialist
2. derm/o, dermat/o
   a. dermatology; medical specialty that diagnoses and treats skin disorders
   b. dermatologist; skin specialist
3. ger/o/nt/o
   a. geriatrics; medical specialty that diagnoses and treats the aged
   b. gerontology; the study of the process and results of aging
   c. gerontologist; specialist in gerontology
4. hem/o, hemat/o
   a. hematology; medical specialty that diagnoses and treats blood disorders
   b. hematologist; a specialist who treats blood disorders
5. neur/o
   a. neurology; medical specialty that diagnoses and treats the nervous system
   b. neurologist; specialist who treats the nervous system
6. oste/o
   a. osteology; medical specialty that diagnoses and treats disorders of the skeletal system; orthopedics
   b. osteologist; a bone specialist or orthopedic surgeon
7. path/o
   a. pathology; study of disease
   b. pathologist; a medical specialist who studies pathology
8. psych/o
   a. psychology; study of the mind
   b. psychiatry; the medical specialty that diagnoses and treats mind disorders
   c. psychiatrist; a medical specialist in psychiatry

EXERCISE 2-4   COMBINING ROOTS AND SUFFIXES THAT DENOTE ADJECTIVES

1. card/i/o
   a. cardiac; refers to the heart
2. hem/o, hemat/o
   a. hemotoxic; destructive of red blood cells
3. derm/o, dermat/o
   a. dermal; adjective denoting skin
   b. dermatic; adjective denoting skin
4. ger/o, geront/o
   a. geriatric; adjective form of *geriatrics*
   b. gerontal; adjective meaning "old-age related"
5. neur/o
   a. neural; adjective meaning "related to the nervous system"
   b. neurotic; adjective form of *neurosis*
6. spin/o
   a. spinal; adjective referring to spinal column
   b. spinous; adjective meaning "having spines"
7. oste/o
   a. osteal; adjective meaning "bone"
   b. osteoid; adjective meaning "resembling bone"

EXERCISE 2-5   MATCHING SUFFIXES WITH MEANINGS

1. G
2. I
3. B
4. M
5. J
6. D
7. C
8. H
9. F
10. E
11. A
12. O
13. N
14. K
15. L

EXERCISE 2-6 ADDING PREFIXES OF TIME OR SPEED

1. anteroom; outer room that leads into another room
2. neoclassic; new classic work
3. postglacial; following the glacial period
4. predominant; important
5. tachometer; instrument used to compute speed based on travel time or distance based on speed

EXERCISE 2-7 ADDING PREFIXES OF DIRECTION

1. abnormal; adjective meaning "away from normal"
2. adjoining; adjective meaning "next to"
3. concentric; having the same center
4. contralateral; the other side
5. diagram; illustration that gives an overall view
6. sympathetic; sharing emotions with another person
7. synthesis; assembling parts into a whole

EXERCISE 2-8 ADDING PREFIXES OF POSITION

1. eccentric; outside the center; unusual
2. ectomorph; slightly built person
3. enslave; to make a slave of
4. endocardial; adjective meaning "inside the heart"
5. epidemic; great number of occurrences of a particular disease
6. exchange; give something in return for another
7. exosphere; the far reaches of the atmosphere
8. extraterrestrial; beyond the earth
9. hypersensitive; highly sensitive
10. hypothesis; a possible explanation underlying the facts
11. infrastructure; the internal framework of a system or organization
12. intercollegiate; participation involving at least two colleges
13. intramural; inside the walls; often applied to sports teams within a school
14. mesosphere; the middle part of the earth's atmosphere
15. metaphysics; beyond physics
16. panorama; a wide expansive view of everything
17. paralegal; a trained assistant to a lawyer
18. retrorocket; a rocket that provides thrust in the direction of motion to slow a vehicle

EXERCISE 2-9 ADDING PREFIXES OF SIZE OR NUMBER

1. biannual; occurring twice a year
2. hemisphere; half of a sphere
3. macrocosm; the universe
4. microscope; a device for viewing objects invisible to the human eye
5. monorail; a railway system on which the vehicle travels on one rail
6. oligarchy; rule by a small group of people
7. quadrilateral; having four sides
8. semiannual; twice a year
9. triangle; three-sided geometric shape
10. unicycle; a vehicle having one wheel

EXERCISE 2-10 CROSSWORD PUZZLE: COMMON SUFFIXES AND PREFIXES

1. across: macro; down: mono
2. hyper
3. logy
4. across: ab; down: anti
5. pan
6. across: inter; down: itis
7. graph
8. pre
9. stenosis
10. tachy
11. scopy
12. meter
13. across: cyte; down: cele
14. dynia
15. ectomy
16. quadri

CHAPTER 2 QUIZ

SUFFIXES

1. -algia, -dynia
2. angiectasis
3. adjective
4. suture of a blood vessel
5. -graphy
6. tumor of the blood vessel
7. surgical repair
8. dermatologist
9. old
10. gerontology is a noun; geriatrics is an adjective

PREFIXES

1. ad-
2. ante-
3. abnormally slow heartbeat
4. beyond
5. hyper-
6. radar used to prevent a collision
7. three
8. the instrument will make visible the objects that are too small to see
9. endocarditis; inflammation of the inside of the heart
10. tachypnea is rapid breathing; dyspnea is difficulty or painful breathing

CHAPTER 3

EXERCISE 3-1   MATCHING

A. PLANES OF THE BODY

1. C   2. B   3. A

B. DIRECTIONAL TERMS

1. F   3. H   5. I   7. A   9. C
2. G   4. J   6. E   8. D   10. B

EXERCISE 3-2   FILL IN THE BLANK

1. distal
2. distal
3. anterior, ventral
4. ventral, anterior
5. superior
6. lateral
7. posterior, dorsal
8. inferior

EXERCISE 3-3   WORD BUILDING

1. hypo-, -ic; hypogastric
2. -al; dorsal
3. -itis; chondritis
4. trans-, -ic; transthoracic
5. -itis; neuritis
6. epi-, -al; epicardial

EXERCISE 3-4   CROSSWORD PUZZLE: THE BODY'S ORGANIZATION

1. umbilicus
2. chromosome
3. organ
4. anterior
5. transverse
6. hypogastric
7. respiratory
8. five
9. epithelial
10. connective
11. digestive
12. posterior
13. cytoplasm

CHAPTER 3 QUIZ

1. lateral
2. toward the back
3. proximal
4. anterior or forward
5. muscle pain
6. False
7. True
8. False
9. True
10. True
11. False
12. True
13. False
14. False
15. True

CHAPTER 4

WORD ELEMENTS EXERCISE: FILL IN THE BLANKS

1. skin
2. fungus
3. cell
4. sweat
5. red
6. dry
7. Latin word meaning "to carry"
8. below
9. sebum (oil; fat)
10. upon
11. white
12. blue
13. dry, scaly (fishlike)
14. skin
15. hornlike
16. skin
17. nail
18. black
19. hair
20. hardening
21. yellow

QUICK CHECK: STRUCTURE OF THE SKIN, HAIR, AND NAILS

SUFFIX	TERM
-ous	subcutaneous
-cytes	melanocytes
-aceous	sebaceous

EXERCISE 4-1   CASE STUDY

1. antibiotic; medication used to kill bacteria or treat an infection
2. impetigo; contagious superficial skin infection that presents with vesicles
3. dermatologist; medical specialist who diagnoses and treats disorders of the skin
4. dermatitis; inflammation of the skin
5. erythematous; redness of the skin
6. pustules; small elevated area of skin that contains pus
7. edema; swelling in the tissues
8. antipruritic medication; medication used to reduce or stop itching
9. pruritus; itching

10. Rewritten version for comparison:

REPORT BY R.A. SMITH, MD (DERMATOLOGIST)

A.J. Farley, MD, who is a family physician with offices at 1008 Harvard Road, Pellston, Michigan, consulted me about his patient, Annabelle Jones, a 29-year-old married woman with two children. Dr. Farley examined her briefly on April 29, 2013, when she visited his office and reported an itching on her forehead. Dr. Farley asked Mrs. Jones whether she had recently acquired a pet to which she might be having an allergic reaction. Mrs. Jones answered no. Dr. Farley prescribed erythromycin, an antibiotic. When she returned to Dr. Farley's office 2 days later, the rash covered her entire face and was erythematous with pustules and marked edema. In addition, pruritus had developed on her feet. Dr. Farley had her admitted to Burnside Hospital for treatment and asked me to consult.

My diagnosis was impetigo, along with an allergic reaction to erythromycin, which I replaced with Cleocin. The patient responded well to the change in antibiotic, and all her symptoms have now disappeared. Dr. Farley and I agreed that Mrs. Jones should be discharged and continue the full course of Cleocin at home. We also agreed that Mrs. Jones be advised about specific side effects and to report any occurrence immediately. I also recommended to Dr. Farley that a follow-up visit by Mrs. Jones to his office in 7 days would be prudent.

R.A. Smith, MD

EXERCISE 4-2   LABELING THE SKIN

1. epidermis
2. dermis
3. subcutaneous layer
4. adipose tissue
5. hair follicle
6. vein
7. nerve
8. artery
9. sudoriferous gland
10. sebaceous gland
11. nerve endings
12. hair

EXERCISE 4-3   WORD BUILDING

1. -itis; dermatitis
2. -oma; melanoma
3. epi-; epidermis
4. -pathy, -osis; onychopathy or onychosis
5. -logy; dermatology
6. -osis; ichthyosis
7. subcutaneous
8. percutaneous
9. intradermal
10. epidermis

EXERCISE 4-4   MATCHING

1. D
2. E
3. I
4. F
5. B
6. C
7. G
8. J
9. H
10. A

EXERCISE 4-5   WORD ANALYSIS

TERM	PREFIX	ROOT(S)	SUFFIX	DEFINITION
1. dermatitis		derma	-itis	inflammation of the skin
2. hematoma	hemat-		-oma	a collection of blood trapped in the tissues
3. dermatomycosis		dermato; myc	-osis	fungus infection of the skin
4. onychia		onych	-ia	inflammation of the fingernail or toenail
5. pachyderma	pachy-	derma		abnormal thickening of the skin
6. onychomalacia		onycho	-malacia	softening of the nails
7. paronychia	par-	onych	-ia	infection around a nail
8. piloid		pil	-oid	hairlike, resembling hair
9. pyoderma	pyo-	derma		a pus-containing skin infection
10. seborrhea		sebo	-rrhea	excessive secretion of sebum

EXERCISE 4-6   WORD BUILDING

1. onycho   myc   osis   onychomycosis
2. dermato   logy   dermatology
3. epi   dermat   itis   epidermatitis
4. sclero   derma   scleroderma
5. onych   ectomy   onychectomy
6. dermato   plasty   dermatoplasty
7. onycho   phagia   onychophagia
8. epi   derm   al   epidermal
9. dermat   osis   dermatosis
10. ep   onych   ium   eponychium

EXERCISE 4-7 SENTENCE COMPLETION

1. hair loss
2. alopecia capitis totalis
3. ecchymosis
4. pityriasis
5. light amplification by stimulated emission of radiation
6. fatty; adipose
7. sudoriferous
8. avascular
9. the skin
10. stratum corneum

EXERCISE 4-8 PRONUNCIATION

There are no right/wrong answers. The student may select any terms from the CD and pronounce them.

EXERCISE 4-9 CROSSWORD PUZZLE: THE INTEGUMENTARY SYSTEM

1. cuticle
2. pustule
3. dermis
4. shingles
5. melanoma
6. adipose
7. scabies
8. necr
9. tinea
10. lesion
11. paronychia
12. melanin
13. alopecia
14. erythematous
15. cry
16. onych
17. vitiligo

CHAPTER 4 QUIZ

1. B
2. B
3. B
4. D
5. D
6. B
7. A
8. C
9. B
10. B
11. keloid
12. fissure
13. cyanosis
14. scleroderma
15. alopecia
16. albinism
17. vitiligo
18. urticaria
19. biopsy
20. polyp

CHAPTER 5

WORD ELEMENTS EXERCISE: FILL IN THE BLANKS

1. swayback, curve
2. joined (yoked) together
3. wrist
4. foot, child
5. bone
6. bones of fingers and toes
7. pain
8. cranium
9. joined together
10. inflammation
11. muscle
12. to visually examine
13. movement
14. correct, straight
15. femur, thighbone
16. softening
17. surgical repair
18. joint
19. pelvis
20. to grow
21. arm
22. finger, toe
23. rib
24. bone marrow
25. electricity
26. thorax, chest
27. humerus, upper arm bone
28. stabilize or fuse
29. porous
30. stiff, fused, closed
31. vertebrae
32. written record of
33. movement
34. both sides
35. calcaneus, heel bone
36. hump
37. neck
38. hand
39. study of
40. cartilage
41. lower back
42. removal of, excision of
43. tumor

QUICK CHECK: STRUCTURE OF THE SKELETAL SYSTEM

1. osteocytes
2. synovial
3. mandible

EXERCISE 5-1   FIGURE LABELING: SKELETON

1. cranium
2. facial bones
3. mandible
4. sternum
5. costal cartilage
6. vertebral column
7. ilium or pelvis
8. pelvis or ilium
9. sacrum
10. calcaneus
11. metatarsals
12. phalanges
13. tarsals
14. tibia
15. fibula
16. patella
17. femur
18. clavicle
19. scapula
20. humerus
21. ribs
22. radius
23. ulna
24. carpals
25. metacarpals
26. phalanges

EXERCISE 5-2   FIGURE LABELING: LONG BONE

1. proximal epiphysis
2. diaphysis
3. distal epiphysis
4. cartilage
5. epiphyseal line
6. spongy bone
7. compact bone
8. medullary cavity
9. yellow marrow
10. periosteum

EXERCISE 5-3   WORD BUILDING

1. osteomyelitis
2. arthroscopy
3. chondromalacia
4. arthrogram
5. arthrodesis
6. kinesiology
7. chondroplasty
8. intercostal
9. osteitis
10. osteosarcoma
11. arthroplasty
12. myelogram
13. chondritis
14. osteoporosis
15. costalgia

EXERCISE 5-4   MATCHING: TERMS OF JOINT MOVEMENT

1. E
2. D
3. B
4. C
5. A
6. F
7. G

EXERCISE 5-5   MATCHING: TYPES OF FRACTURES

1. C
2. H
3. F
4. G
5. D
6. E
7. A
8. B

EXERCISE 5-6   CHOOSING THE RIGHT TERM

1. b. chondroma
2. c. osteomyelitis
3. a. arthrolysis
4. d. osteogenesis
5. a. manubrium
6. d. kyphosis
7. c. closed reduction
8. d. comminuted fracture
9. a. xiphoid process

EXERCISE 5-7   WRITING DESCRIPTIONS TO FIT MEDICAL TERMS

1. a physician who treats and diagnoses skeletal disorders
2. unable to flex or move her wrist much
3. a wrist bone was broken in several places
4. hip bone was broken and pressed into another part of the bone
5. realignment
6. a treatment using elastics or pulley and weights

EXERCISE 5-8   CROSSWORD PUZZLE: THE SKELETAL SYSTEM

1. osteoplasty
2. maxilla
3. arthroscope
4. ROM
5. mandible
6. arthrodynia
7. CT
8. arthritis
9. carpals
10. phalanges
11. chondr
12. crani
13. across: calcaneus; down: coccyx
14. costalgia

CHAPTER 5 QUIZ

1. C
2. B
3. C
4. D
5. A
6. A
7. D (all the terms are conditions except for diaphysis)
8. B (all are bones in the upper extremity except for the fibula)
9. D (all are bones in the lower extremity except for the ulna)
10. A (all are bones except for deltoid)
11. A (all are abnormal curvatures of the spine except for sclerosis)
12. B (all are parts of the spine except for parietal)
13. D (all are bones except for diaphragm)
14. B (all are fractures except for insertion)
15. thoracotomy
16. arthritis
17. arthrocentesis
18. orthopedics
19. set, repair, or realign broken bones
20. orthopedic surgeon

CHAPTER 6

WORD ELEMENTS EXERCISE: IDENTIFYING WORD ELEMENTS AND THEIR MEANINGS

1. root — ligament
2. root — tendon
3. root — tone
4. suffix — paralysis
5. root — muscle
6. root — movement
7. suffix — partial or incomplete paralysis
8. root — strength
9. root — muscle
10. prefix — four
11. root — fibrous membrane
12. root — fiber
13. prefix — half
14. prefix — beside, beyond, near

QUICK CHECK: THE THREE TYPES OF MUSCLES

TYPE	WHERE LOCATED
1. skeletal or striated	found throughout the skeletal system (voluntary)
2. smooth	attached to organs throughout the body (involuntary)
3. cardiac	the heart

EXERCISE 6-1   DEFINING TERMS THAT NAME MUSCLE MOVEMENTS

1. turning inward
2. bending backward
3. movement away from midline
4. movement toward midline
5. bending the sole of the foot
6. turning upward
7. turning a body part on its own axis
8. turning outward
9. opening the angle of a joint
10. closing the angle of a joint
11. turning downward

EXERCISE 6-2   CASE STUDY

1. flexion (closing the angle of a joint); extension (opening the angle of a joint); rotation (turning a body part on its own axis); abduction (movement away from midline)
2. inflammation of a tendon
3. range of motion
4. nonsteroidal anti-inflammatory drug

EXERCISE 6-3   WRITE THE ABBREVIATION

1. EMG
2. CTD
3. DMD
4. ROM
5. DTR
6. IM
7. MG
8. RICE

EXERCISE 6-4   WORD BUILDING

1. tenotomy
2. neurologist
3. paraplegia
4. myocele
5. hemiparesis
6. fasciitis
7. kinesialgia
8. fibromyalgia
9. myopathy; musculopathy
10. myositis

EXERCISE 6-5   FILL IN THE BLANK

1. skeletal, smooth, cardiac
2. orthopedic surgeons, neurologist
3. paraplegic is a person who has paralysis of both legs and the lower part of the body (para- is a prefix meaning "alongside" and -plegia means "paralysis"); a hemiplegic has total paralysis of one side of the body (hemi- means "half")
4. a- is a prefix meaning "without"; my/o is the combining form meaning "muscle"; troph is a root meaning "nutrition or growth"; -ic is an adjective suffix
5. muscles that contract and produce movement
6. epicondylitis
7. electromyography
8. a group of inherited muscle disorders that cause muscle weakness
9. RICE: rest, ice, compression, elevation
10. ligament

EXERCISE 6-6   TRUE OR FALSE

1. True
2. False; it is a type of muscular dystrophy
3. True
4. False; it is epicondylitis
5. True
6. False; weakness or partial paralysis
7. True
8. False; attach muscles to bones
9. True

EXERCISE 6-7   CROSSWORD PUZZLE: THE MUSCULAR SYSTEM

1. deltoid
2. paresis
3. atrophy
4. quadri
5. fibromyalgia
6. DMD
7. antagonist
8. hemi
9. tendon
10. plegia
11. fascia
12. atony
13. epicondylitis
14. IM
15. hamstring
16. my
17. ROM
18. across: SLR; down: smooth
19. myocardium

CHAPTER 6 QUIZ

1. C
2. C
3. B
4. D
5. A
6. A
7. C
8. plantar flexion
9. asthenia
10. myocele
11. plantar fasciitis
12. EMG
13. tenoplasty, tenontoplasty, tendinoplasty, tendoplasty
14. myology
15. myodynia, myalgia
16. a muscle that counteracts the action of another muscle
17. weakness or slight paralysis of a muscle
18. deep tendon reflex
19. rest, ice, compression, elevation
20. moving away from a central point

CHAPTER 7

WORD ELEMENTS EXERCISE: FILL IN THE BLANKS

1. weakness, loss of movement
2. outer layer or covering
3. referring to the mind
4. paralyzed
5. memory
6. physician; to treat
7. suffix meaning "morbid or unreasonable fear"
8. brain
9. the cerebrum; also, the brain in general
10. water
11. a membrane
12. ganglia (singular: ganglion)
13. suffix meaning "morbid attraction to" or "impulse toward"
14. in connection with the nervous system, refers to the spinal cord and medulla oblongata
15. a nerve cell; nervous system
16. spider
17. to split
18. head
19. referring to the mind
20. like
21. the cerebellum
22. referring to the spinal cord
23. speech
24. glue

QUICK CHECK: MAIN PARTS OF THE NERVOUS SYSTEM

1. brain and spinal cord
2. homeostasis
3. brain stem

EXERCISE 7-1   FIGURE LABELING: NEURON

1. dendrites
2. cell body
3. nucleus
4. axon covered with myelin sheath
5. axon branch
6. myelin sheath
7. muscle

EXERCISE 7-2   CASE STUDY

1. transient ischemic attack; sometimes called a ministroke
2. cerebrovascular accident
3. dys- means "difficult"; -phasia means "speak"
4. partial or incomplete paralysis
5. hemiparesis means "partially paralyzed on half the body"; hemiplegia means "complete paralysis on half the body"
6. hemi- means "half"; -plegia means "paralysis"

EXERCISE 7-3   WORD PARTS

1. neur/o
2. myel/o
3. -tomy
4. cephal/o
5. -phasia
6. schiz/o
7. psych/o, -phrenia, ment/o

EXERCISE 7-4   WORD ELEMENTS

1. psych–root
   -osis–suffix
   a condition of the mind
2. electro–root
   encephalo–root
   -graphy–suffix
   the process of recording an electrical record of the brain
3. astro–root
   cyt–root
   -oma–suffix
   a tumor of brain cells
4. cerebro–root
   vascul–root
   -ar–suffix
   adjective referring to blood vessels in the brain
5. hemi–root
   -plegia–suffix
   paralysis on one side of the body
6. hydro-root
   cephal–root
   -us–suffix
   fluid on the brain
7. encephal–root
   -itis–suffix
   inflammation of the brain
8. epi–prefix
   dur–root
   -al–suffix
   adjective referring to the outer surface of the brain
9. psych–root
   iatr–root
   -ist–suffix
   a specialist who treats disorders of the mind
10. meningi–root
    -oma–suffix
    tumor of the meninges

EXERCISE 7-5   MATCHING

1. K
2. F
3. C
4. N
5. H
6. J
7. E
8. B
9. M
10. G
11. D
12. A
13. L
14. I

EXERCISE 7-6   SPELL CHECK

1. aphasia
2. schizophrenia
3. neurotransmitters
4. subdural hematoma

EXERCISE 7-7 WRITE THE ABBREVIATION

1. IQ	7. CVA	13. ADHD
2. PTSD	8. PERRLA	14. ECT
3. PNS	9. LP	15. EEG
4. TENS	10. SAD	16. ICP
5. CNS	11. TIA	17. LOC
6. MS	12. OBS	18. OCD

EXERCISE 7-8 CROSSWORD PUZZLE: THE NERVOUS SYSTEM

1. phobia	7. OCD	13. schizophrenia
2. cerebrum	8. depression	14. subarachnoid
3. delusions	9. bipolar	15. sedative
4. psychologist	10. LOC	16. across: midbrain; down: myelin
5. brain stem	11. pons	17. neuroglia
6. hallucination	12. MRI	

CHAPTER 7 QUIZ

1. transient ischemic attack	8. C	17. poliomyelitis
2. pupils equal, round, and reactive to light and accommodation	9. A	18. dementia
	10. B	19. multiple sclerosis
	11. A	20. myelomeningocele
3. lumbar puncture	12. B	21. cerebral thrombosis
4. electroencephalography	13. C	22. ataxia
5. multiple sclerosis	14. C	23. epilepsy
6. organic brain syndrome	15. C	24. syncope
7. D	16. hyperesthesia	25. neuralgia

CHAPTER 8

WORD ELEMENTS EXERCISE: FILL IN THE BLANKS

1. endocrine system or glands	8. extremities
2. pituitary gland	9. gland
3. adrenal glands	10. thyroid gland
4. suffix used in the formation of names of chemical substances	11. enlargement
5. suffix meaning "nourishment" or "stimulation"	12. sugar, glucose, glycogen
	13. to separate or secrete
6. tumor	14. parathyroid gland
7. pancreas	15. calcium

QUICK CHECK: A FEW FACTS ABOUT GLANDS

1. hypophysis
2. on top of the kidneys
3. the fluids surrounding tissues

EXERCISE 8-1   DEFINING ABBREVIATIONS

1. follicle-stimulating hormone
2. fasting blood sugar
3. prolactin
4. antidiuretic hormone
5. thyroid-stimulating hormone
6. diabetes mellitus
7. melanocyte-stimulating hormone
8. hemoglobin A1c (reflects average long-term glucose levels for 2 to 3 months before glucose blood level is drawn)
9. luteinizing hormone
10. non–insulin-dependent diabetes mellitus
11. insulin-dependent diabetes mellitus
12. growth hormone
13. adrenocorticotrophic hormone
14. blood sugar

EXERCISE 8-2   FIGURE LABELING: THE ENDOCRINE SYSTEM

1. pineal
2. pituitary (hypophysis)
3. thyroid
4. parathyroids
5. thymus
6. adrenals
7. pancreatic islets
8. ovaries
9. testes

EXERCISE 8-3   CASE STUDY

1. If your answer is "I have no idea," there are at least two people with the same answer: you and the author of this textbook.
2. difficulty speaking
3. goiter, thyromegaly
4. thyroid-stimulating hormone
5. The examining physician discovered a nodule on the right side of the patient's neck and noted that her eyes were bulging.

EXERCISE 8-4   SPELL CHECK

1. endocrinologist
2. hypoglycemic
3. insulin
4. diabetes mellitus

EXERCISE 8-5   DISORDERS AND SYMPTOMS OF THE ENDOCRINE SYSTEM

1. endogenous
2. acromegaly
3. diabetes mellitus (DM)
4. thyromegaly
5. hyperglycemia
6. polyuria
7. glycosuria
8. Cushing's syndrome

EXERCISE 8-6   WORD BUILDING: THE ENDOCRINE SYSTEM

1. adrenomegaly
2. adrenalectomy
3. adrenopathy
4. hypothyroidism
5. thyroiditis
6. thyroidotomy
7. thyromegaly
8. pancreatoma
9. pancreatitis
10. pancreatogenic

EXERCISE 8-7   CROSSWORD PUZZLE: THE ENDOCRINE SYSTEM

1. thyroid
2. testosterone
3. ovary
4. across: GH; down: glycosuria
5. across: hypoglycemic; down: hypoglycemia
6. FBS
7. pituitary
8. insulin
9. Graves
10. Cushing
11. hormone
12. goiter
13. gigantism
14. adenoma
15. testes
16. parathyroids
17. adrenal
18. LH

CHAPTER 8 QUIZ

1. A	9. D	17. M
2. B	10. D	18. J
3. B	11. K	19. B
4. C	12. G	20. C
5. B	13. I	21. L
6. A	14. A	22. H
7. D	15. E	
8. A	16. F	

CHAPTER 9

WORD ELEMENTS EXERCISE: FILL IN THE BLANKS

1. ven/o	10. -gram	19. brady-
2. cardi/o	11. -emia	20. varic/o
3. angi/o or vas/o	12. my/o	21. coron/o
4. endo-	13. -stenosis	22. -ectasis
5. tachy-	14. hem/o, hemat/o	23. vas/o or angi/o
6. thromb/o	15. arteri/o	24. electr/o
7. peri-	16. phleb/o	25. ventricul/o
8. ather/o	17. valv/o, valvul/o	26. isch
9. atri/o	18. aort/o	

QUICK CHECK: BLOOD VESSELS

1. veins
2. heart
3. red blood cells

EXERCISE 9-1   FIGURE LABELING: THE BLOOD FLOW THROUGH THE HEART

1. superior and inferior venae cavae	5. pulmonary valve	10. left ventricle
2. right atrium	6. pulmonary arteries	11. aortic valve
3. tricuspid valve	7. pulmonary veins	12. aorta
4. right ventricle	8. left atrium	
	9. mitral or bicuspid valve	

EXERCISE 9-2   CASE STUDY

1. pain in the chest due to ischemia
2. shortness of breath
3. high blood pressure
4. electrocardiogram; record of the heart's electrical activity
5. aspirin—anticoagulant affect; antiarrhythmics—decrease abnormal atrial heart beats; diuretics—decrease fluid volume by increasing urine volume output; vasodilators—increase diameter of blood vessels to help decrease blood pressure and increase blood flow
6. heart attack, lack of blood supply (infarction) to the heart muscle (my/o means "muscle"; cardi/o means "heart")
7. irregular atrial contractions; frequently a rapid irregular rhythm

EXERCISE 9-3   WORD BUILDING: THE CARDIOVASCULAR SYSTEM

1. cardiogenic
2. atriotomy
3. erythrocyte
4. hemophilia
5. vasospasm
6. thrombectomy
7. vasodilation
8. cardiomegaly
9. arteriostenosis
10. atheroma
11. leukocyte
12. valvectomy
13. cardiac
14. hemolysis, erythrolysis
15. interventricular
16. anemia
17. myocardium
18. atherectomy
19. arrhythmia

EXERCISE 9-4   SPELLING

1. thrombocytopenia
2. oxygen
3. myocardial
4. ischemia
5. arterectomy
6. atrioventricular
7. leukemia
8. atherosclerosis
9. semilunar
10. diastolic

EXERCISE 9-5   MATCHING

1. D
2. C
3. H
4. J
5. I
6. E
7. A
8. F
9. B
10. G

EXERCISE 9-6   WRITE THE ABBREVIATION

1. CAD
2. HDL
3. ICU
4. CHF
5. MI
6. EKG or ECG
7. PTCA
8. RBC
9. AV
10. SOB
11. P
12. CCU
13. HTN
14. A-fib
15. CABG
16. SA
17. TIA
18. DIC
19. CP
20. LDL
21. Hb
22. HR
23. BP
24. WBC

EXERCISE 9-7   CROSSWORD PUZZLE: THE CARDIOVASCULAR SYSTEM

1. coagulation
2. thrombocyte
3. venules
4. arterioles
5. vasoconstriction
6. thrombus
7. edema
8. plasma
9. CHF
10. aortic
11. ischemia
12. capillaries
13. ather
14. erythrocyte
15. hematology
16. leukemia
17. dyscrasia
18. Hb
19. phagocytosis
20. emia

CHAPTER 9 QUIZ

1. C
2. C
3. B
4. A
5. B
6. B
7. D
8. A
9. A
10. C
11. A
12. B
13. B
14. D
15. B
16. D
17. D
18. D
19. D
20. D

CHAPTER 10

WORD ELEMENTS EXERCISE: FILL IN THE BLANKS

1. immune system
2. ingest or engulf
3. protection
4. enlargement
5. lymph node, usually palatine tonsil
6. spleen
7. without
8. lymph nodes
9. lymph vessels
10. lymph or lymphatic system
11. thymus
12. resembling

QUICK CHECK: A FEW KEY TERMS

1. fluid balance
2. tonsils, spleen, thymus gland, and appendix
3. immunization (or vaccination)

EXERCISE 10-1   CASE STUDY

1. disease of the lymph nodes
2. splenomegaly
3. an infectious disease caused by a virus
4. example of a rewritten report (see the following)

BRIEF HISTORY: Fatigue was preventing a 16-year-old boy from keeping up with schoolwork and after-school sports activities. His throat was sore, and he noticed "lumps" in his neck and groin. He also suffered from a fever, loss of appetite, and stomach pain.

OFFICE VISIT: A physician's examination and blood tests revealed lymphadenopathy in the cervical, axillary, and inguinal areas; an erythematous throat; and an enlarged spleen.

DIAGNOSIS AND TREATMENT PLAN: The diagnosis was mononucleosis. The prescribed treatment consisted of analgesics, an increase in fluid intake, and rest.

EXERCISE 10-2   MATCHING

1. E
2. G
3. J
4. H
5. A
6. B
7. C
8. I
9. D
10. F

EXERCISE 10-3   WORD BUILDING: THE LYMPHATIC SYSTEM AND IMMUNITY

1. adenitis
2. lymphoma
3. thymomegaly
4. lymphangiitis or lymphangitis
5. lymphadenopathy
6. immunologist
7. lymphography
8. phagocytosis

EXERCISE 10-4   WRITING THE ABBREVIATION

1. RA
2. RIA
3. HLA
4. SLE
5. AIDS
6. CBC
7. HIV

EXERCISE 10-5   CROSSWORD PUZZLE: THE LYMPHATIC SYSTEM AND IMMUNITY

1. phag
2. leuk
3. hemolysis
4. chemotherapy
5. splen

6. erythema
7. autoimmune
8. thymus
9. immunity
10. Hodgkin

11. AIDS
12. emia
13. aden

CHAPTER 10 QUIZ

1. True
2. False; the tonsils are one of four protective organs in the immune system.
3. False; a reaction to poison ivy is an example of dermatitis.

4. True
5. False; hemolysis is the destruction of red blood cells.
6. True
7. True
8. True

9. False; Peyer's patches are located on the walls of the small intestine.
10. True

CHAPTER 11

WORD ELEMENTS EXERCISE: CHOOSING AN ELEMENT

1. -phonia
2. trache/o
3. thorac/o, thorac/i, thoracic/o
4. bronch/o, bronchi/o
5. -pnea

6. laryng/o
7. sinus/o
8. pleur/o
9. pneum/o, pneumon/o
10. nas/o, rhin/o
11. -oxia

12. pharyng/o
13. phren/o
14. pulmon/o
15. or/o

QUICK CHECK: DEFINING COMPLEX TERMS BY DECIPHERING WORD ELEMENTS

nas/o, nose; pharyng/o, pharynx; -al, adjective suffix

EXERCISE 11-1   FIGURE LABELING: THE RESPIRATORY SYSTEM

1. nares
2. nasal cavity
3. pharynx
4. nasopharynx
5. oropharynx
6. laryngopharynx
7. epiglottis

8. larynx (vocal cords)
9. esophagus
10. trachea
11. left lung
12. right lung
13. right bronchus
14. mediastinum

15. terminal bronchiole
16. alveolar duct
17. alveoli
18. capillaries
19. diaphragm

EXERCISE 11-2   CASE STUDY

1. A
2. E
3. If you did understand, you have probably been exposed to a localized version of "clinical" culture, which you might be wise to question rather than rely on.
4. In your rewritten version, include answers to questions you might want to ask the writer. If possible, discuss and compare your version with classmates to discover similarities and differences with their versions.

EXERCISE 11-3 MATCHING

1. E	7. B	13. O
2. D	8. J	14. H
3. C	9. K	15. M
4. F	10. L	16. Q
5. A	11. R	17. I
6. G	12. N	18. P

EXERCISE 11-4 DEFINITIONS

1. inspiration	4. sinusitis	7. pleurotomy
2. hemoptysis	5. dysphonia	8. pleuralgia
3. thoracopathy	6. pneumothorax	9. pleurocele

EXERCISE 11-5 WORD BUILDING

1. bronchitis	4. sinusitis	7. bradypnea
2. bronchiectasis	5. epiglottitis	8. dyspnea
3. laryngitis	6. tachypnea	9. orthopnea

EXERCISE 11-6 CASE STUDY

1. A. crackling sounds caused by mucus in airways; abnormal breath sounds heard with a stethoscope
   B. discomfort in breathing that is brought on or aggravated by lying flat

EXERCISE 11-7 FILL IN THE BLANKS WITH MEANINGS OF ABBREVIATIONS

1. respiratory rate
2. chest X-ray
3. tonsils and adenoids (also tonsillectomy and adenoidectomy)
4. expiratory reserve volume (as measured with test equipment)
5. tidal volume (as measured with test equipment)
6. cystic fibrosis
7. shortness of breath
8. tuberculosis
9. arterial blood gas
10. chronic obstructive pulmonary disease
11. carbon dioxide
12. inspiratory reserve volume (as measured with test equipment)
13. oxygen
14. pulmonary function test
15. residual volume (as measured with test equipment)
16 total lung capacity (as measured with test equipment)

EXERCISE 11-8 CROSSWORD PUZZLE: THE RESPIRATORY SYSTEM

1. bronchiole	8. sputum	15. pharynx
2. emphysema	9. pulmonology	16. bronchitis
3. pnea	10. trachea	17. rhinitis
4. laryngitis	11. mediastinum	18. alveolus
5. ABG	12. atelectasis	19. bronchoscope
6. asthma	13. bronchus	20. thoracentesis
7. pneumonia	14. larynx	

CHAPTER 11 QUIZ

1. C	8. B	15. A
2. B	9. D	16. B
3. C	10. B	17. C
4. B	11. C	18. C
5. C	12. D	19. B
6. D	13. C	
7. B	14. B	

CHAPTER 12

WORD ELEMENTS EXERCISE: DEFINING WORD ELEMENTS

1. eat or swallow
2. common bile duct
3. mouth
4. sigmoid colon
5. abdomen
6. intestine
7. abdomen
8. rectum
9. stone
10. salivary glands
11. liver
12. pylorus
13. bile, gall
14. bile duct
15. esophagus
16. vomit
17. device for visual examination
18. tongue
19. jejunum
20. stomach
21. lip
22. ileum
23. pancreas
24. cheek
25. gallbladder
26. digestion
27. colon
28. teeth
29. eating, swallowing
30. duodenum
31. anus and rectum
32. gums
33. visual examination

QUICK CHECK: KEY TERMS

1. gallbladder
2. secretion of enzymes and acids to aid the digestion process
3. duodenum, jejunum, and ileum

EXERCISE 12-1   FIGURE LABELING: THE DIGESTIVE SYSTEM

1. mouth
2. pharynx
3. esophagus
4. stomach
5. duodenum
6. small intestine
7. cecum
8. ascending colon
9. transverse colon
10. descending colon
11. sigmoid colon
12. rectum
13. anus
14. parotid gland
15. sublingual gland
16. submandibular glands
17. liver
18. gallbladder
19. pancreas

EXERCISE 12-2   CASE STUDY

1. shortness of breath
2. blood pressure
3. HTN stands for hypertension, which is signaled by high blood pressure. Hypertension and shortness of breath may accompany each other; smoking and excessive caffeine intake may be related to both conditions.
4. white blood cell
5. Endo- means "within" or "inside"; -scopy means "look" or "see." Thus, endoscopy may be defined as looking inside by means of an instrument called an endoscope.

EXERCISE 12-3   WORD BUILDING

1. oral
2. stomatitis
3. buccal
4. cheilosis
5. gingivectomy
6. glossotomy
7. lingual
8. gastrodynia, gastralgia
9. pharyngeal
10. enteritis
11. duodenal
12. jejunal
13. ileitis
14. colectomy
15. rectocele
16. anal
17. proctologist
18. hepatomegaly
19. bilirubin
20. cholecystectomy

EXERCISE 12-4   ABBREVIATIONS AND ACRONYMS

1. barium enema
2. bowel movement
3. gastrointestinal
4. irritable bowel syndrome
5. gastroesophageal reflux disease

EXERCISE 12-5   CROSSWORD PUZZLE: THE DIGESTIVE SYSTEM

1. dysphagia
2. peritonitis
3. saliva
4. stomatitis
5. polyp
6. alimentary
7. bulimia
8. cirrhosis
9. flatus
10. ulcer
11. melena
12. across: gastr; down: gloss
13. sial
14. eructation
15. anorexia
16. hyperemesis
17. buccal
18. cecum
19. jejunum
20. anus

CHAPTER 12 QUIZ

MATCHING

1. B
2. F
3. I
4. G
5. H
6. D
7. E
8. A
9. C
10. J

MULTIPLE CHOICE

11. B
12. C
13. C
14. A
15. C
16. C
17. B
18. D
19. B
20. A

CHAPTER 13

WORD ELEMENTS EXERCISE: FILL IN THE BLANKS

1. urine
2. night
3. little, few
4. suffix meaning "condition" or "state"
5. glomerulus
6. kidney
7. urethra
8. stone
9. prefix meaning "much" or "many"
10. pus
11. pelvis
12. ureter
13. bladder

QUICK CHECK: A FEW KEY POINTS

1. kidneys, ureters, urinary bladder, and urethra
2. cholecyst/o
3. hilum

EXERCISE 13-1   FIGURE LABELING: THE URINARY SYSTEM

1. right kidney
2. right ureter
3. urethra
4. left kidney
5. left ureter
6. urinary bladder

EXERCISE 13-2   CASE STUDY

1. urologist
2. dysuria
3. hematuria
4. urinalysis
5. KUB
6. calculi
7. urinary bladder
8. UTI
9. calculi
10. antibiotic
11. cystoscopy

EXERCISE 13-3   DEFINITIONS

1. incision into the kidney
2. condition of stones in the kidney
3. filtration to remove wastes from the kidney
4. continuous ambulatory peritoneal dialysis
5. pus in the urine
6. plastic repair of the ureter
7. urinary tract infection
8. suture repair of the ureter
9. around the urethra
10. enlarged kidney

EXERCISE 13-4   MATCHING TERMS WITH DEFINITIONS

1. G
2. D
3. K
4. A
5. B
6. J
7. H
8. F
9. E
10. R
11. P
12. M
13. N
14. Q
15. L
16. I
17. C
18. O

EXERCISE 13-5   WORD BUILDING

1. nephritis
2. pyelonephritis
3. nephrolithiasis
4. nephrotomy
5. urolith
6. uremia
7. urinalysis
8. polyuria
9. hematuria
10. anuria

EXERCISE 13-6   TRUE OR FALSE

1. True
2. False; the renal fascia is a thin layer of connective tissue that forms each kidney's outer covering.
3. False; two tubes are the ureters.
4. True
5. True
6. True
7. False; one who studies
8. False; nephrotomy
9. False; ureterotomy
10. False; cystitis

EXERCISE 13-7   FILL IN THE BLANKS WITH THE APPROPRIATE ABBREVIATIONS

ABBREVIATION

1. IVP
2. KUB
3. CAPD
4. BUN
5. GFR
6. ESRD
7. PSA
8. UA
9. UTI
10. BPH

EXERCISE 13-8   CROSSWORD PUZZLE: THE URINARY SYSTEM

1. dysuria
2. dialysis
3. IVP
4. nephron
5. pyuria
6. hematuria
7. BUN
8. diuretic
9. bladder
10. enuresis
11. cystectomy
12. UA
13. nephroptosis
14. ureters
15. uremia
16. void
17. anuria
18. cystitis
19. ren
20. nocturia

CHAPTER 13 QUIZ

1. renal transplant
2. nephropexy
3. pyelolithotomy
4. ureterectomy
5. cystoscopy
6. drug used to kill bacterial growth
7. drug used to decrease spasms of the bladder
8. blood urea nitrogen
9. bedwetting
10. overgrowth of the kidney

MULTIPLE CHOICE

11. D	13. D	15. A
12. B	14. A	16. C

CHAPTER 14

WORD ELEMENTS EXERCISE: CONVERTING WORDS TO WORD ROOTS

1. mast/o, mamm/o
2. spermat/o, sperm/o
3. salping/o
4. vas/o
5. circum/o
6. oophor/o, oo, ovari/o
7. colp/o, vagin/o
8. prostat/o
9. amni/o
10. nat/o
11. uter/o, hyster/o, metr/o
12. vulv/o
13. orch/o, orchi/o, orchid/o, test/o
14. cervic/o
15. balan/o
16. gonad/o
17. gynec/o
18. lact/o
19. men/o
20. ovari/o, oophor/o, oo

QUICK CHECK: A FEW TERMS SOMETIMES OVERLOOKED

1. to produce sperm
2. lactation
3. gestation

EXERCISE 14-1   FIGURE LABELING: THE MALE REPRODUCTIVE SYSTEM

1. testis
2. epididymis
3. scrotum
4. ductus (vas) deferens
5. ejaculatory duct
6. urethra
7. penis
8. glans penis
9. prepuce (foreskin)
10. seminal vesicle
11. prostate
12. bulbourethral gland
13. urinary bladder

EXERCISE 14-2   FIGURE LABELING: THE FEMALE REPRODUCTIVE SYSTEM

1. fallopian tube
2. ovary
3. uterus
4. urinary bladder
5. clitoris
6. labium minora
7. labium majora
8. cervix
9. rectum
10. anus
11. vagina
12. urethra

EXERCISE 14-3   DECIPHERING MEDICAL DOCUMENTS

1. second pregnancy, 1 child or live birth; see also question 8
2. transabdominal puncture of the amniotic sac to remove amniotic fluid for testing
3. within the uterus
4. It provides a starting point for an investigation, but the unanswered questions it implies would make an investigator's job very difficult, if not impossible.
5. Given the vagueness of the report, the word "remarkable" is unremarkable (in the sense in which it is used).
6. One might select a host of adjectives to end a sentence describing the tone of this document. However, the list would not include *clear*, *competent*, *helpful*, *professional*, or *worthy of its title*, that being "Medical Document."
7. The answer to this question is subjective, of course. If the document is an indication of the level of care, I cannot imagine anyone thinking that the care was very good at any point during the pregnancy.
8. Reexamine your answer to question 1 and compare it to answers given by your classmates. HINT: Given that the opening remark is a sentence fragment, is it possible to know whether this woman was gravida II, para I before or after she lost this baby? If it was before, which one might surmise, what does the term "remarkable" then signify?

EXERCISE 14-4   BUILDING MEDICAL TERMS

1. hysteropexy
2. hysterectomy
3. hysterorrhexis
4. hysterorrhaphy
5. metropathy
6. metritis
7. metrorrhagia
8. vaginal
9. vaginocele
10. vaginitis
11. vaginolabial or labiovaginal
12. colposcopy
13. colporrhaphy
14. prostatectomy
15. prostatic
16. prostatitis
17. vesiculopathy
18. vesiculitis
19. orchitis
20. orchiopathy
21. orchialgia, orchodynia

EXERCISE 14-5   SURGICAL PROCEDURE TERM IDENTIFICATION

1. fallopian tube
2. uterus
3. fallopian tube
4. vagina
5. breast
6. ovary
7. testis
8. vas deferens
9. glans penis
10. breast

EXERCISE 14-6   MATCHING TERMS WITH DEFINITIONS

1. D
2. O
3. E
4. I
5. A
6. G
7. C
8. M
9. B
10. K
11. N
12. F
13. H
14. L
15. J

EXERCISE 14-7   THE MEANINGS OF ABBREVIATIONS

1. sexually transmitted disease
2. dysfunctional uterine bleeding
3. in vitro fertilization
4. venereal disease
5. last menstrual period
6. hysterosalpingogram
7. transurethral resection of the prostate
8. estimated date of confinement (due date)
9. dilation and curettage
10. hormone replacement therapy
11. intrauterine device
12. gonorrhea
13. herpes simplex virus
14. obstetrics
15. pelvic inflammatory disease
16. benign prostatic hypertrophy
17. premenstrual syndrome
18. cesarean section
19. total abdominal hysterectomy
20. gynecology

EXERCISE 14-8   CROSSWORD PUZZLE: THE REPRODUCTIVE SYSTEM

1. vulv
2. gonorrhea
3. cervix
4. endometriosis
5. laparoscopy
6. hymen
7. oophor
8. cystocele
9. vasectomy
10. menarche
11. colposcope
12. areola
13. perineum
14. across: prostatitis; down: phimosis
15. TURP
16. orchitis
17. vas
18. oviduct
19. gynec

CHAPTER 14 QUIZ

1. A
2. B
3. A
4. D
5. B
6. B
7. C
8. A
9. D
10. False; gestation
11. True
12. False; fertilization
13. False; in vitro fertilization
14. False; ovulation
15. True
16. True
17. False; obstetrics
18. False; dysmenorrhea
19. False; Pap smear

CHAPTER 15

WORD ELEMENTS EXERCISE: DEFINING WORD ELEMENTS RELATED TO THE EYE

1. retina
2. tears or lacrimal sac
3. suffix for vision
4. light, eye, vision
5. eye
6. middle layer of the eye containing muscles and blood vessels
7. two, double
8. tears, lacrima
9. tear, lacrimal apparatus
10. suffix for eye vision
11. iris
12. eye
13. lens
14. old age
15. eyelid
16. conjunctiva (plural: conjunctivae)
17. pupil
18. cornea
19. sclera (also means hard)
20. hard, cornea

QUICK CHECK: A FEW KEY SYNONYMS

1. orbit, eyelids, conjunctiva, and lacrimal
2. palpebrae
3. tears

WORD ELEMENTS EXERCISE: DEFINING WORD ELEMENTS RELATED TO THE EAR

1. sound
2. ear
3. hearing
4. tympanic membrane (eardrum)
5. eardrum
6. ear
7. stapes
8. ear

QUICK CHECK: A FEW KEY SYNONYMS

1. malleus, incus, and stapes
2. eustachian tube
3. cochlea

WORD ELEMENTS EXERCISE: ABBREVIATIONS

1. intracapsular cataract extraction
2. both ears
3. otitis media
4. decibel
5. posterior vitreous detachment (referring to the vitreous body)
6. right ear
7. right eye
8. left eye
9. American Sign Language
10. left ear
11. extracapsular cataract extraction
12. extraocular movement
13. electroretinography
14. intraocular pressure
15. both eyes

EXERCISE 15-1   FIGURE LABELING: THE EYE

1. sclera
2. cornea
3. iris
4. lens
5. ciliary body
6. vitreous humor
7. fovea centralis
8. retina
9. choroid

EXERCISE 15-2   OPERATIVE REPORT

1. middle ear infection or inflammation
2. incision into the tympanic membrane
3. earwax
4. medication given to combat the growth of bacteria

EXERCISE 15-3   MATCHING TERMS WITH DEFINITIONS: EYE

1. J
2. G
3. E
4. D
5. H
6. A
7. F
8. I
9. C
10. B

EXERCISE 15-4   MATCHING TERMS WITH DEFINITIONS: EAR

1. C
2. G
3. D
4. I
5. B
6. J
7. E
8. A
9. H
10. F

EXERCISE 15-5   FILL IN THE BLANK

1. cataract
2. presbycusis
3. diplopia
4. vertigo
5. tinnitus
6. pinna
7. hordeolum
8. otalgia
9. astigmatism
10. keratitis
11. xerophthalmia
12. antiemetic
13. otosclerosis
14. blepharoptosis
15. audiometry

EXERCISE 15-6   CROSSWORD PUZZLE: EYE AND EAR

1. labyrinth
2. strabismus
3. audiologist
4. retina
5. OD
6. kerat
7. OS
8. ophthalmoscope
9. dacryocyst
10. AS
11. refraction
12. OU
13. iris
14. ossicles
15. incus
16. ot
17. ophthalm
18. cerumen

CHAPTER 15 QUIZ

1. B
2. A
3. D
4. C
5. A
6. D
7. B
8. C
9. A
10. D
11. staped
12. tympanitis, myringitis
13. glaucoma
14. eustachian tube
15. OD
16. mastoiditis
17. conductive
18. labyrinthotomy
19. AS
20. cochlea

Glossary of Word Elements

a-	without	balan/o	glans penis
ab-	away from	bi-	two or both
abdomin/o	abdomen	bi/o	life
-ac	pertaining to	blephar/o	eyelid
acous/o, acust/o	hearing	brachi/o	arm
acr/o	extremity or topmost	brady-	slow
ad-	to, toward, or near	bronch/o, bronchi/o	bronchus (airway)
aden/o	gland	bucc/o	cheek
adip/o	fat	bulb/o	bulblike
adren/o, adrenal/o	adrenal	calcane/o	heel
-al	pertaining to	calc/i	calcium
albin/o	albino	cardi/o	heart
-alges, -algia	pain	carp/o	wrist
alimen/o	digestive tract	-cele	pouching or hernia
alveol/o	alveolus (air sac)	-centesis	puncture for
amni/o	amnion		aspiration
amphi-	on both sides	cephal/o	head
an-	without	cerebell/o	cerebellum
ana-	up, apart	cerebr/o	largest part of the
andr/o	male		brain, cerebrum
-aneous	converts noun to	cerv/o, cervic/o	neck
	adjective: pertaining to	cheil/o	lip
angi/o	vessel	chem/o	chemical
ankyl/o	crooked	chir/o	hand
ante-	before	cholangi/o	bile duct
anter/o	anterior	chol/o, chole/o	bile
anti-	against or opposed to	cholecyst/o	gallbladder
aort/o	aorta	choledoch/o	common bile duct
appendic/o	appendix	chondr/o	cartilage
-ar	pertaining to	-cidal, -cide	to kill
arachn/o	spider	circum/o	around
arteri/o	artery	cirrh/o	yellow
arthr/o	joint	coagul/o	clotting
-ary	pertaining to	col/o, colon/o	colon (large intestine)
-asthen	weakness	colp/o	vagina
astr/o	star-shaped	con-	with, together
ather/o	fatty, lipid, paste	condyl-	rounded end surface of
atri/o	atrium		a bone
audi/o, audit/o	hearing	conjunctiv/o	conjunctiva
aur/o, auricul/o	ear	contra-	against or opposed to
auto-	self	corne/o	cornea
bacteri/o	bacteria	coron/o	circle or crown

cortic/o	outer layer or covering	erythr/o	red
cost/o	rib	esophag/o	esophagus
crani/o	skull	esthesi/o	sensation
-crasia	blending, mixture	eu-, ex-, ex/o	out or away
crin/o	to secrete	extra-	outside
cry/o	to freeze	fasci/o	fibrous membrane
crypt-	hidden	femur/o	femur, thighbone
-cusis	hearing	fibr/o	fiber
cutane/o	skin	gangli/o, ganglion/o	ganglia (singular: ganglion)
cyan/o	blue		
cyst/o	bladder or sac	gastr/o	stomach
cyt/o, -cyte	cell	gen-, -genesis	origin or production
dacry/o	tear	-genic	pertaining to origin
dacryocyst/o	lacrimal sac	ger/o, geront/o	aged
dactyl/o	finger, toe	gingiv/o	gums
de-	from, down, or not	gli/o	glue
dent/i, dent/o	teeth	-globin	protein
derm/o, dermat/o	skin	glomerul/o	glomerulus
-desis	binding	gloss/o	tongue
di-	two	gluc/o, glyc/o	sugar (glucose)
dia-	across or through	gonad/o	gonad
-dilator	increase diameter, open up	-gram	record
		-graph	instrument for recording
dipl-, dipl/o	two, double		
dips/o	thirst	-graphy	process of recording
dors/o	dorsal	gyn/o, gynec/o	female
duoden/o	duodenum	hem/o, hemat/o	blood
dur/o	dura	hemi-	half
-dynia	painful	hep/o, hepat/o	liver
dys-	painful, difficult, or faulty	herni/o	hernia
		hormon/o	hormone
ec-, ecto	out or away	humer/o	humerus, upper arm bone
-ectasia	dilation of a tubular structure		
		hydr/o	water
-ectasis	dilation of a tubular structure	hyper-	above or excessive
		hypn/o	sleep
-ectomy	excision or removal	hypo-	below or deficient
-edema	collection of watery fluid in tissues	hypophys/o	pituitary gland
		hyster/o	uterus
electr/o	electricity	-ia	condition of
-emesis	vomiting	iac, -ian	specialist
-emetic	pertaining to vomiting	-iasis	formation or presence of
-emia	blood condition	-iatric	medical specialty
encephal/o	entire brain	-iatrist	specialist
en-, endo-	within	iatr/o	treatment
endocrin/o	endocrine	-iatry	medical specialty
enter/o	small intestine	-ic, -ical	pertaining to
-eous	upon, following, subsequent to	ichthy/o	fish scales, very dry
		-ics	medical specialty
epi-	upon	ile/o	ileum
erythemat/o	redness	immun/o	safe

-ine	suffix used in the formation of names of chemical substances
infra-	inside or below
inguin/o	inguinal
inter-	between
intra-	within
-iole	smaller
-ion	condition
ir/o, irid/o, irit/o	iris (colored circle)
isch/o	to hold back
-ism	condition of
-ist	one who specializes in
-itis	inflammation
-ium	structure or tissue
jaund/o	yellow
jejun/o	jejunum
kerat/o	cornea
kine-, kinesi/o, -kinesia	movement
kyph/o	humpbacked
labi/o	lips
labyrinth/o	labyrinth
lacrim/o	tear
lact/o	milk
lapar/o	abdomen
laryng/o	larynx (voice box)
-lepsy	seizure
leuk/o	white
ligament/o	ligament
-lipid	fatty
lith/o, -lith	stone
-lithiasis	condition of having stones
-logist	one who specializes in the study or treatment of
-logy	study of
lord/o	bent
lumb/o	loin (lower back)
lymph/o, lymphat/o	clear fluid
lymphaden/o	lymph nodes
lymphangi/o	lymph vessels
-lysis	breakdown or dissolution
macro-	large
-malacia	softening
mamm/o	breast
-mania	condition of abnormal impulse toward or frenzy
mast/o	breast

-megaly	enlargement
melan/o	black
men/o	month (menstruation)
mening/o	membrane (meninges)
ment/o	referring to the mind
meso-	middle, mean
meta-	beyond, after, or change
-meter	instrument for measuring
metr/o	uterus
-metry	process of measuring
micro-	small
-mnesia	memory
mono-	one
muc/o	mucus
muscul/o	muscle
my/o	muscle
myc/o	fungus
myel/o	bone marrow or spinal cord
myring/o	eardrum or tympanic membrane
narc/o	stupor or sleep
nas/o	nose
nat/o	birth
necr/o	dead
neo-	new
nephr/o	kidney
neur/o	nerve
noct/o	night
ocul/o	eye
-oid	resembling
-ole	small
olig-, oligo-	scanty
-oma	tumor
onc/o	tumor
-one	chemical compound
onych/o	nail
oo	ovary, egg
oophor/o	ovary
ophthalm/o	eye
-opia	eye, vision
-opsia	vision
-opsy	process of viewing
opt/o	eye
or/o	mouth
orch/o, orchi/o, orchid/o	testis or testicle
orth/o-	straight, normal, or correct
-ory	pertaining to

-osis	abnormal condition or increase	-pnea	breathing
osse/o	bone, bony	pneum/o	air or lung
oste/o	bone	-poiesis	formation
ot/o	ear	poly-	many
-otic	pertaining to	-porosis	porous
-ous	pertaining to	post-	after
ov/i, ov/o	egg	poster/o	posterior
ovari/o	ovary	pre-	before
ox/o, -oxia	oxygen	presby/o	old age
pan-	all	proct/o	rectum and anus
pancreat/o	pancreas	prostat/o	prostate gland
para-	alongside of or abnormal	proxim/o	proximal
		prurit/o	to itch
parathyr/o, parathyroid/o	parathyroid	psych/o	mind
		-ptosis	falling or downward displacement
-paresis	weakness, loss of movement	-ptysis	spitting
		pulmon/o	lung
pariet/o	a wall of the body	pupil/o	pupil
path/o, -pathy	disease	py/o	pus
pector/o	chest	pyel/o	pelvis
pedicul/o	lice	pylor/o	pylorus
ped/o	foot, child	pyret/o	fever
pelv/o	pelvis	quadri-	four
-penia	abnormal reduction, deficiency	rect/o	rectum
		ren/o	kidney
-pepsia	digestion	retin/o	retina
peri-	around	retro-	behind, backward
-pexy	suspension or fixation	rheum/o, rheumat/o	to flow
phac/o, phak/o	lens	rhin/o	nose
phag/o, -phagia	eat or swallow	-rrhage, -rrhagia	to burst forth (usually blood)
phalang/o	bones of fingers and toes		
pharm/o, pharmacy/o	drug	-rrhaphy	suture
		-rrhea	discharge
pharyng/o	pharynx or throat	-rrhexis	rupture
phas/o, -phasia	speech	salping/o	uterine or fallopian tube
-phil	attraction for	sarc/o	flesh
phleb/o	vein	scab/o	to scratch
-phobia	condition of abnormal fear or sensitivity	schiz/o	split
		scler/o	hard or sclera
phon/o, -phonia	voice	-sclerosis	hardness
phot/o	light	scoli/o	twisted
phren/o	diaphragm, mind	-scope	instrument for examination
-phylaxis	protection		
-physis	to grow	-scopy	process of examination
pil/o	hair	seb/o	sebaceous
-plasia	formation	semi-	half
-plasty	surgical repair or reconstruction	-septic	decay or breaking
		sial/o	salivary glands
-plegia	paralysis	sigmoid/o	sigmoid colon
pleur/o	pleura	sinus/o	sinus

-spasm	involuntary contraction	**-tomy**	incision
sperm/o, spermat/o-	sperm	**ton/o**	tone or tension
sphygm/o	pulse	**tonsill/o**	tonsil
spin/o	thorn	**trache/o**	trachea (windpipe)
spir/o	breathing	**trans-, trans/o**	across or through
splen/o	spleen	**tri-**	three
spondyl/o	vertebra	**-tripsy**	crushing
staped/o	stapes	**troph/o, -trophy,**	nourishment or
-stasis	stop or stand	**tropin**	development
sten/o	narrow	**tympan/o**	eardrum or tympanic
-stenosis	narrowed, block		membrane
stern/o	chest	**-ular**	converts a root or noun
steth/o	chest		to an adjective
sthen/o	strength	**-um**	singular noun ending
stomat/o	mouth	**uni-**	one
-stomy	creation of an opening	**ur/o, urin/o**	urine
sub-	below or under	**ureter/o**	ureter
sudor/o	sweat gland	**urethr/o**	urethra
super/o, super-,	above or excessive	**-us**	condition
supra-		**uter/o**	uterus
sym-	together	**uve/o**	uvea
syn-	together or with	**vagin/o**	vagina
tachy-	fast	**valv/o, valvul/o**	valve
temper/o	temper	**varic/o**	swollen, twisted vein
tend/o, tendin/o	tendon	**vas/o, vascul/o**	vessel
tens-	pressure	**ven/o**	vein
test/o, testost/o	testis or testicle	**ventricul/o**	ventricle (belly or
tetra-	four		pouch)
thorac/i, thorac/o,	chest	**-version**	to turn
thoracic/o		**vertebr/o**	vertebra
thromb/o	clot	**vesic/o**	bladder or sac
thym/o	thymus gland	**vulv/o**	vulva
thyr/o, thyroid/o	thyroid gland	**xanth/o**	yellow
	(shield)	**xer/o**	dry
tom/o	to cut	**-y**	adjective suffix
-tome	cutting instrument	**zyg/o**	yoke, to join

APPENDIX C

Glossary of Medical Abbreviations

ABOUT ABBREVIATIONS

Abbreviations can be useful. However, their usefulness has limits beyond which lie confusion and, possibly, danger as well.

The usefulness of an abbreviation is mostly associated with time saved, often measurable in seconds. The confusion it may engender, on the other hand, can last for hours or days, during which a patient's life may hang in the balance.

Keep those facts in mind when choosing between a word and its abbreviation in any given circumstance, especially if you feel a rush of importance when you use an abbreviation that will baffle an ordinary mortal—in other words, anyone whose specialty differs from yours.

A	anterior; assessment	**AMA**	antimitochondrial antibody
A&P	auscultation and percussion	**AML**	acute myelogenous leukemia
A&W	alive and well		
a.c.	before meals	**amt**	amount
a.m.	morning; before noon	**Amu**	atomic mass unit
ACL	anterior cruciate ligament	**ANA**	antinuclear antibody
ACTH	adrenocorticotrophin hormone	**ANS**	autonomic nervous system
		AP	anteroposterior
AD	right ear (spell out right ear)	**APAP**	acetaminophen
ad lib.	as desired	**Apgar (*ap'gär*)**	appearance, pulse, grimace, activity, respiration
ADH	antidiuretic hormone		
ADHD	attention deficit hyperactivity disorder	**aq**	water
		ARF	acute renal failure; acute rheumatic fever
A-fib	atrial fibrillation		
Ag	antigen; [L.] *argentum*, silver	**As**	arsenic
AID	artificial insemination donor	**AS**	[L.] *auris sinistra*, left ear (spell out left ear)
AIDS (*ādz*)	acquired immunodeficiency syndrome	**ASA**	acetylsalicylic acid (aspirin); antisperm antibodies
AIH	artificial insemination by husband; artificial insemination, homologous	**ASD**	atrial septal defect
		ASHD	arteriosclerotic heart disease
AJCCS	American Joint Committee on Cancer Staging (criteria)	**ASL**	American Sign Language
		AST	aspartate aminotransferase (enzyme)
AKA	above-knee amputation		
Al	aluminum	**at. wt.**	atomic weight
alb	albumin	**ATP**	adenosine 5′-triphosphate
ALL	acute lymphocytic leukemia	**Au**	[L.] *aurum*, gold
ALS	amyotrophic lateral sclerosis	**AU**	[L.] *auris utraque*, each ear, both ears (spell out both ears)
ALT	alanine aminotransferase (enzyme)		

AV, A-V	arteriovenous; atrioventricular	**c̄**	with
AVN	atrioventricular node	**C&S**	culture and sensitivity
AW	atomic weight	**C. diff**	*Clostridium difficile*
ax.	axis	**c/o**	complains of
b	blood (subscript)	**CA**	cancer; carcinoma; cardiac
B	barometric pressure		arrest; chronologic age;
	(subscript); boron		croup-associated (virus);
Ⓑ	bilateral		cytosine arabinoside; cancer
b.i.d.	[L.] *bis in die*, twice a day		antigen; carbohydrate antigen
Ba	barium	**ca.**	[L.] *circa*, about,
BADL	basic activities of daily living		approximately
BAEP	brainstem auditory evoked	**CABG**	coronary artery bypass graft
	potential	**CAD**	coronary artery disease
BAER	brainstem auditory evoked	**cal**	calorie (small)
	response	**Cal**	calorie (large)
BBB	blood–brain barrier	**CAM**	complementary and
BCC	basal cell carcinoma		alternative medicine
BD	bipolar disorder	**cap**	capsule
BE	barium enema	**CAPD**	continuous ambulatory
B-E	below-the-elbow amputation		peritoneal dialysis
Bi	Bismuth	**CAT (kat)**	computerized axial
BiPAP	bilevel positive airway		tomography
	pressure	**CBC**	complete blood (cell) count
BKA	below-knee amputation	**CC**	chief complaint
BM	bowel movement	**cc**	cubic centimeter (use the
BMI	body mass index		metric equivalent mL)
BMP	basic metabolic panel	**CCK**	cholecystokinin
BP	blood pressure; boiling	**CCU**	cardiac care unit; coronary
	point; British Pharmacopoeia		care unit; critical care unit
BPH	benign prostatic hypertrophy;	**Cd**	cadmium
	benign prostatic hyperplasia	**CEA**	carcinoembryonic antigen
Br	bromine	**CF**	complement fixation; cystic
BRAT	diet of banana, rice cereal,		fibrosis; coupling factor
	applesauce, toast	**CHF**	congestive heart failure
BRCA	breast cancer antigen	**CHO**	carbohydrate
BRP	bathroom privileges	**CI**	color index
BS	blood sugar	**CIB**	[L.] *cibus*, food
BSA	body surface area	**CIS**	carcinoma in situ
BT	bleeding time	**CJD**	Creutzfeldt-Jakob disease
BTU	British thermal unit	**Cl**	chlorine
BUN	blood urea nitrogen	**CL**	cardiolipin
BUN:Cr	blood urea nitrogen to	**CLIA**	Clinical Laboratory
	creatinine ratio		Improvement Amendments
Bx	biopsy	**CLL**	chronic lymphocytic
C	calorie (large); carbon;		leukemia
	Celsius; centigrade; cervical;	**cm**	centimeter
	clearance rate, renal	**Cm**	curium
	(as subscript); compliance;	**CMC**	carpometacarpal
	concentration; cylindrical	**CML**	chronic myelogenous
	lens; cytidine		leukemia
c	calorie (small); capillary	**CMP**	comprehensive metabolic
	blood (subscript); centi		panel

CMV	controlled mechanical ventilation; cytomegalovirus	**dB**	decibel
CNS	central nervous system	**DC, D/C**	discharge; discontinue (spell out discharge or discontinue)
Co	cobalt	**D-dimer**	fibrin degradation product
CO	cardiac output	**DDS**	doctor of dental surgery
CO₂	carbon dioxide	**def**	decayed, extracted, or filled (deciduous teeth)
CoA	coenzyme A	**DEF**	decayed, extracted, or filled (permanent teeth)
COG	center of gravity		
COPD	chronic obstructive pulmonary disease	**df**	decayed and filled (deciduous teeth)
CP	cerebral palsy; chest pain; costophrenic	**DF**	decayed and filled (permanent teeth)
CPPB	continuous (or constant) positive pressure breathing	**DIC**	disseminated intravascular coagulation
CPPV	continuous positive-pressure ventilation	**DJD**	degenerative joint disease
		DKA	diabetic ketoacidosis
CPR	cardiopulmonary resuscitation	**DM**	diabetes mellitus
cps	cycles per second	**DMD**	Duchenne muscular dystrophy
Cr	chromium; creatinine		
CR	conditioned reflex; crown-rump length	**dmf**	decayed, missing, or filled (deciduous teeth)
CRD	chronic respiratory disease	**DMF**	decayed, missing, or filled (permanent teeth)
CRP	cross-reacting protein		
CRST	calcinosis cutis, Raynaud phenomenon, sclerodactyly, and telangiectasia syndrome	**DNA**	deoxyribonucleic acid
		DNR	do not resuscitate
		DOA	dead on arrival
CS	cesarean section	**DPI**	dry powder inhaler
CSD	cat scratch disease	**DPT**	dipropyltryptamine; diphtheria, pertussis, and tetanus (vaccines)
CSF	cerebrospinal fluid		
CT	computed tomography		
CTA	computed tomographic angiography	**dr**	dram
CTD	cumulative trauma disorder	**DRE**	digital rectal examination
CTS	carpal tunnel syndrome	**DRG**	diagnosis-related group
cu mm, mm³	cubic millimeter	**DSA**	digital subtraction angiography
CV	cardiovascular		
CVA	cerebrovascular accident	**dsDNA**	double-stranded DNA
CVP	central venous pressure	**DT**	delirium tremens; duration of tetany
CVS	chorionic villus sampling		
CXR	chest X-ray	**DTP**	diphtheria and tetanus toxoids and pertussis vaccine; distal tingling on percussion (Tinel sign)
Cys	cysteine		
Cyt	cytosine		
d	deci-; day		
D	dead space gas (subscript); deciduous; deuterium; diffusing capacity; dihydrouridine (in nucleic acids); diopter; [L.] *dexter*, right (opposite of left); vitamin D potency of cod liver oil	**DTR**	deep tendon reflex
		DUB	dysfunctional uterine bleeding
		DVT	deep vein thrombosis
		EB, EBV	Epstein-Barr virus
		ECCE	extracapsular cataract extraction
D&C	dilation and curettage	**ECF**	extracellular fluid
D&E	dilation and evacuation	**ECG**	electrocardiogram

echo	echocardiogram	FHR	fetal heart rate
ECT	electroconvulsive therapy	FHT	fetal heart tones
ECU	emergency care unit	fl oz	fluid ounce
EDC	estimated date of confinement	FOBT	fecal occult blood test
EDD	estimated date of delivery	Fr	francium; French (gauge, scale)
EEG	electroencephalogram		
EENT	eye, ear, nose, and throat	FRC	functional residual capacity (of lungs)
EGD	esophagogastroduode-noscopy		
		Fru	fructose
EGR	electroretinopathy	FS	frozen section
EKG	[German] *Elektrokardio-gramme*, electrocardiogram	FSH	follicle-stimulating hormone
		FU	fluorouracil
ELISA (*ĕ-lī'să*)	enzyme-linked immunosorbent assay	FUO	fever of unknown origin
		FVC	forced vital capacity
EM	electron microscopy	Fw	F wave (fibrillary wave, flutter wave)
EMG	electromyogram		
EMS	emergency medical services	Fx	fracture
ENT	ear, nose, and throat	g	gram
EOM	extraocular movement; extraocular muscles	Ga	gallium
		GAD	generalized anxiety disorder
EP	electrophysiology	GB	gallbladder
EPAP	expiratory positive airway pressure	GBS	gallbladder X-ray series
		GC	gonococcus, gonorrhea
EPS	electrophysiologic study	GERD (*gĕrd*)	gastroesophageal reflux disease
ER	endoplasmic reticulum; emergency room; estrogen receptor		
		GFR	glomerular filtration rate
		GH	glenohumeral; growth hormone
ERBF	effective renal blood flow		
ERV	expiratory reserve volume	GI	gastrointestinal; gingival index
ESP	extrasensory perception		
ESR	electron spin resonance; erythrocyte sedimentation rate	GIST (*jist*)	gastrointestinal stromal tumor
		gm	gram
ESRD	end-stage renal disease	gr	grain
ESWL	extracorporeal shock wave lithotripsy	gt	drop
		gt.	[L.] *gutta*, a drop
ETOH	ethyl alcohol	GTT	glucose tolerance test
EUS	endoscopic ultrasonography	gtt.	[L.] *guttae*, drops
F	Fahrenheit; Faraday constant; fertility factor; field of vision; fluorine; force; fractional concentration; free energy	GU	genitourinary
		GVHD	graft-versus-host disease
		Gy	gray (unit of absorbed dose of ionizing radiation)
		GYN	gynecology
FB	foreign body	h	hecto-; hour
FBS	fasting blood sugar	H	henry; hydrogen; hyperopia; hyperopic
Fe	[L.] *ferrum*, iron		
FEF	forced expiratory flow	H&H	hemoglobin and hematocrit
FET	forced expiratory time	H&P	history and physical
FEV	forced expiratory volume	*H. pylori*	*Helicobacter pylori*
FGT	female genital tract	h. s., HS	[L.] *hora somni*, at bedtime
FH	family history	H$^+$	hydrogen ion

HAART (*hart*)	highly active antiretroviral therapy		**ICCE**	intracapsular cataract extraction
HAV	hepatitis A virus		**ICD**	*International Classification of Diseases*; implantable cardioverter defibrillator
Hb	hemoglobin			
HbA1c	hemoglobin A1c			
HBV	hepatitis B virus		**ICF**	intracellular fluid
HCG, hCG	human chorionic gonadotropin		**ICP**	intracranial pressure
			ICU	intensive care unit
HCI	hydrochloric acid		**ID**	intradermal
HCT, Hct	hematocrit		**IDDM**	insulin-dependent diabetes mellitus
HCV	hepatitis C virus			
HD	Huntington's disease		**IF**	initiation factor; intrinsic factor
HDL	high-density lipoprotein			
He	helium		**IFN**	interferon
HEENT	head, eyes, ears, nose, and throat		**Ig**	immunoglobulin
			IgG	immunoglobulin G
Hg	[L.] *hydrargyrum*, mercury		**IgM**	immunoglobulin M
Hgb	hemoglobin		**IH**	infectious hepatitis
HGH	human (pituitary) growth hormone		**IL**	interleukin
			IM	internal medicine; intramuscular(ly); infectious mononucleosis
HHV	human herpesvirus			
HIPAA (*hip′ă*)	Health Insurance Portability and Accountability Act of 1996			
			IMP	impression
			INR	international normalized ratio (prothrombin time)
HIV	human immunodeficiency virus			
			IOP	intraocular pressure
HLA	human leukocyte antigen		**IP**	interphalangeal; intraperitoneal(ly); inpatient
HMO	health maintenance organization			
			IPAP	inspiratory positive airway pressure
hpf, HPF	high-power field			
HPI	history of present illness		**IPPV**	intermittent positive pressure ventilation
HPV	human papillomavirus			
HR	heart rate		**IPV**	inactivated poliovirus vaccine
HRT	hormone replacement therapy			
HSG	hysterosalpingogram		**IQ**	intelligence quotient
HSV	herpes simplex virus		**Ir**	iridium
HSV-1	herpes simplex virus type 1		**IRV**	inspiratory reserve volume
HSV-2	herpes simplex virus type 2		**ISMP**	Institute for Safe Medication Practices
Ht	height			
HTN	hypertension		**ITP**	idiopathic thrombocyto-penic purpura; inosine 5′-triphosphate
Hx	medical history			
Hz	hertz			
I	inspired gas (subscript); iodine		**IU**	international unit
			IUCD	intrauterine contraceptive device
I&D	incision and drainage			
I&O	(fluid) intake and output		**IUD**	intrauterine device
I, II, III, IV, V, VI, VII, VIII, IX, X	uppercase Roman numerals 1 to 10		**IV**	intravenous
			IVF	in vitro fertilization
			IVP	intravenous pyelogram
IBD	inflammatory bowel disease		**IVU**	intravenous urogram
IBS	irritable bowel syndrome		**J**	joule

JCAHO	Joint Commission on Accreditation of Healthcare Organizations
k	kilo-
K	[Modern L.] *kalium*, potassium; Kelvin
kcal	kilocalorie
kg	kilogram
KJ	knee jerk
KS	Kaposi's sarcoma
KUB	kidneys, ureters, bladder
kV	kilovolt
L	inductance; left; [L.] *limes*, boundary, limit; liter; lumbar
Ⓛ	left
L&W	living and well
LA	lupus antibody; lupus anticoagulant
LASER (*lā'zĕr*)	light amplification by stimulated emission of radiation
LASIK (*lā'sik*)	laser in situ keratomileusis
lb	pound
LBT	lupus band test
LC	lethal concentration
LD	lethal dose
LDL	low-density lipoprotein
LE	left eye; lower extremity; lupus erythematosus
LEEP (*lĕp*)	loop electrosurgical excision procedure
LES	lower esophageal sphincter
LFA	left frontoanterior (fetal position)
LFP	left frontoposterior (fetal position)
LFT	left frontotransverse (fetal position)
LH	luteinizing hormone
Li	lithium
LLQ	left lower quadrant
LMA	left mentoanterior (fetal position)
LMP	left mentoposterior (fetal position); last menstrual period
LMT	left mentotransverse (fetal position)
LOA	left occipitoanterior (fetal position)
LOC	level of consciousness
LOP	left occipitoposterior (fetal position)
LOT	left occipitotransverse (fetal position)
LP	lumbar puncture
lpf, LPF	low-power field
Lr	lawrencium
LSA	left sacroanterior (fetal position)
LSP	left sacroposterior (fetal position)
LST	left sacrotransverse (fetal position)
LTB	laryngotracheobronchitis
LTH	luteotropic hormone
LTM	long-term memory
LUQ	left upper quadrant
LVET	left ventricular ejection time
LVH	left ventricular hypertrophy
lytes	electrolytes
Ⓜ	mass; meter; milli-; minim; molar; moles (per liter)
M	mega-, meg-; molar; moles (per liter); morgan; myopic; myopia
m	murmur
mA	milliampere
MA	mental age
MAC (*mak*)	monitored anesthesia care
MAP	morning-after pill
mA-S	milliampere-second
Mb	myoglobin
MBC	maximum breathing capacity
MCH	mean cell hemoglobin
MCHC	mean cell hemoglobin concentration
MCP	metacarpophalangeal
MCV	mean corpuscular (cell) volume
MD	medical doctor; muscular dystrophy
MDI	metered-dose inhaler
MEDLARS	Medical Literature Analysis and Retrieval System
MEP	maximal expiratory pressure
meq, mEq	milliequivalent
MET	metabolic equivalent of task
MEV	million electron volts (10 ev)
mg	milligram
Mg	magnesium
MG	myasthenia gravis

MHA	microhemagglutination		**mV**	millivolt
MHC	major histocompatibility complex		**MVP**	mitral valve prolapse
			MVV	maximal voluntary ventilation
MHz	megahertz		**MW**	molecular weight
MI	myocardial infarction		**My**	myopia
MICU (*mik′yū*)	medical intensive care unit		**mμ**	millimicron
MID	minimal infecting dose		**N**	Newton; nitrogen; normal concentration
MIP	maximum inspiratory pressure		**n**	normal (small caps)
MIS (*mis*)	minimally invasive surgery		**Na**	[Modern L.] *natrium*, sodium
MJD	Machado-Joseph disease			
ml or mL	milliliter		**NA**	Nomina Anatomica
MLD	minimal lethal dose		**NAD**	nicotinamide adenine dinucleotide; no acute distress
mm	millimeter			
mm³	cubic millimeter			
mmol	millimole		**NCV**	nerve conduction velocity
MMPI	Minnesota Multiphasic Personality Inventory		**Ne**	neon
			NE	norepinephrine; not examined
MMR	measles-mumps-rubella (vaccine)		**NEEP**	negative end-expiratory pressure
Mn	manganese			
MO	medical officer; mineral oil		**NF**	National Formulary
MODS (*mods*)	multiple organ dysfunction syndrome		**ng**	nanogram
			NG	nasogastric
mol	mole		**NGT**	nasogastric tube
mol wt	molecular weight		**Ni**	nickel
MOM	milk of magnesia		**NICU** (*nik′yū*)	neonatal intensive care unit
mono	infectious mononucleosis		**NIDDM**	non–insulin-dependent diabetes mellitus
MOPP	Mustargen (mechlorethamine hydrochloride), Oncovin (vincristine sulfate), procarbazine hydrochloride, and prednisone			
			NK	natural killer (cell)
			NKA	no known allergies
			NKDA	no known drug allergy
mor. sol.	[L.] *more solito*, as usual, as customary		**nm**	nanometer
			noc.	night
MPD	maximal permissible dose		**NPO**	nothing by mouth
MRA	magnetic resonance angiography		**NREM**	nonrapid eye movement (sleep)
mrd, MRD	minimal reacting dose		**nRNA**	nuclear ribonucleic acid
MRI	magnetic resonance imaging		**NSAID**	nonsteroidal anti-inflammatory drug
mRNA	messenger ribonucleic acid			
MRSA	methicillin-resistant *Staphylococcus aureus*		**NSR**	normal sinus rhythm
			O	[L.] *oculus*, eye; opening (in formulas for electrical reactions); oxygen; objective
MS	multiple sclerosis; morphine sulfate; musculoskeletal			
ms, msec	millisecond		**o-**	ortho-
MSG	monosodium glutamate		**Ø**	none; negative
MSH	melanocyte-stimulating hormone		**O&P**	ova and parasites
			O₂	oxygen
MTP	metatarsophalangeal (joint)		**OA**	osteoarthritis
MUGA (*myŭ′ga*)	multiple-gated acquisition (imaging)		**OB**	obstetrics
			OB/GYN	obstetrics and gynecology

OBS	organic brain syndrome	PDA	patent ductus arteriosus
OC	oral contraceptive	PDLL	poorly differentiated
OCD	obsessive-compulsive		lymphocytic lymphoma
	disorder	PE	physical examination;
OCP	oral contraceptive pill		pulmonary embolism;
OD	right eye (spell out right eye)		polyethylene
OH	occupational history	PEFR	peak expiratory flow rate
OM	otitis media	PEG (*peg*)	percutaneous endoscopic
OMS	organic mental syndrome		gastrostomy
OP	osmotic pressure; outpatient	per	by or through
OPV	oral poliovirus vaccine	PERRLA	pupils equal, round,
OR	operating room		and reactive to light and
ORIF	open reduction, internal		accommodation
	fixation	PET	positron emission
OS	[L.] *oculus sinister*, left eye		tomography
	(spell out left eye)	PF	peak flow
OT	occupational therapy	PFT	pulmonary function test
OTC	over the counter	PG	prostaglandin
	(nonprescription drug)	pH	hydrogen ion concentration;
OU	both eyes (spell out both eyes)		p (power) of $[H^+]_{10}$;
OXT	oxytocin		potential of hydrogen
oz	ounce	PH	past history
p	pico-; pupil	PI	present illness
p-	para-	PICC	peripherally inserted central
P	partial pressure; peta-;		catheter
	phosphorus, phosphoric	PICU (*pik'yū*)	pediatric intensive care unit
	residue; plasma	PID	pelvic inflammatory disease
	concentration; pressure;	PIH	pregnancy-induced
	para (obstetric history);		hypertension
	plan; posterior; pulse;	PIP (*pip*)	proximal interphalangeal
	blood group (PI antigen)		(joint)
p̄	after	PKU	phenylketonuria
p.c.	[L.] *post cibum*, after a meal	PLT	platelet
p.m.	after noon	PM	postmortem
p24	HIV antibody	PMH	past medical history
PA	posterior-anterior	PMN	polymorphonuclear
PaCO₂	partial pressure of carbon		(leukocyte)
	dioxide	PMS	premenstrual syndrome
PACS (*paks*)	picture archival	PND	paroxysmal nocturnal
	communications system		dyspnea; postnasal drip
PACU (*pak'yū*)	postanesthetic care unit	PNPB	positive-negative pressure
PALS (*pals*)	pediatric advanced life		breathing
	support	PNS	peripheral nervous system
PaO₂	partial pressure of arterial	PO	[L.] *per os*, by mouth
	oxygen	PO₂, Po₂	partial pressure of oxygen
Pap	Papanicolaou (smear)	POMP	prednisone, Oncovin
PAR	postanesthetic recovery		(vincristine sulfate),
Pb	[L.] *plumbum*, lead		methotrexate, and Purinet-
PCO₂	partial pressure of carbon		hol (6-mercaptopurine)
	dioxide	POR	problem-oriented medical
PD	prism diopter; panic disorder		record

post-op, postop	postoperative	**QNS**	quantity not sufficient
PPBS	postprandial blood sugar	**Qo₂**	oxygen consumption
ppm	parts per million	**qt**	quart
PPPPPP	pain, pallor, pulselessness, paresthesia, paralysis, prostration	**r**	racemic; roentgen
		R	gas constant (8.315 joules); organic radical; Reamur (scale); [L.] *recipe*, take; resistance determinant (plasmid); resistance (electrical); resistance (unit; in the cardiovascular system); resolution; respiration; respiratory (exchange ratio); respiratory rate; roentgen
PPV	positive pressure ventilation		
PR	per rectum; progesterone receptor		
pre-op, preop	preoperative		
PRL	prolactin		
PRN	as needed		
pro time	prothrombin time		
PSA	prostate-specific antigen		
PSG	polysomnography	Ⓡ	right
psi	pounds per square inch	**Ra**	radium
PSV	pressure-supported ventilation	**RA**	rheumatoid arthritis
pt	patient	**RAI**	radioactive iodine
PT	physical therapy; prothrombin time	**RBC**	red blood cell; red blood count
PTA	plasma thromboplastin antecedent; phosphotungstic acid; prior to admission	**RBF**	renal blood flow
		RD	reaction of degeneration; reaction of denervation
PTCA	percutaneous transluminal coronary angioplasty	**RDA**	recommended daily allowance
		rDNA	ribosomal deoxyribonucleic acid
PTH	parathyroid hormone		
PT-INR	prothrombin time international normalized ratio	**RDS**	respiratory distress syndrome
PTP	posttransfusion purpura	**REM (rem)**	rapid eye movement (sleep); reticular erythematous mucinosis
PTSD	posttraumatic stress disorder		
PTT	partial thromboplastin time		
Pu	plutonium	**RF**	release factor; rheumatoid factor
PUD	peptic ulcer disease		
PUO	pyrexia of unknown origin	**RFA**	right frontoanterior (fetal position)
PUVA (pū-vă)	psoralen ultraviolet A		
PV	per vagina	**RFP**	right frontoposterior (fetal position)
PVD	posterior vitreous detachment		
Px	physical examination	**RFT**	right frontotransverse (fetal position)
Q	volume of blood flow		
q	every	**Rh**	Rhesus (Rh blood group); rhodium
q.d.	every day, daily (spell out every day or daily)		
		RH	releasing hormone
q.i.d.	four times a day	**RhD**	rhesus antigen D typing
q.o.d.	every other day (spell out every other day)	**RIA**	radioimmunoassay
		RICE	rest, ice, compression, elevation
q.s.	[L.] *quantum satis*, as much as is enough; [L.] *quantum sufficiat*, as much as may suffice; quantity sufficient		
		RLL	right lower lobe
		RLQ	right lower quadrant
		RMA	right mentoanterior (fetal position)
q2h	every 2 hours		
qh	every hour	**RML**	right middle lobe

RMP	right mentoposterior (fetal position)	**sat. sol.**	saturated solution
RMT	right mentotransverse (fetal position)	**sc**	subcutaneous(ly)
		SC	sternoclavicular; subcutaneous(ly) (spell out subcut or subcutaneously)
Rn	radon		
RNA	ribonucleic acid	**SCC**	squamous cell carcinoma
RNase	ribonuclease	**Se**	selenium
RNP	ribonucleoprotein	**SERM** (*serm*)	selective estrogen receptor modulator
R/O	rule out		
ROA	right occipitoanterior (fetal position)	**SGOT**	serum glutamic-oxaloacetic transaminase (aspartate aminotransferase)
ROM	range of motion		
ROP	right occipitoposterior (fetal position)	**SGPT**	serum glutamic-pyruvic transaminase (alanine aminotransferase)
ROS	review of symptoms		
ROT	right occipitotransverse (fetal position)	**SH**	serum hepatitis; social history
		Si	silicon
rpm	revolutions per minute	**SIDS** (*sids*)	sudden infant death syndrome
rRNA	ribosomal ribonucleic acid		
Rs	resolution	**Sig:**	label; instruction to patient
RSA	right sacroanterior (fetal position)	**SIMV**	spontaneous intermittent mandatory ventilation; synchronized intermittent mandatory ventilation
RSP	right sacroposterior (fetal position)		
RST	right sacrotransverse (fetal position)	**SIRS** (*sĕrs*)	systemic inflammatory response syndrome
RTC	return to clinic	**SK**	streptokinase
RTO	return to office	**SL**	sublingual
RUQ	right upper quadrant	**SLE**	systemic lupus erythematosus
RV	residual volume		
RVH	right ventricular hypertrophy	**SLR**	straight leg raising
		SMAC (*smak*)	sequential multiple analyzer computer
Rx	[L.] *recipe* (the first word on a prescription), take; prescription; treatment		
		Sn	[L.] *stannum*, tin
S	[L.] *sinister*, left; sacral; saturation of hemoglobin (percentage of; followed by subscript O_2 or CO_2); siemens; spherical; spherical lens; sulfur; Svedberg unit; subjective	**SOAP** (*sōp*)	subjective data, objective data, assessment, and plan (problem-oriented medical record)
		SOB	shortness of breath
		sol., soln.	solution
		sp.	species
		sp. gr.	specific gravity
s̄	without	**SPECT**	single-photon emission computed tomography
SA	sinoatrial		
SAB	spontaneous abortion	**SPF**	sun protection factor
SAD (*sad*)	seasonal affective disorder	**SpGr**	specific gravity
SaO₂	oxygen saturation of arterial (oxyhemoglobin)	**spm**	suppression and mutation
		spp.	species (plural)
SARS (*sarz*)	severe acute respiratory syndrome	**SQ**	subcutaneous (spell out subcut or subcutaneously)
sat.	saturated	**Sr**	strontium

SR	systems review	**TKA**	total knee arthroplasty
ssDNA	single-stranded deoxyribonucleic acid	**TKR**	total knee replacement
		Ti	titanium
ssp.	subspecies	**TIA**	transient ischemic attack
ST	scapulothoracic	**TIBC**	total iron-binding capacity
stat, STAT	[L.] *statim*, immediately, at once	**tinct.**	tincture
		TKO	to keep (venous infusion line) open
STD	sexually transmitted disease		
STM	short-term memory	**Tl**	thallium
STSG	split-thickness skin graft	**TLC**	thin-layer chromatography; total lung capacity; tender loving care
sub-Q	subcutaneous (spell out subcut or subcutaneously)		
SUI	stress urinary incontinence	**TLV**	threshold-limit value
suppos	suppository	**TM**	transport maximum; tympanic membrane
SV	stroke volume		
SVT	supraventricular tachycardia	**TMJ**	temporomandibular joint
Sx	symptom	**TMT**	tarsometatarsal
t	metric ton	**TNF**	tumor necrosis factor
T	temperature, absolute (Kelvin); tension (intraocular); tera-; tesla; tetanus (toxoid); thoracic; tidal (volume) (subscript); tocopherol; transverse (tubule); tritium; tumor (antigen)	**TNM**	tumor, node, metastasis (tumor staging)
		t-PA, tPA, TPA	tissue plasminogen activator
		TPN	total parenteral nutrition
		TPR	temperature, pulse, and respirations
		Tr	treatment
		tr.	tincture
T&A	tonsillectomy and adenoidectomy	**tRNA**	transfer ribonucleic acid
		TRUS (*trŭs*)	transrectal ultrasound
T&C	type and crossmatch	**TSH**	thyroid-stimulating hormone
t.i.d.	three times a day	**TSS**	toxic shock syndrome
T_3	3,5,5′-triiodothyronine	**TTP**	thrombotic thrombocytopenic purpura
T_4	tetraiodothyronine (thyroxine)		
		TU	toxic unit
TA	Terminologia Anatomica	**TURP**	transurethral resection of the prostate
tab	tablet		
TAB	therapeutic abortion	**TV**	tidal volume
TAF	tumor angiogenesis factor	**Tx**	treatment; traction
TAH	total abdominal hysterectomy	**U**	unit; uranium; uridine (in polymers); urinary (concentration)
TB	tuberculosis		
Tc	technetium		
TCN	talocalcaneonavicular (joint)	**UA**	urinalysis
		UCHD	usual childhood diseases
Td	tetanus-diphtheria (toxoids, adult type)	**UGI**	upper gastrointestinal
		UGIS	upper gastrointestinal series
TEDS	thromboembolic disease stockings	**ung.**	[L.] *unguentum*, ointment
		u-PA	urokinase
TEE	transesophageal echocardiogram	**URI**	upper respiratory infection
		US, U/S	ultrasound
TENS (*tens*)	transcutaneous electrical nerve stimulation	**UTI**	urinary tract infection
		UV	ultraviolet
THR	total hip replacement	**v**	venous (blood); volt

V	vanadium; vision; visual (acuity); volt; volume (frequently with subscripts denoting location, chemical species, and conditions)	**wk**	week
		WN	well-nourished
		WNL	within normal limits
		WNV	West Nile virus
		Wt	weight
V̇	ventilation; gas flow (frequently with subscripts indicating location and chemical species); ventilation	**x**	times; for
		X-ray	radiography
		y/o or y.o.	year old
		yr	year
V/Q	ventilation/perfusion	**β**	beta, second in a series; blood (subscript)
VA	viral antigen		
V-A	ventriculoatrial	**γ**	gamma; Ostwald solubility coefficient; the third in a series; heavy chain class corresponding to IgG
VATS (*vats*)	video-assisted thoracic surgery		
VC	vision, color; vital capacity		
VCE	vagina, (ecto)cervix, endocervical canal	**Δ**	delta; change; heat
		μ	mu; micro-; heavy chain class corresponding to IgM
VCU, VCUG	voiding cystourethrogram		
V_D	(physiologic) dead space	**μl, μL**	microliter
VD	venereal disease	**μm**	micrometer
VDRL	Venereal Disease Research Laboratory (test)	**μμ**	micromicro-
		Σ	sigma; reflection coefficient; standard deviation; 1 millisecond (0.001 sec)
VHDL	very-high-density lipoprotein		
VLDL	very-low-density lipoprotein		
V_max	maximal velocity	**Ω**	omega; ohm
VP	vasopressin; Voges-Proskauer	**#**	number; pound
VS	volumetric solution; vital signs	**<**	less than (spell out less than)
Vt	tidal volume	**>**	greater than (spell out greater than)
W	watt; [German] *Wolfram*, tungsten	**×**	times; for
w.a.	while awake	**↑**	increased
WBC	white blood cell; white blood count	**↓**	decreased
		°	degree; hour
WDLL	well-differentiated lymphocytic (or lymphatic) lymphoma	**μg**	microgram
		^{123}I	iodine-123 (radioisotope)
		^{125}I	iodine-125
WDWN	well-developed, well-nourished	**^{131}I**	iodine-131
		^{99m}Tc	technetium-99m

APPENDIX D

ISMP's List of Error-Prone Abbreviations, Symbols, and Dose Designations

The abbreviations, symbols, and dose designations found in this table have been reported to ISMP through the USP-ISMP Medication Error Reporting Program as being frequently misinterpreted and involved in harmful medication errors. They should NEVER be used when communicating medical information. This includes internal communications, telephone/verbal prescriptions, computer-generated labels, labels for drug storage bins, medication administration records, as well as pharmacy and prescriber computer order entry screens.

The Joint Commission (TJC) has established a National Patient Safety Goal that specifies that certain abbreviations must appear on an accredited organization's do-not-use list; we have highlighted these items with a double asterisk (**). However, we hope that you will consider others beyond the minimum TJC requirements. By using and promoting safe practices and by educating one another about hazards, we can better protect our patients.

Abbreviations	Intended Meaning	Misinterpretation	Correction
μg	Microgram	Mistaken as "mg"	Use "mcg"
AD, AS, AU	Right ear, left ear, each ear	Mistaken as OD, OS, OU (right eye, left eye, each eye)	Use "right ear," "left ear," or "each ear"
OD, OS, OU	Right eye, left eye, each eye	Mistaken as AD, AS, AU (right ear, left ear, each ear)	Use "right eye," "left eye," or "each eye"
BT	Bedtime	Mistaken as "BID" (twice daily)	Use "bedtime"
cc	Cubic centimeters	Mistaken as "u" (units)	Use "mL"
D/C	Discharge or discontinue	Premature discontinuation of medications if D/C (intended to mean "discharge") has been misinterpreted as "discontinued" when followed by a list of discharge medications	Use "discharge" and "discontinue"
IJ	Injection	Mistaken as "IV" or "intrajugular"	Use "injection"
IN	Intranasal	Mistaken as "IM" or "IV"	Use "intranasal" or "NAS"
HS	Half-strength	Mistaken as bedtime	Use "half-strength" or "bedtime"
hs	At bedtime, hours of sleep	Mistaken as half-strength	

Abbreviations	Intended Meaning	Misinterpretation	Correction
IU**	International unit	Mistaken as IV (intravenous) or 10 (ten)	Use "units"
o.d. or OD	Once daily	Mistaken as "right eye" (OD [oculus dexter]), leading to oral liquid medications administered in the eye	Use "daily"
OJ	Orange juice	Mistaken as OD or OS (right or left eye); drugs meant to be diluted in orange juice may be given in the eye	Use "orange juice"
Per os	By mouth, orally	The "os" can be mistaken as "left eye" (OS [oculus sinister])	Use "PO," "by mouth," or "orally"
q.d. or QD**	Every day	Mistaken as q.i.d., especially if the period after the "q" or the tail of the "q" is misunderstood as an "i"	Use "daily"
qhs	Nightly at bedtime	Mistaken as "qhr" or every hour	Use "nightly"
qn	Nightly or at bedtime	Mistaken as "qh" (every hour)	Use "nightly" or "at bedtime"
q.o.d. or QOD**	Every other day	Mistaken as "q.d." (daily) or "q.i.d. (four times daily) if the "o" is poorly written	Use "every other day"
q1d	Daily	Mistaken as q.i.d. (four times daily)	Use "daily"
q6PM, etc.	Every evening at 6 PM	Mistaken as every 6 hours	Use "6 PM nightly" or "6 PM daily"
SC, SQ, sub q	Subcutaneous	SC mistaken as SL (sublingual); SQ mistaken as "five every;" the "q" in "sub q" has been mistaken as "every" (e.g., a heparin dose ordered "sub q 2 hours before surgery" misunderstood as every 2 hours before surgery)	Use "subcut" or "subcutaneously"
ss	Sliding scale (insulin) or half (apothecary)	Mistaken as "55"	Spell out "sliding scale;" use "one-half" or "½"
SSRI	Sliding scale regular insulin	Mistaken as selective-serotonin reuptake inhibitor	Spell out "sliding scale (insulin)"
SSI	Sliding scale insulin	Mistaken as Strong Solution of Iodine (Lugol's)	
i/d	One daily	Mistaken as "tid"	Use "1 daily"
TIW or tiw	3 times a week	Mistaken as "3 times a day" or "twice in a week"	Use "3 times weekly"
U or u**	Unit	Mistaken as the number 0 or 4, causing a 10-fold overdose or greater (e.g., 4U seen as "40" or 4u seen as "44"); mistaken as "cc" so dose given in volume instead of units (e.g., 4u seen as 4cc)	Use "unit"

Dose Designations and Other Information	Intended Meaning	Misinterpretation	Correction
Trailing zero after decimal point (e.g., 1.0 mg)**	1 mg	Mistaken as 10 mg if the decimal point is not seen	Do not use trailing zeros for doses expressed in whole numbers
"Naked" decimal point (e.g., .5 mg)**	0.5 mg	Mistaken as 5 mg if the decimal point is not seen	Use zero before a decimal point when the dose is less than a whole unit
Drug name and dose run together (especially problematic for drug names that end in "l" such as Inderal 40 mg; Tegretol 300 mg)	Inderal 40 mg Tegretol 300 mg	Mistaken as Inderal 140 mg Mistaken as Tegretol 1300 mg	Place adequate space between the drug name, dose, and unit of measure
Numerical dose and unit of measure run together (e.g., 10 mg, 100 mL)	10 mg 100 mL	The "m" is sometimes mistaken as a zero or two zeros, risking a 10- to 100-fold overdose	Place adequate space between the dose and unit of measure
Abbreviations such as mg. or mL. with a period following	Mg; mL	The period is unnecessary and could be mistaken as the number 1 if written poorly	Use mg, mL, etc., without a terminal period
Large doses without properly placed commas (e.g., 100000 units; 1000000 units)	100,000 units 1,000,000 units	100000 has been mistaken as 10,000 or 1,000,000; 1000000 has been mistaken as 100,000	Use commas for dosing units at or above 1,000, or use words such as 100 "thousand" or 1 "million" to improve readability

Drug Name Abbreviations	Intended Meaning	Misinterpretation	Correction
ARA A	vidarabine	Mistaken as cytarabine (ARA C)	Use complete drug name
AZT	zidovudine (Retrovir)	Mistaken as azathioprine or aztreonam	Use complete drug name
CPZ	Compazine (prochlorperazine)	Mistaken as chlorpromazine	Use complete drug name
DPT	Demerol-Phenergan-Thorazine	Mistaken as diphtheria-pertussis-tetanus (vaccine)	Use complete drug name
DTO	Diluted tincture of opium, or deodorized tincture of opium (Paregoric)	Mistaken as tincture of opium	Use complete drug name
HCl	hydrochloric acid or hydrochloride	Mistaken as potassium chloride (the "H" is misinterpreted as "K")	Use complete drug name unless expressed as a salt of a drug
HCT	hydrocortisone	Mistaken as hydrochlorothiazide	Use complete drug name
HCTZ	hydrochlorothiazide	Mistaken as hydrocortisone (seen as HCT250 mg)	Use complete drug name
MgSO4**	magnesium sulfate	Mistaken as morphine sulfate	Use complete drug name
MS, MSO4**	morphine sulfate	Mistaken as magnesium sulfate	Use complete drug name
MTX	methotrexate	Mistaken as mitoxantrone	Use complete drug name
PCA	procainamide	Mistaken as patient-controlled analgesia	Use complete drug name
PTU	propylthiouracil	Mistaken as mercaptopurine	Use complete drug name
T3	Tylenol with codeine No. 3	Mistaken as liothyronine	Use complete drug name
TAC	triamcinolone	Mistaken as tetracaine, Adrenalin, cocaine	Use complete drug name
TNK	TNKase	Mistaken as "TPA"	Use complete drug name
ZnSO4	zinc sulfate	Mistaken as morphine sulfate	Use complete drug name

Stemmed Drug Names	Intended Meaning	Misinterpretation	Correction
"Nitro" drip	nitroglycerin infusion	Mistaken as sodium nitroprusside infusion	Use complete drug name
"Norflox"	norfloxacin	Mistaken as Norflex	Use complete drug name
"IV Vanc"	intravenous vancomycin	Mistaken as Invanz	Use complete drug name

Symbols	Intended Meaning	Misinterpretation	Correction
ℨ	Dram	Symbol for dram mistaken as "3"	Use the metric system
ℳ	Minim	Symbol for minim mistaken as "mL"	
x3d	For 3 days	Mistaken as "three doses"	Use "for 3 days"
> and <	Greater than and less than	Mistaken as opposite of intended; mistakenly use incorrect symbol; "< 10" mistaken as "40"	Use "greater than" or "less than"
/ (slash mark)	Separates two doses or indicates "per"	Mistaken as the number 1 (e.g., "25 units/10 units" misread as "25 units and 110 units")	Use "per" rather than a slash mark to separate doses
@	At	Mistaken as "2"	Use "at"
&	And	Mistaken as "2"	Use "and"
+	Plus or and	Mistaken as "4"	Use "and"
°	Hour	Mistaken as a zero (e.g., q2° seen as q 20)	Use "hr," "h," or "hour"

**These abbreviations are included on TCJ's "minimum list" of dangerous abbreviations, acronyms, and symbols that must be included on an organization's "Do Not Use" list effective January 1, 2004. Visit www.jointcommission.org for more information about this TJC requirement.

Reprinted with permission from the Institute for Safe Medication Practices. List originally appeared at www.ismp.org. Report medication errors or near misses to the ISMP Medication Errors Reporting Program (MERP) at 1-800-FAIL-SAF(E) or online at www.ismp.org.

Commonly Prescribed Drugs and Their Applications

This list has been selected to be representative of the most commonly prescribed drugs in the United States and Canada for the year 2009 (see references). The list is arranged alphabetically by generic drug name (lower case), followed by representative trade names (uppercase) for the United States and Canadian markets. Combination products have their individual ingredients listed. The final column lists a commonly used classification for the drug.

Generic Name	Trade Name United States	Trade Name Canada	Classification
abacavir/lamivudine/ zidovudine	TRIZIVIR	TRIZIVIR	Combination Product
acetaminophen/codeine	TYLENOL WITH CODEINE	RATIO-EMTEC, TYLENOL WITH CODEINE	Combination Product
acetaminophen/ hydrocodone	ANEXSIA, LORTAB, NORCO, VICODIN, ZYDONE	NOT AVAILABLE	Combination Product
acetaminophen/oxycodone	ENDOCET, PERCOCET, ROXICET, TYLOX	ENDOCET, PERCOCET, RATIO-OXYCOCET	Combination Product
acetaminophen/tramadol	ULTRACET	TRAMACET	Combination Product
acyclovir	ZOVIRAX	ZOVIRAX	Antiviral
adalimumab	HUMIRA	HUMIRA	Immunomodulators
adapalene	DIFFERIN	DIFFERIN	Retinoid
albuterol (salbutamol)	PROVENTIL, VENTOLIN, PROAIR HFA	AIROMIR, APO-SALVENT, RATIO-SALBUTAMOL HFA, VENTOLIN, VOLMAX	β2-Agonist
alendronate	FOSAMAX, FOSAMAX PLUS D	FOSAMAX, NOVO-ALENDRONATE	Bisphosphonate
alfuzosin	UROXATRAL	XATRAL	α-Blocker
allopurinol	LOPURIN, ZURINOL, ZYLOPRIM	ALLOPRIN, APO-ALLOPURINOL, PURINOL, ZYLOPRIM	Xanthine Oxidase Inhibitor
alprazolam	XANAX	APO-ALPRAZ, GEN-ALPRAZOLAM, XANAX	Benzodiazepine
amantadine	SYMMETREL	SYMMETREL	Antiviral
amiodarone	CORDARONE, PACERONE	CORDARONE	Antiarrhythmic
amitriptyline	AMITID, AMITRIL, ELAVIL, EMITRIP, ENDEP	APO-AMITRIPTYLINE, LEVATE	Tricyclic Antidepressant
amlodipine	NORVASC	NORVASC	Calcium Channel Blocker
Amlopidine + benazepril	LOTREL	LOTREL	Calcium channel blocker
amlodipine/atorvastatin	CADUET	CADUET	Combination Product
amlodipine/benazepril	LOTREL	—	Combination Product

(continued)

Generic Name	Trade Name United States	Trade Name Canada	Classification
amoxicillin	AMOXIL, DISPERMOX, LAROTID, POLYMOX, TRIMOX	AMOXIL, APO-AMOXI, GEN-AMOXICILLIN, NOVAMOXIN, ZIMAMOX	Penicillin
amoxicillin/clavulanate	AUGMENTIN	AUGMENTIN, CLAVULIN	Combination Product
Amphetamine + dextroamphetamine	ADDERALL XR	NOT AVAILABLE	amphetamine
amphetamine mixed salts	ADDERALL, ADDERALL XR	ADDERALL XR	Indirect-Acting Sympathomimetic
anastrozole	ARIMIDEX	ARIMIDEX	Antineoplastic
aripiprazole	ABILIFY	NOT AVAILABLE	Atypical Antipsychotic
aspirin	ASCRIPTIN, BUFFERIN, ECOTRIN	ASAPHEN, BUFFERIN, ECOTRIN, NOVASEN, RIVASA	Nonsteroidal Anti-Inflammatory Drug (NSAID)
atazanavir	REYATAZ	REYATAZ	Antiretroviral Agent (protease inhibitor)
atenolol	TENORMIN	APO-ATENOL, NOVO-ATENOL, PMS-ATENOLOL, RATIO-ATENOLOL, TENORMIN	Cardioselective β-Blocker
atenolol/chlorthalidone	TENORETIC	TENORETIC	Combination Product
atomoxetine	STRATTERA	STRATTERA	Selective Norepi-nephrine Reuptake Inhibitor (SNRI)
atorvastatin	LIPITOR	LIPITOR	HMG-CoA Reductase Inhibitor
atropine	ISOPTO ATROPINE	ISOPTO ATROPINE	Anticholinergic
azathioprine	AZASAN, IMURAN	IMURAN	Immunosuppressant
azelastine	ASTELIN, OPTIVAR	NOT AVAILABLE	Antihistamine
azithromycin	ZITHROMAX	ZITHROMAX	Macrolide
baclofen	LIORESAL	LIORESAL	Skeletal Muscle Relaxant
benazepril	LOTENSIN	LOTENSIN	Angiotensin-Converting Enzyme (ACE) Inhibitor
benazepril/hydro-chlorothiazide	LOTENSIN HCT	NOT AVAILABLE	Combination Product
benzonatate	TESSALON	TESSALON	Local Anesthetic
benztropine	COGENTIN		Anticholinergic
bicalutamide	CASODEX	CASODEX	Antiandrogen
bimatoprost	LUMIGAN	LUMIGAN	Prostaglandin
bisoprolol	ZEBETA	MONOCOR	Cardioselective β-Blocker
brimonidine	ALPHAGAN	ALPHAGAN	Central Sympatholytic
budesonide	PULMICORT, RHINOCORT AQUA, PULMICORT RESPULES	PULMICORT NEBUAMP, ENTOCORT, PULMICORT, RHINOCORT AQUA	Glucocorticoid
Budesonide + formoterol	SYMBICORT	SYMBICORT	Anti-inflammatory
bumetanide	BUMEX	BURINEX	Loop Diuretic
Buprenorphine + naloxone	SUBOXONE	SUBOXONE	opioid
bupropion	WELLBUTRIN, ZYBAN, WELLBUTRIN SR, WELLBUTRIN XL	WELLBUTRIN SR, WELLBUTRIN XL	Atypical Antidepressant
buspirone	BUSPAR	BUSPAR, BUSPIREX	Anxiolytic

Generic Name	Trade Name United States	Trade Name Canada	Classification
butalbital/acetaminophen/ caffeine	FIORICET	NOT AVAILABLE	Combination Product
butorphanol	STADOL		Opiate Agonist
cabergoline	DOSTINEX	DOSTINEX	Endocrine and Metabolic Agents
caffeine	CAFCIT, VIVARIN	CAFCIT	Methylxanthine
calcitonin	MIACALCIN	APO-CALCITONIN, CALCIMAR	Endocrine and Metabolic Agent
calcitriol	ROCALTROL	ROCALTROL	Vitamins
calcium acetate	PHOSLO	PHOSLO	Minerals
candesartan	ATACAND	ATACAND	Angiotensin Receptor Blocker (ARB)
capecitabine	XELODA	XELODA	Antineoplastic
captopril	CAPOTEN	CAPOTEN, CAPTOPRIL	Angiotensin-Converting Enzyme (ACE) Inhibitor
carbamazepine	TEGRETOL	TEGRETOL	Anticonvulsant
carbidopa/levodopa	SINEMET	SINEMET	Combination Product
carisoprodol	SOMA	NOT AVAILABLE	Skeletal Muscle Relaxant
carvedilol	COREG	DILATREND, EUCARDIC, PROREG	β-Blocker
cefadroxil	DURICEF, ULTRACEF	DURICEF	Cephalosporin
cefdinir	OMNICEF	OMNICEF	Cephalosporin
cefprozil	CEFZIL	CEFZIL	Cephalosporin
cefuroxime	CEFTIN, KEFUROX, ZINACEF	CEFTIN, KEFUROX, ZINACEF	Cephalosporin
celecoxib	CELEBREX	CELEBREX	COX-2 Inhibitor
cephalexin	CEFANEX, KEFLEX, KEFTAB	APO-CEPHALEX, CEPOREX, NOVO-LEXIN	Cephalosporin
cetirizine	ZYRTEC	ALLERGY RELIEF, REACTINE	Antihistamine
cetirizine/pseudoephedrine	ZYRTEC-D	REACTINE ALLERGY AND SINUS	Combination Product
chlorhexidine gluconate	PERIDEX, PERIOGARD	DENTICARE	Mouth and Throat Products
chlorpheniramine	ALLERGY, CHLOR-TRIMETON	CHLOR-TRIPOLON	Antihistamine
cholestyramine	LOCHOLEST, QUESTRAN		Bile Acid Sequestrant
ciclopirox	PENLAC	LOPROX, STIEPROX	Antifungal
cilazapril	NOT AVAILABLE	INHIBACE	Angiotensin-Converting Enzyme (ACE) Inhibitor
cilostazol	PLETAL	PLETAL Inhibitor	Platelet Aggregation
ciprofloxacin	CILOXAN, CIPRO	CILOXAN, CIPRO	Fluoroquinolone
ciprofloxacin/ dexamethasone	CIPRODEX	CIPRODEX	Combination Product
citalopram	CELEXA	CELEXA	Selective Serotonin Reuptake Inhibitor (SSRI)
clarithromycin	BIAXIN, BIAXIN XL	BIAXIN	Macrolide
clavulanate	2	2	β-Lactamase Inhibitor
clindamycin	CLEOCIN	DALACIN	Lincosamide
clindamycin/benzoyl peroxide	BENZACLIN, DUAC	NOT AVAILABLE	Combination Product

(continued)

Generic Name	Trade Name United States	Trade Name Canada	Classification
clobetasol	CORMAX, EMBELINE, TEMOVATE	DERMASONE, DERMOVATE, TEMOVATE	Glucocorticoid
clonazepam	KLONOPIN	APO-CLONAZEPAM, PMS-CLONAZEPAM, RIVOTRIL	Benzodiazepine
clonidine	CATAPRES	CATAPRES, DIXARIT	Central Sympatholytic
clopidogrel	PLAVIX	PLAVIX	Platelet Aggregation Inhibitor
clorazepate	TRANXENE	TRANXENE	Benzodiazepine
clotrimazole/betamethasone	LOTRISONE	LOTRIDERM	Combination Product
clozapine	CLOZARIL	CLOZARIL	Atypical Antipsychotic
colchicine	1		Agents for Gout
conjugated estrogens (equine)	PREMARIN	CES, CONGEST, PREMARIN	Estrogen
conjugated estrogens/ medroxyprogesterone	PREMPHASE, PREMPRO	NOT AVAILABLE	Combination Product
cyclobenzaprine	FLEXERIL		Skeletal Muscle Relaxant
cyclosporine	GENGRAF, NEORAL, SANDIMMUNE, RESTASIS	NEORAL, SANDIMMUNE	Immunosuppressant
desloratadine	CLARINEX	AERIUS	Antihistamine
desmopressin	DDAVP, MINIRIN	DDAVP, MINIRIN, OCTOSTIM	Vasopressin Analogue
desoximetasone	TOPICORT	TOPICORT	Glucocorticoid
dexamethasone	DECADRON, DEXAMETH, DEXONE, HEXADROL	HEXADROL	Glucocorticoid
dexmethylphenidate	FOCALIN XR	NOT AVAILABLE	CNS Stimulant
dextroamphetamine	DEXEDRINE	DEXEDRINE	Indirect-Acting Sympathomimetic
diazepam	DIASTAT, VALCAPS, VALIUM, VAZEPAM	APO-DIAZEPAM, DIAZEMULS, E-PAM, VALIUM	Benzodiazepine
diclofenac	CATAFLAM, SOLARAZE, VOLTAREN	DICLOTEC, VOLTAREN	Nonsteroidal Anti-Inflammatory Drug (NSAID)
diclofenac/misoprostol	ARTHROTEC	ARTHROTEC	Combination Product
dicyclomine	BENTYL	BENTYLOL	Anticholinergic
didanosine	VIDEX	VIDEX	Antiretroviral Agents
digoxin	DIGITEK, LANOXICAPS, LANOXIN	LANOXIN	Cardiac Glycoside
diltiazem	CARDIZEM, CARTIA, DILACOR, DILTIA, TAZTIA, TIAZAC	APO-DILTIAZ, CARDIZEM, RATIO-DILTIAZEM CD, TIAZAC	Calcium Channel Blocker
diphenoxylate/atropine	LOMOTIL	LOMOTIL	Combination Product
dipyridamole/aspirin	AGGRENOX	AGGRENOX	Antiplatelet Agent
divalproex	SEE VALPROIC ACID		
docusate	COLACE	COLACE, SOFLAX	Stool Softener
donepezil	ARICEPT	ARICEPT	Cholinesterase Inhibitor
dorzolamide/timolol	COSOPT	COSOPT	Combination Product
doxazosin	CARDURA	CARDURA	β-Blocker
doxepin	ADAPIN, SINEQUAN, ZONALON	SINEQUAN, TRIADAPIN, ZONALON	Tricyclic Anti-depressant (TCA)
doxycycline	ADOXA, DORYX, MONODOX, VIBRAMYCIN, VIBRA-TABS	DORYX, VIBRAMYCIN, VIBRA-TABS	Tetracycline

Generic Name	Trade Name United States	Trade Name Canada	Classification
Drospirenone + ethinyl estradiol	YAZ	YAZ	birth control agent
duloxetine	CYMBALTA	NOT AVAILABLE	Atypical Antidepressant
dutasteride	AVODART	AVODART	5α-Reductase Inhibitor
econazole	SPECTAZOLE	ECOSTATIN	Antifungal
efavirenz	SUSTIVA	SUSTIVA	Reverse Transcriptase Inhibitor
eletriptan	RELPAX	RELPAX	5-HT1 Receptor Agonist
emtricitabine/tenofovir	TRUVADA	TRUVADA	Antiretroviral Agent
enalapril	VASOTEC	VASOTEC	Angiotensin-Converting Enzyme (ACE) Inhibitor
enfuvirtide	FUZEON	FUZEON	Antiretroviral Agent
enoxaparin	LOVENOX	LOVENOX	Low-Molecular-Weight Heparin (LMWH)
epinephrine	EPIPEN	EPIPEN	Vasopressor
epoetin alfa	EPOGEN, PROCRIT	EPREX	Recombinant Human Erythropoietin
erythromycin	E-MYCIN, ERY-TAB, ILOSONE, ILOTYCIN	ILOSONE, ILOTYCIN	Macrolide
escitalopram	LEXAPRO	CIPRALEX	Selective Serotonin Reuptake Inhibitor (SSRI)
esomeprazole	NEXIUM	NEXIUM	Proton Pump Inhibitor (PPI)
estradiol	CLIMARA, ESTRACE, ESTRADERM, VIVELLE, VIVELLE DOT, VAGIFEM	CLIMARA, ESTRACE, ESTRADERM, ESTRADOT	Estrogen
eszopiclone	LUNESTA	NOT AVAILABLE	Sedatives and Hypnotics
etanercept	ENBREL	ENBREL	Disease-Modifying Antirheumatic Drug (DMARD)
Ethinyl + norgestimate	ORTHO-TRI-CYCLEN	ORTHO-TRI-CYCLEN	Birth control agent
Ethinyl estradiol + norethindrone	LOESTRIN 24 FE	LOESTRIN 24 FE	Birth control agent
ethinyl estradiol/desogestrel	APRI, MIRCETTE, KARIVA	MARVELON	Combination Product
ethinyl estradiol/drospirenone	YASMIN	YASMIN	Combination Product
ethinyl estradiol/norelgestromin	ORTHO EVRA	NOT AVAILABLE	Combination Product
ethinyl estradiol/norethindrone	BREVICON, ESTROSTEP, FEMHRT, LOESTRIN, MICROGESTIN, MICRONOR, OVCON, NECON 1/35	BREVICON, FEMHRT, LOESTRIN, MICRONOR, SYNPHASIC	Combination Product
ethinyl estradiol/norgestimate	ORTHO-CYCLEN, TRI-CYCLEN, TRINESSA, TRI-SPRINTEC	CYCLEN, TRI-CYCLEN	Combination Product
ethinyl estradiol/norgestrel	CRYSELLE, OGESTREL, OVRAL	OVRAL	Combination Product

(continued)

Generic Name	Trade Name United States	Trade Name Canada	Classification
etodolac	LODINE	ULTRADOL	Nonsteroidal Anti-Inflammatory Drug (NSAID)
etonogestrel/ethinyl estradiol	NUVARING	NUVARING	Combination Product
exenatide	BYETTA	NOT AVAILABLE	Incretin Mimetic Agent
ezetimibe	ZETIA	EZETROL	Cholesterol Absorption Inhibitor
ezetimibe/simvastatin	VYTORIN	NOT AVAILABLE	Combination Product
famciclovir	FAMVIR	FAMVIR	Antiviral
famotidine	PEPCID	PEPCID	H_2-Receptor Antagonist (H_2RA)
felodipine	PLENDIL	PLENDIL, RENEDIL	Calcium Channel Blocker
fenofibrate	TRICOR	LIPIDIL	Fibric Acid Derivative
fentanyl	ACTIQ, DURAGESIC, SUBLIMAZE	DURAGESIC, SUBLIMAZE	Opiate Agonist
ferrous sulfate	FEOSOL	NIFEREX	Trace Element
fexofenadine	ALLEGRA	ALLEGRA	Antihistamine
fexofenadine/ pseudoephedrine	ALLEGRA-D	ALLEGRA-D	Combination Product
filgrastim	NEUPOGEN	NEUPOGEN	Granulocyte-Colony Stimulating Factor (G-CSF)
finasteride	PROPECIA, PROSCAR	PROPECIA, PROSCAR	5β-Reductase Inhibitor
flecainide	TAMBOCOR	TAMBOCOR	Antiarrhythmic
fluconazole	DIFLUCAN	APO-FLUCONAZOLE, DIFLUCAN	Antifungal
fluocinonide	LIDEX	LYDERM, LIDEX	Glucocorticoid
fluoxetine	PROZAC	PROZAC	Selective Serotonin Reuptake Inhibitor (SSRI)
fluticasone	FLONASE, FLOVENT	FLONASE	Glucocorticoid
fluvastatin	LESCOL, LESCOL XL	LESCOL, LESCOL XL	HMG-CoA Reductase Inhibitor
fluvoxamine	LUVOX	LUVOX	Selective Serotonin Reuptake Inhibitor (SSRI)
folic acid	FOLVITE	FOLICARE	Vitamins
fosinopril	MONOPRIL	MONOPRIL	Angiotensin-Converting Enzyme (ACE) Inhibitor
furosemide	LASIX	APO-FUROSEMIDE, LASIX, NOVO-SEMIDE	Loop Diuretic
fusidic acid	NOT AVAILABLE	FUCIDIN	Antibacterial
gabapentin	NEURONTIN	NEURONTIN, PMS-GABAPENTIN	Anticonvulsant
gemfibrozil	LOPID	LOPID	Fibric Acid Derivative
gentamicin	GARAMYCIN	GARAMYCIN	Aminoglycoside
glatiramer	COPAXONE	COPAXONE	Immunosuppressant
glimepiride	AMARYL	AMARYL	Oral Antidiabetic
glipizide	GLUCOTROL, GLUCOTROL XL	NOT AVAILABLE	Oral Antidiabetic

Generic Name	Trade Name United States	Trade Name Canada	Classification
glyburide (glibenclamide)	DIABETA, MICRONASE	APO-GLYBURIDE, DIABETA, GEN-GLYBE, NOVO-GLYBURIDE	Oral Antidiabetic
glyburide/metformin	GLUCOVANCE	NOT AVAILABLE	Combination Product
griseofulvin	GRIFULVIN V	FULVICIN U/F	Antifungal
hydralazine	APRESOLINE	APRESOLINE	Vasodilator
hydrochlorothiazide	ESIDRIX, HYDRODIURIL, ORETIC	APO-HYDRO, ESIDRIX, HYDRODIURIL, NOVO-HYDRAZIDE	Thiazide and Related Diuretics
hydrochlorothiazide/ bisoprolol	ZIAC	ZIAC	Combination Product
hydrochlorothiazide/ irbesartan	AVALIDE	AVALIDE	Combination Product
hydrochlorothiazide/ lisinopril	PRINZIDE, ZESTORETIC	PRINZIDE, ZESTORETIC	Combination Product
hydrochlorothiazide/ losartan	HYZAAR	HYZAAR	Combination Product
hydrochlorothiazide/ triamterene	DYAZIDE, MAXZIDE	APO-TRIAZIDE, DYAZIDE	Combination Product
hydrochlorothiazide/ valsartan	DIOVAN HCT	DIOVAN HCT	Combination Product
hydrocodone/ chlorpheniramine	TUSSIONEX	TUSSIONEX	Combination Product
hydrocodone/ibuprofen	VICOPROFEN	VICOPROFEN	Combination Product
hydrocortisone	CORT-DOME, CORTEF, DERMOLATE	CORTATE, CORTEF	Glucocorticoid
hydromorphone	DILAUDID, PALLADONE	DILAUDID, PALLADONE	Opiate Agonist
hydroxychloroquine	PLAQUENIL	PLAQUENIL	Antimalarial
hydroxyzine	ATARAX, VISTARIL	APO-HYDROXYZINE, ATARAX	Antihistamine
hyoscyamine	LEVSIN	LEVSIN	Anticholinergic
ibandronate	BONIVA	NOT AVAILABLE	Bisphosphonates
ibuprofen	ADVIL, MOTRIN	ADVIL, APO-IBUPROFEN	Nonsteroidal Anti-Inflammatory Drug (NSAID)
imatinib	GLEEVEC		Antineoplastic
imipramine	TOFRANIL	TOFRANIL	Tricyclic Antidepressant (TCA)
imiquimod	ALDARA	ALDARA	Immunomodulator
indapamide	LOZOL	LOZIDE, GEN-INDAPAMIDE, PMS-INDAPAMIDE	Thiazide and Related Diuretics
indomethacin	INDOCIN		Nonsteroidal Anti-Inflammatory Drug (NSAID)
Influenza virus vaccine	FLUVIRIN	FLUVIRIN, FLUVIRAL	antiviral
influenza virus vaccine	FLUZONE		Vaccine
insulin	HUMULIN, NOVOLIN	HUMULIN, NOVOLIN GE NPH	Insulin
insulin aspart	NOVOLOG	NOVORAPID	Insulin
insulin glargine	LANTUS	LANTUS	Insulin
insulin lispro	HUMALOG	HUMALOG	Insulin
interferon beta-1a	AVONEX	AVONEX, REBIF	Immunomodulator
interferon beta-1b	BETASERON	BETASERON	Immunomodulator
ipratropium	ATROVENT	ATROVENT	Anticholinergic

(continued)

Generic Name	Trade Name United States	Trade Name Canada	Classification
ipratropium/albuterol	COMBIVENT	COMBIVENT	Combination Product
irbesartan	AVAPRO	AVAPRO	Angiotensin Receptor Blocker (ARB)
isosorbide mononitrate	IMDUR, ISMO, ISOTRATE, MONOKET	IMDUR	Nitrate
itraconazole	SPORANOX	SPORANOX	Antifungal
ketoconazole	NIZORAL	NIZORAL	Antifungal
labetalol	NORMODYNE, TRANDATE	TRANDATE	β-Blocker
lamivudine/zidovudine	COMBIVIR	COMBIVIR	Combination Product
lamotrigine	LAMICTAL	LAMICTAL	Anticonvulsant
lansoprazole	PREVACID	PREVACID	Proton Pump Inhibitor (PPI)
latanoprost	XALATAN	XALATAN	Prostaglandin
leflunomide	ARAVA	ARAVA	Disease-Modifying Antirheumatic Drug (DMARD)
levalbuterol	XOPENEX	NOT AVAILABLE	β2-Agonist
levetiracetam	KEPPRA	KEPPRA	Anticonvulsant
levofloxacin	LEVAQUIN, QUIXIN	LEVAQUIN	Fluoroquinolone
levothyroxine	LEVOTHROID, LEVOXYL, SYNTHROID, UNITHROID	ELTROXIN, SYNTHROID	Thyroid Hormone
lidocaine	LIPODERM	DERMA E ALPHA LIPODERM	Topical anesthetic
lidocaine	LIDODERM, XYLOCAINE	XYLOCAINE	Local Anesthetic
Lisdexamfetamine dimesylate	VYVANSE	VYVANSE	Central nervous system stimulant
lisinopril	PRINIVIL, ZESTRIL	APO-LISINOPRIL, PRINIVIL, ZESTRIL	Angiotensin-Converting Enzyme (ACE) Inhibitor
lithium	ESKALITH, LITHANE, LITHOBID, LITHOTABS	CARBOLITH, DURALITH, LITHANE, LITHIZINE	Antimanic
lopinavir	2	2	Protease Inhibitor
lopinavir/ritonavir	KALETRA	KALETRA	Combination Product
losartan	COZAAR	COZAAR	Angiotensin Receptor Blocker (ARB)
lovastatin	ALTOCOR, MEVACOR	MEVACOR	HMG-CoA Reductase Inhibitor
meclizine	ANTIVERT, BONINE	ANTIVERT	Anticholinergic
medroxyprogesterone	CYCRIN, PROVERA	MEPROGEST, PROVERA, RATIO-MPA	Progestin
megestrol	MEGACE	MEGACE	Progestin
meloxicam	MOBIC	MOBICOX	Nonsteroidal Anti-Inflammatory Drug (NSAID)
memantine	NAMENDA	EBIXA	NMDA Receptor Antagonist
mercaptopurine	PURINETHOL	PURINETHOL	Antineoplastic Agent
mesalamine	ASACOL, PENTASA	ASACOL, MESASAL, PENTASA, QUNITASA, SALOFALK	Nonsteroidal Anti-Inflammatory Drug (NSAID)
methadone	METHADOSE, DOLOPHINE	METADOL	Opioid Analgesic
metaxolone	SKELAXIN	SKELAXIN	Muscle relaxant

Generic Name	Trade Name United States	Trade Name Canada	Classification
metformin	GLUCOPHAGE, GLUCOPHAGE XR	APO-METFORMIN, GEN-METFORMIN, GLUCOPHAGE, NOVO-METFORMIN, PMS-METFORMIN, RATIO-METFORMIN	Oral Antidiabetic
methadone	METHADOSE, DOLOPHINE	METADOL	Opioid Analgesic
methocarbamol	ROBAXIN	ROBAXIN	Skeletal Muscle Relaxant
methotrexate	RHEUMATREX, TREXALL	RHEUMATREX	Antineoplastic
methylphenidate	CONCERTA, RITALIN	CONCERTA, PMS-METHYLPHENIDATE, RITALIN	Indirect-Acting Sympathomimetic
methylprednisolone	MEDROL	MEDROL	Glucocorticoid
metoclopramide	MAXOLON, REGLAN	MAXERAN	Prokinetic Antiemetic
metolazone	MYKROX, ZAROXOLYN	ZAROXOLYN	Thiazide and Related Diuretics
metoprolol	LOPRESSOR, TOPROL-XL	BETALOC, LOPRESSOR, NOVO-METOPROL	Cardioselective β-Blocker
metronidazole	FLAGYL, METROGEL, NORITATE	APO-METRONIDAZOLE, FLAGYL, METROGEL, NORITATE	Antibacterial Antiprotozoal
midodrine	PROAMATINE	AMATINE	Vasopressor
minocycline	DYNACIN, MINOCIN	MINOCIN, ULTRAMYCIN	Tetracycline
mirtazapine	REMERON	REMERON	Atypical Antidepressant
misoprostol	CYTOTEC	CYTOTEC	Prostaglandin
modafinil	PROVIGIL	ALERTEC	Central Nervous System (CNS) Stimulant
mometasone	ELOCON, NASONEX	ELOCON, NASONEX	Glucocorticoid
montelukast	SINGULAIR	SINGULAIR	LTD_4 Receptor Antagonist
morphine	MS CONTIN, MSIR, ORAMORPH	MS CONTIN, MSIR	Opiate Agonist
moxifloxacin	AVELOX, VIGAMOX	AVELOX	Fluoroquinolone
mupirocin	BACTROBAN	BACTROBAN	Antibacterial $\beta2$-Agonist
mycophenolate mofetil	CELLCEPT	CELLCEPT	Immunosuppressant
nabumetone	RELAFEN		Nonsteroidal Anti-Inflammatory Drug (NSAID)
nadolol	CORGARD	CORGARD	β-Blocker
naproxen	ALEVE, ANAPROX, NAPRELAN, NAPROSYN	ANAPROX, APO-NAPROXEN, NAPROSYN, NAXEN	Nonsteroidal Anti-Inflammatory Drug (NSAID)
nebivolol	BYSTOLIC	BYSTOLIC	β-Blocker
nicotine	HABITROL, NICODERM, NICORETTE, NICOTROL	HABITROL, NICODERM, NICORETTE, NICOTROL	Ganglionic Stimulant
nicotinic acid	NIASPAN	NIASPAN	Vitamin
nifedipine	ADALAT, NIFEDICAL XL, PROCARDIA XL, PROCARDIA ER	ADALAT XL, APO-NIFED	Calcium Channel Blocker
nisoldipine	SULAR	NOT AVAILABLE	Calcium Channel Blocker

(continued)

Generic Name	Trade Name United States	Trade Name Canada	Classification
nitrofurantoin	FURADANTIN, MACROBID, MACRODANTIN	MACROBID, MACRODANTIN	Antibacterial
nitroglycerin	NITRO-DUR, NITROSTAT, TRANSDERM-NITRO	NITRO-DUR, NITROSTAT, TRANSDERM-NITRO	Nitrate
nortriptyline	AVENTYL, PAMELOR	AVENTYL	Tricyclic Antidepressant (TCA)
nystatin	MYCOSTATIN, NILSTAT	NILSTAT	Antifungal
ofloxacin	FLOXIN, OCUFLOX	FLOXIN, OCUFLOX	Fluoroquinolone
olanzapine	ZYPREXA	ZYPREXA	Atypical Antipsychotic
olmesartan	BENICAR	NOT AVAILABLE	Angiotensin Receptor Blocker (ARB)
olmesartan/hydro-chlorothiazide	BENICAR HCT	NOT AVAILABLE	Combination Product
olopatadine	PATANOL	PATANOL	Antihistamine
omeprazole	PRILOSEC	LOSEC	Proton Pump Inhibitor (PPI)
ondansetron	ZOFRAN	ZOFRAN	5-HT$_3$ Antagonist
oseltamivir	TAMIFLU	TAMIFLU	Antiviral
oxandrolone	ANAVAR, OXANDRIN	NOT AVAILABLE	Androgen
oxcarbazepine	TRILEPTAL	TRILEPTAL	Anticonvulsant
oxybutynin	DITROPAN, DITROPAN XL	DITROPAN, DITROPAN XL, APO-OXYBUTYNIN	Anticholinergic
oxycodone	OXYCONTIN, OXYIR, M-OXY	OXYCONTIN, OXY-IR	Opiate Agonist
pantoprazole	PROTONIX	PANTOLOC	Proton Pump Inhibitor (PPI)
paroxetine	PAXIL, PAXIL CR	PAXIL, PAXIL CR	Selective Serotonin Reuptake Inhibitor (SSRI)
peginterferon alfa-2a	PEGASYS	PEGASYS	Immunomodulator
penicillin v	V-CILLIN K, VEETIDS	APO-PEN VK, V-CILLIN K	Penicillin
phenazopyridine	PYRIDIUM	PYRIDIUM	Urinary Analgesic
phenobarbital	LUMINAL	PMS-PHENOBARBITAL	Barbiturate
phentermine	FASTIN, IONAMIN	FASTIN, IONAMIN	Indirect-Acting Sympathomimetic
phenytoin	DILANTIN	DILANTIN	Hydantoin
pimecrolimus	ELIDEL	ELIDEL	Immunomodulator
pioglitazone	ACTOS	ACTOS	Oral Antidiabetic
piroxicam	FELDENE	FELDENE	Nonsteroidal Anti-Inflammatory Drug (NSAID)
polyethylene glycol (peg)	COLYTE, MIRALAX	COLYTE, PEGLYTE	Laxative
potassium chloride	K-TAB, K-DUR, KLOR-CON	KAY CIEL	Electrolytes
pramipexole	MIRAPEX	MIRAPEX	Antiparkinson Agent
pravastatin	PRAVACHOL	APO-PRAVASTATIN, LIN-PRAVASTATIN, PRAVACHOL	HMG-CoA Reductase Inhibitor
prednisolone	ORAPRED, PEDIAPRED, PRED FORTE	PEDIAPRED, PRED FORTE	Glucocorticoid
prednisone	DELTASONE	DELTASONE	Glucocorticoid
pregabalin	LYRICA	LYRICA	Anticonvulsant
primidone	MYSOLINE		Anticonvulsant
prochlorperazine	COMPAZINE	STEMETIL	Phenothiazine

Generic Name	Trade Name United States	Trade Name Canada	Classification
progesterone	CRINONE, PROCHIEVE, PROGESTASERT, PROMETRIUM	CRINONE, GESTEROL, PROMETRIUM	Progestin
promethazine	ANERGAN, PHENERGAN, PRO-METHEGAN, PHENADOZ	HISTANTIL, PHENERGAN	Phenothiazine
promethazine/codeine	PHENERGAN WITH CODEINE	NOT AVAILABLE	Combination Product
propafenone	RYTHMOL	RYTHMOL	Antiarrhythmic
propranolol	BETACHRON, INDERAL	APO-PROPRANOLOL, DETENSOL, INDERAL	β-Blocker
quetiapine	SEROQUEL	SEROQUEL	Atypical Antipsychotic
quinapril	ACCUPRIL	ACCUPRIL, ACCUPRO	Angiotensin-Converting Enzyme (ACE) Inhibitor
quinine	QUALAQUIN	NOVO-QUININE	Antimalarial
rabeprazole	ACIPHEX	PARIET	Proton Pump Inhibitor (PPI)
raloxifene	EVISTA	EVISTA	Selective Estrogen Receptor Modulator (SERM)
ramipril	ALTACE	ALTACE, RAMACE	Angiotensin-Converting Enzyme (ACE) Inhibitor
ranitidine	ZANTAC	APO-RANITIDINE, GEN-RANITIDINE, NOVO-RANITIDINE, ZANTAC	H_2-Receptor Antagonist (H_2RA)
ribavirin	REBETOL, VIRAZOLE	VIRAZOLE	Antiviral
risedronate	ACTONEL	ACTONEL	Bisphosphonate
risperidone	RISPERDAL	RISPERDAL	Atypical Antipsychotic
ritonavir	NORVIR	NORVIR	Protease Inhibitor
ropinirole	REQUIP	REQUIP	Antiparkinson Agent
rosiglitazone	AVANDIA	AVANDIA	Oral Antidiabetic
rosuvastatin	CRESTOR	CRESTOR	HMG-CoA Reductase Inhibitor
salbutamol (see albuterol)	—	—	—
salmeterol/fluticasone	ADVAIR	ADVAIR	Combination Product
sertraline	ZOLOFT	APO-SERTRALINE, ZOLOFT	Selective Serotonin Reuptake Inhibitor (SSRI)
sildenafil	REVATIO	REVATIO	Different mfr. Viagra
sildenafil	VIAGRA	VIAGRA	Phosphodiesterase Type 5 (PDE5) Inhibitor
simvastatin	ZOCOR	APO-SIMVASTATIN, GEN-SIMVASTATIN, ZOCOR	HMG-CoA Reductase Inhibitor
sitagliptin	JANUVIA	JANUVIA	Antidiabetic agent
sodium fluoride	ETHEDENT, PHARMAFLUR	PREVIDENT	Trace Elements
solifenacin	VESICARE	VESICARE	antispasmodic
sotalol	BETAPACE	ZIMSOTALOL	β-Blocker
spironolactone	ALDACTONE	ALDACTONE, NOVO-SPIROTON	Potassium-Sparing Diuretic
sucralfate	CARAFATE	SULCRATE	Cytoprotective
sumatriptan	IMITREX		$5\text{-}HT_{1B/1D}$ Agonist

(continued)

Generic Name	Trade Name United States	Trade Name Canada	Classification
tacrolimus	PROGRAF, PROTOPIC	PROGRAF, PROTOPIC	Immunosuppressant
tadalafil	CIALIS	CIALIS	Impotence Agent
tamoxifen	NOLVADEX	NOLVADEX, TAMOFEN, TAMONE	Antiestrogen
tamsulosin	FLOMAX	FLOMAX	β-Blocker
telithromycin	KETEK	KETEK	Ketolide
telmisartan	MICARDIS	MICARDIS	Angiotensin Receptor Blocker (ARB)
telmisartan/hydro-chlorothiazide	MICARDIS HCT	MICARDIS PLUS	Combination Product
temazepam	RESTORIL	APO-TEMAZEPAM, RESTORIL	Benzodiazepine
tenofovir	VIREAD	—	Reverse Transcriptase Inhibitor
terazosin	HYTRIN	HYTRIN	β-Blocker
terbinafine	LAMISIL	LAMISIL	Antifungal
terconazole	TERAZOL 7, TERAZOL 3	TERAZOL 7, TERAZOL 3	Antifungal
teriparatide	FORTEO	FORTEO	Parathyroid Hormone
testosterone	ANDRODERM, ANDROGEL, DELATESTRYL, STRIANT, TESTIM	ANDRODERM, DELATESTRYL, MALOGEN	Androgen
tetracycline	ACHROMYCIN, SUMYCIN	ACHROMYCIN	Tetracycline
thalidomide	THALOMID	NOT AVAILABLE	Immunomodulators
thyroid desiccated	ARMOUR THYROID	THYROIDINUM	Thyroid Hormone
timolol	BLOCADREN, TIMOPTIC	BLOCADREN, TIMOPTIC	β-Blocker
tiotropium	SPIRIVA	SPIRIVA	Anticholinergic
tizanidine	ZANAFLEX	ZANAFLEX	Central Sympatholytic
tobramycin/ dexamethasone	TOBRADEX	TOBRADEX	Combination Product
tolterodine	DETROL, DETROL LA	DETROL, DETROL LA	Anticholinergic
topiramate	TOPAMAX	TOPAMAX	Anticonvulsant
torsemide	DEMADEX	DEMADEX	Loop Diuretic
tramadol	ULTRAM, ULTRAM ER	ZYTRAM XL	Opiate Agonist
trandolapril/verapamil	TARKA	TARKA	Combination Product
travoprost	TRAVATAN	TRAVATAN	Prostaglandin Agonist
trazodone	DESYREL	APO-TRAZODONE, DESYREL	Atypical Antidepressant
tretinoin	RENOVA, RETIN-A, VESANOID	RENOVA, RETIN-A, VESANOID	Retinoid
triamcinolone	ARISTOCORT, AZMACORT, KENALOG, NASACORT	ARISTOCORT, AZMACORT, KENALOG	Glucocorticoid
triamterene	DYRENIUM	2	Potassium-Sparing Diuretic
trimethoprim/polymyxin B	POLYTRIM	POLYTRIM	
trimethoprim/ sulfamethoxazole	BACTRIM, COTRIM, SEPTRA, SULFATRIM	APO-SULFATRIM DS, BACTRIM	Combination Product
valacyclovir	VALTREX	VALTREX	Antiviral
valproic acid (divalproex)	DEPAKENE, DEPAKOTE	APO-DIVALPROEX, DEPAKENE, DEPROIC, EPIVAL, RATIO-DIVALPROEX	Anticonvulsant
valsartan	DIOVAN	DIOVAN	Angiotensin Receptor Blocker (ARB)

Generic Name	Trade Name United States	Trade Name Canada	Classification
vardenafil	LEVITRA	LEVITRA	Impotence Agent (Phosphodiesterase Type 5 Inhibitors)
varenicline	CHANTIX	CHAMPIX	Smoking cessation agent
venlafaxine	EFFEXOR		Selective Serotonin Reuptake Inhibitor (SSRI)
verapamil	CALAN, COVERA, ISOPTIN, VERELAN	VERELAN	Calcium Channel Blocker
warfarin	COUMADIN	APO-WARFARIN, COUMADIN, TARO-WARFARIN	Anticoagulant
ziprasidone	GEODON	NOT AVAILABLE	Atypical Antipsychotic
zolmitriptan	ZOMIG	ZOMIG	$5\text{-HT}_{1B/1D}$ Agonist
zolpidem	AMBIEN, AMBIEN CR	NOT AVAILABLE	Benzodiazepine Receptor Agonist
zonisamide	ZONEGRAN	ZONEGRAN	Anticonvulsant

[1]Not sold under any trade name. Available under the generic name.
[2]Only available in combination products. Not available as a single entity.
Adapted from Stedman TL. *Stedman's Medical Dictionary for the Health Professions and Nursing*. 7th ed. Philadelphia, PA: Lippincott Williams & Wilkins; 2011.

References:
www.drugs.com
www.level1health.com
www.pharmacists.ca/content
Accessed in January 2011

Index

Page numbers followed by an "*f*" indicates figures; page numbers followed by a "*t*" indicates tables.